DKA — 4 hours af[ter] [...]
started (average) [...]
slower in hyperosmolar —

To alleviate 2,3 diphosphoglycerate df.

Pharmacy — KCl 20 meq KH₂PO₄ 20 meq

Coat IV tubing + containers
c̄ sterile albumin for
all insulin included —

6-60 profile 4h after therapy started

Calculate osmolality — If calculated
osmolality > 310 get measured
also calcul record anion gap —

used faster method of lactate (serum)
determin if is lactic acidosis
is > 4 - 5 mM — + HbA1c
(Methodology?)

Contact Residency program from
one hospital

Need a pediatrist —

Need a doppler to check
pulses and get brachial/pedal
systolic

DIABETES MELLITUS

Production Editor: *Alexander Noble*
Assistant Editor for ADA: *William S. Niquette*
Art Director: *Don Sellers*
Acquisitions Editor: *Kathy Regiec*
Director of Publications, ADA: *Caroline Stevens*

DIABETES MELLITUS
VOLUME V

Harold Rifkin, M.D.
Philip Raskin, M.D.
EDITORS

Robert J. Brady Company, Bowie, Maryland
A Prentice-Hall Publishing and Communications Company.

ISSN 0146-2792

ISBN 0-87619-747-0

Prentice-Hall International, Inc., London
Prentice-Hall of Australia, Pty., Ltd., Sydney
Prentice-Hall of India Private Limited, New Delhi
Prentice-Hall of Japan, Inc., Tokyo
Prentice-Hall of Southeast Asia Pte. Ltd., Singapore
Whitehall Books, Limited, Petone, New Zealand

Printed in the United States of America

82 83 84 85 86 87 88 89 90   10 9 8 7 6 5 4 3 2

CONTENTS

LONG-TERM PROBLEMS

SPECIAL PROBLEMS AND RELATED
CLINICAL ISSUES

INTRODUCTION

Since the publication of the previous editions of "Diabetes Mellitus—Diagnosis and Treatment," there have been increasing advances along several fronts in the battle against diabetes mellitus. Thus, in preparing Volume V, we have attempted to bring together leading authorities in the field of diabetes to discuss in a clear and unambiguous manner, those concepts regarding the nature of the disease and its management that have stood the "test of time" and those that are now just emerging.

Because of the explosion of new ideas in the past five years, this edition includes many topics not covered in the preceding volumes. These include a fuller discussion of somatostatin as well as other neurogastrointestinal peptide hormones, insulin receptors, and newer concepts regarding the genetics of the disease. We have also added separate chapters on the foot in diabetes and the dental manifestation of the disease. Finally in regard to therapy, chapters on glycosylated hemoglobin and alternative methods of treatment have been added.

The editors and the members of the Committee on Professional Education trust that this volume will accomplish the goal of providing an up-to-date review of the state of the art in diabetes mellitus. Hopefully, those who become familiar with its contents should be able to deliver optimal care to their diabetic patients.

The editors wish to thank Harry Hansen and Caroline Stevens of the American Diabetes Association, Inc. for their advice and support during the inception and production of this volume. They also gratefully acknowledge the editorial and technical assistance of William S. Niquette for the American Diabetes Association, Inc. and Alexander Noble for the Robert J. Brady Company.

Harold Rifkin, M.D.
Philip Raskin, M.D.
Editors

CONTRIBUTORS

Carol E. Anderson, Fellow, Division of Medical Genetics, Harbor-UCLA Medical Center, Torrance, California

Ronald A. Arky, M.D., Professor of Medicine, Harvard Medical School at Mount Auburn Hospital

Gurunanjappa S. Bale, Ph.D., Senior Research Assistant, Statistical Bureau, Metropolitan Life Insurance Company

Peter H. Bennett, M.B., F.R.C.P., F.F.C.M., National Institute of Arthritis, Metabolism, and Digestive Diseases: Epidemiology and Field Studies Branch

Sheldon J. Bleicher, M.D., Chairman, Department of Internal Medicine, The Brooklyn-Cumberland Hospital Center; Professor of Medicine, Downstate Medical Center, State University of New York

Robert F. Bradley, M.D., President, Joslin Diabetes Foundation, Inc.; Associate Clinical Professor of Medicine, Harvard Medical School, Boston, Massachusetts

Paul W. Brand, F.R.C.S., Chief, Rehabilitation Branch, U.S. Public Health Service Hospital, Carville, Louisiana; Clinical Professor of Surgery and Orthopedic Surgery, Louisiana State University Medical School, New Orleans, Louisiana

George F. Cahill, Jr., M.D., Director of Research, Howard Hughes Medical Institute; Professor of Medicine, Harvard Medical School, Boston, Massachusetts

Joan I. Casey, M.D., F.R.C.P. (C), Division of Infectious Diseases, Montefiore Hospital, Albert Einstein College of Medicine, Bronx, New York

John K. Davidson, M.D., Ph.D., Professor of Medicine, Director, Diabetes Unit, Emory University School of Medicine, Atlanta, Georgia

Jørn Ditzel, M.D., Ph.D., Aalborg Regional Hospital, Aalborg, Denmark

Allan L. Drash, M.D., Children's Hospital of Pittsburgh, Division of Endocrinology; Professor of Pediatrics, University of Pittsburgh School of Medicine; Director, Division of Pediatric Endocrinology, Metabolism and Diabetes Mellitus

Max Ellenberg, M.D., Clinical Professor of Medicine, The Mount Sinai School of Medicine

Paul S. Entmacher, M.D., Vice-President and Chief Medical Director, Metropolitan Life Insurance Company

Stefan S. Fajans, M.D., Professor of Internal Medicine; Head, Division of Endocrinology and Metabolism; Director, The Metabolism Research Unit; Director, Michigan Diabetes Research and Training Center, The University of Michigan, Ann Arbor, Michigan

Philip Felig, M.D., C.N.H. Long Professor and Vice Chairman, Department of Internal Medicine; Chief, Section of Endocrinology, Yale University School of Medicine, New Haven, Connecticut

Rudolf Flückiger, Ph.D., Cell Biology Laboratory, Diabetes Unit, Children's Hospital Medical Center, Boston, Massachusetts

Daniel W. Foster, M.D., Department of Internal Medicine, University of Texas Health Science Center at Dallas, Dallas, Texas

Norbert Freinkel, M.D., Kettering Professor of Medicine; Professor of Biochemistry; Chief, Section of Endocrinology and Metabolism; Director of the Center for Endocrinology, Metabolism and Nutrition, Northwestern University Medical School, Chicago, Illinois

Gerald J. Friedman, M.D., F.A.C.P., Chief, Diabetes and Metabolism, Beth Israel Medical Center; Attending Physician in Medicine, Beth Israel Medical Center, Bellevue Hospital, University Hospital; Clinical Professor of Medicine, Mount Sinai School of Medicine, City University of New York

Kenneth H. Gabbay, M.D., Chief, Diabetes Unit, Children's Hospital Medical Center; Associate Professor of Pediatrics, Harvard Medical School, Boston, Massachusetts

John A. Galloway, M.D., Clinical Research Division, Eli Lilly and Company; Professor of Medicine, Indiana University School of Medicine, Indianapolis, Indiana

Lawrence M. Gartner, M.D., Professor of Pediatrics; Director of Division of Neonatology; Director of the Rose F. Kennedy Clinical Research Unit at the Albert Einstein College of Medicine

J.E. Gerich, M.D., Professor of Medicine and Physiology, Mayo Medical School; Director, Endocrine Research Unit, Mayo Clinic, Rochester, Minnesota

Robert S. Gilgor, M.D., Assistant Professor of Medicine, Division of Dermatology, Department of Medicine, Duke University Medical Center, Durham, North Carolina

Frederick C. Goetz, M.D., Section of Endocrinology and Metabolism, Department of Medicine, University of Minnesota, Minneapolis

Robert Gottsegen, D.D.S., Professor of Dentistry; Director, Division of Periodontics, School of Dental and Oral Surgery, Columbia University, New York

Jeffrey B. Halter, M.D., Associate Director, Geriatric Research, Education and Clinical Center, Seattle VA Medical Center, Seattle, Washington; Assistant Professor of Medicine, University of Washington

Paul Henkind, M.D., Ph.D., Professor and Chairman, Department of Ophthalmology, Albert Einstein College of Medicine, Montefiore Hospital and Medical Center, Bronx, New York

Dorothy M. Kahkonen, M.D., Staff physician, Division of Metabolic Diseases, Henry Ford Hospital, Detroit; Clinical Instructor of Internal Medicine, University of Michigan Medical School

Harvey C. Knowles, Jr., M.D., University of Cincinnati Medical Center, Cincinnati, Ohio

Veikko A. Koivisto, M.D., Research Associate, Department of Internal Medicine, Yale University School of Medicine, New Haven, Connecticut

Orville G. Kolterman, M.D., Assistant Professor of Medicine, University of Colorado School of Medicine, Denver, Colorado

Robert A. Kreisberg, M.D., Professor of Medicine; Chairman, Department of Medicine; University of South Alabama College of Medicine, Mobile, Alabama

Gerald S. Lazarus, M.D., F.A.C.P., J. Lamar Callaway Professor of Dermatology; Chief, Division of Dermatology, Department of Medicine, Duke University Medical Center, Durham, North Carolina

Philip M. LeCompte, M.D., Gastroenterology Department, Lemuel Shattuck Hospital; Pathologist Emeritus, Faulkner Hospital, Boston, Massachusetts; Lecturer, Tufts University School of Medicine

Marvin E. Levin, M.D., Associate Professor of Clinical Medicine; Associate Director Metabolism Clinic, Washington University School of Medicine; Attending Physician, The Jewish Hospital, St. Louis, Missouri

Philip D. Lief, M.D., Associate Professor of Medicine, Albert Einstein College of Medicine; Attending Physician, Renal Division, Montefiore Hospital and Medical Center, New York

William McBride, M.D., F.R.C.P. (C), Instructor of Medicine, Section of Gastroenterology, Yale University School of Medicine, New Haven, Connecticut

J. Denis McGarry, Ph.D., Department of Internal Medicine and Biochemistry, University of Texas Health Science Center at Dallas, Dallas, Texas

Donald E. McMillan, M.D., Sansum Medical Research Foundation, Santa Barbara, California

Daniel H. Mintz, M.D., Professor of Medicine; Chairman, Department of Medicine, University of Miami School of Medicine

Michele Muggeo, M.D., Professor of Medicine, Department of Medicine, University of Padova, Padova, Italy

Mary Jo O'Sullivan, M.D., Associate Professor of Obstetrics and Gynecology, University of Miami School of Medicine

Stephen Podolsky, M.D., Chief, Endocrinology and Metabolism Section, Boston VA Outpatient Clinic; Consultant in Diabetes, Medical Service, West Roxbury VA Medical Center; Assistant Clinical Professor of Medicine, Harvard Medical School, Boston, Massachusetts

Daniel Porte, Jr., M.D., Chief, Division of Endocrinology and Metabolism, Seattle VA Medical Center, Seattle, Washington; Director, Diabetes Research Center, University of Washington

Stanley G. Rabinowitz, M.D., Department of Medicine, Northwestern University Medical School, Chicago, Illinois

Richard K. Raker, M.D., Assistant Professor of Pediatrics and Staff Neonatologist, The Albert Einstein College of Medicine; Chief, Newborn Services, New Rochelle Hospital Medical Center

Philip Raskin, M.D., Clinical Investigator, Dallas VA Medical Center; Associate Professor, Department of Internal Medicine, University of Texas Health Science Center at Dallas, Dallas, Texas

Harold Rifkin, M.D., Clinical Professor of Medicine, Albert Einstein College of Medicine; Principal Consultant, Diabetes Research and Training Center, Albert Einstein College of Medicine—Montefiore Hospital and Medical Center; Attending Physician, Montefiore Hospital Medical Center, Lenox Hill Hospital, Bellevue Hospital, and University Hospital, New York

David L. Rimoin, M.D., Ph.D., Professor of Pediatrics and Medicine; Chief, Division of Medical Genetics, Harbor-UCLA Medical Center, Torrance, California

R.A. Rizza, M.D., Assistant Professor of Medicine, Mayo Medical School; Consultant in Endocrinology, Mayo Clinic, Rochester, Minnesota

Herbert Ross, M.D., Assistant Clinical Professor of Medicine, Albert Einstein College of Medicine; Associate Attending Physician, in Medicine and Endocrinology, Montefiore Hospital and Medical Center, New York

Jerome I. Rotter, M.D., Assistant Professor of Medicine and Pediatrics, Division of Medical Genetics, Harbor-UCLA Medical Center, Torrance, California

Jesse Roth, M.D., Chief, Diabetes Branch, National Institute of Arthritis, Metabolism and Digestive Diseases, National Institutes of Health, Bethesda, Maryland

Arthur H. Rubenstein, M.D., Professor and Associate Chairman, Department of Medicine, University of Chicago, Chicago, Illinois

Holbrooke S. Seltzer, M.D., Chief of Metabolism, VA Hospital; Professor of Internal Medicine, The University of Texas Southwestern Medical School, Dallas, Texas

Robert S. Sherwin, Associate Professor of Medicine, The Department of Internal Medicine, Yale University School of Medicine, New Haven, Connecticut

Jay S. Skyler, M.D., Associate Professor of Medicine and Pediatrics, University of Miami School of Medicine, Miami, Florida

Howard M. Spiro, M.D., Professor of Medicine, Yale University School of Medicine, New Haven, Connecticut

A. Denise Stevens, BSN, MAT, Director of Nursing, Joslin Diabetes Foundation, Inc., Boston, Massachusetts

Karl E. Sussman, M.D., Clinical Investigator, Denver VA Medical Center; Professor of Medicine, University of Colorado School of Medicine, Denver, Colorado

Roger H. Unger, M.D., Senior Medical Investigator, Dallas VA Medical Center; Professor of Internal Medicine, The University of Texas, Southwestern Medical School, Dallas, Texas

Wylie W. Vale, M.D., The Salk Institute, San Diego, California

Joseph B. Walsh, M.D., Assistant Professor and Director of Retinal Service, Department of Ophthalmology, Albert Einstein College of Medicine, Montefiore Hospital and Medical Center, Bronx, New York

Kelly M. West, M.D., Professor of Biostatistics and Epidemiology; Clinical Professor of Medicine, University of Oklahoma Health Sciences Center, Oklahoma City, Oklahoma

Fred W. Whitehouse, M.D., Chief, Division of Metabolic Diseases, Henry Ford Hospital, Detroit; Clinical Professor of Internal Medicine, University of Michigan Medical School

1

On the Etiology of Diabetes Mellitus

Norbert Freinkel, M.D.

GENERAL CONSIDERATIONS OF ETIOLOGICAL HETEROGENEITY

Explosive developments in the past five years have clearly indicated that "primary" or "idiopathic" diabetes represents a syndrome characterized by absolute or relative insulin insufficiency but mediated by a number of different causes.*[1-5] In the least, insulin-dependent diabetes mellitus, IDDM, (i.e., Type I, formerly designated as juvenile-onset or ketosis-prone diabetes) and noninsulin-dependent diabetes mellitus, NIDDM, (i.e., Type II, formerly designated as maturity-onset or ketosis-resistant diabetes) represent wholly different entities rather than simple quantitative gradations of insulinopenia. A number of observations have underscored this distinction. First, studies in monozygotic twins are particularly compelling. In the most impressive series, concordance obtained for 50 percent of the 64

---

*"Secondary" forms of diabetes mellitus, that is, conditions associated with diabetes mellitus or impaired glucose tolerance in which the etiological relationship is known (as in certain endocrinopathies, or pancreatic disease, or following the administration of certain drugs, etc.), are not included in the present analysis. However, the distinction may be arbitrary: genetic determinants may render individuals particularly vulnerable to environmental agents with diabetogenic capabilities (see above), and various subgroups of "primary" diabetes mellitus may be added to the list of "secondary" disorders as these environmental factors are increasingly identified.

1

monozygotic pairs in which the diagnosis of diabetes was made before the age of 40 vis-à-vis 93 percent for the 31 pairs in which the index twin became diabetic after 40.[6] Difference could not be ascribed to variation in the duration of observation since the risk for diabetes in the group under the age of 40 appeared to be confined entirely to the 3-year interval following the appearance of disease in the index twin. Second, IDDM is associated with certain patterns in the histocompatibility antigens (HLA) which are coded for by genes on the sixth chromosome.[7] In Caucasians, there is a higher prevalence of HLA-B8, −Bw 15, −B18, −Dw3 and−Dw4 and a lower prevalence of HLA-B7 and−Dw2; altered HLA frequencies also obtain in nonwhite races, but with somewhat different distribution. By contrast, HLA patterns do not deviate from the normal in NIDDM. Third, immunologic phenomena are readily demonstrable in some IDDM, especially early in the course of the disease. These include lymphocytic infiltrates in the islets and evidence for cell-mediated immune reactions[8] as well as circulating antibodies directed at islet cell plasma membranes[9] or cytoplasmic components.[10] Associations with other autoimmune diseases are not uncommon. These properties do not appear to characterize NIDDM. Finally, seasonal variations and clusterings in association with certain childhood viral epidemics may attend the onset of IDDM, whereas NIDDM does not display such clear correlations with environmental variables.

ETIOLOGICAL FACTORS IN NONINSULIN-DEPENDENT DIABETES MELLITUS (NIDDM)

The high concordance rates for NIDDM in monozygotic twins, even when they are geographically separated, suggests that intrinsic factors are of greatest etiological significance in this population. Unfortunately, however, the site and nature of these intrinsic determinants have not yet been identified. Postulated genetic markers for primary defects in the periphery, such as abnormalities in basement membranes, circulating insulin antagonists, or inappropriate feedback of contrainsulin hormones, have not withstood the test of time. By analogy to animal models, the inborn defect(s) in NIDDM probably reside in some aspect of islet function. Possibilities include limitations in islet replication, insulin biosynthesis and storage, or any of the components of stimulus-secretion coupling. Some reduction in islet B cells appears at autopsy in most NIDDM and could concord with replicative restrictions or accelerated senescence of islet cells; one subject with NIDDM has been described in whom biosynthesis of a structurally-modified insulin with diminished biological potency could be implicated;[11] and many display sluggish secretory response to glucose but not to certain other nonnutrient secretogogues, as if coupling between stimulus and secretion were compromised.[2, 3] The variable patterns of insulin secretion in NIDDM are strongly suggestive of etiological heterogeneity, and the differences between nonobese and obese NIDDM are particularly noteworthy in this regard. Total secretion of insulin is most frequently attenuated in the lean, whereas the obese more often display exuberant insulin release. The distinction has some prognostic significance insofar as carbohydrate tolerance may undergo progressive deterioration in the insulinopenic NIDDM, whereas the insulinoplethoric do not seem to progress to more severe diabetes mellitus.[3]

The delineation of a new subgroup of NIDDM with unique genetic properties, i.e., maturity-onset type of diabetes in young people (MODY), has provided some of the best evidence for etiological heterogeneity.[2, 3] Direct transmission in three generations has been identified in MODY and the ratio of nondiabetic to diabetic offspring conforms almost 1:1. Accordingly, genetic transmission as an autosomal dominant with strong penetrance has been invoked; inheritance via X-linked dominance has been excluded by virtue of demonstrated male-to-male transmission.[5] Despite the fact that MODY may well represent the only monogenic type of diabetes mellitus that has been delineated in man, the underlying intrinsic defect has not been identified even in this group. MODY should constitute an ideally circumscribed population on which to focus etiological inquiries. However, such inquiries may necessitate better and more specific tools for pinpointing discrete steps in intrinsic islet function than are currently available. For the moment, it can only be concluded that environmental modifications may not appreciably modify the incidence of any type of NIDDM in view of the strong genetic overlay. Such manipulations should, however, modify the severity, and perhaps even the time of appearance, a concept that affords ample justification for attempts at weight reduction in all forms of NIDDM which are attended by obesity.

ETIOLOGICAL FACTORS IN INSULIN-DEPENDENT DIABETES MELLITUS (IDDM)

The less constant genetic pattern in IDDM than in NIDDM (see above) suggests that environmental factors may exert a greater etiological impact. Since the HLA region is close to the site of immune response genes in man, the associations between IDDM and HLA have been construed as evidence that immunological mechanisms are important in the pathogenesis of IDDM. It seems unlikely that the HLA antigens are implicated directly since the specific HLA correlations differ in various racial groups. Moreover, even in white populations, HLA-B8 and HLA-Bw15 seem to confer additive risks for IDDM and display differing associations with HLA-Dw3 and Dw4 and with islet cell antibodies, insulin antibodies, and antipancreatic cell-mediated immunity.[4] Thus, it seems more probable that the correlations between HLA and IDDM reflect linkage disequilibria between genes determining vulnerabilities to IDDM and those coding for HLA antigens. That premise has been reinforced by the recent report that an allele at the genetic locus for properdin factor B (i.e., Bf[F 1]), which is closely linked to the major histocompatibility complex, appears to be a codominantly inherited trait in IDDM which occurs more frequently than any single or combination of HLA antigens.[12]

What, then, is the environmental factor to which IDDM are genetically vulnerable and what is the nature of the genetic vulnerability? With regard to the former, mounting evidence implicates viruses in some instances.[1] A syndrome simulating IDDM in man has been produced by inoculating genetically susceptible mice with the M variant of encephalomyocarditis virus (a murine picornavirus which is similar to the Coxsackie viruses of man). Insular changes in appropriate laboratory animals have also been produced by four viruses of human origin: reovirus, Type 3; Coxsackie virus B4, Venezuelan-encephalitis virus, and rubella virus. Most important, in a fatal case of human diabetic ketoacidosis, a virus, related to a diabetogenic variant of Coxsackie virus B4, has been isolated from the patient's pancreas, and recovered again from susceptible inbred mice after inoculation had produced hyperglycemia, beta cell necrosis, and localization of virus in the beta cells coincident with rising virus-antibody titers.[13]

Chemicals may also be contributory. A recent review cites approximately 20 cases of IDDM following ingestion of the rodenticide, Vacor.[1] However, the impact of chemicals may be mediated in a complex fashion. For example, the hyperglycemia and insulitis that can be elicited in selective inbred strains of mice by repeated subdiabetogenic injections of streptozotocin may be accompanied by activation of latent C-type retroviruses in the beta cell and can be modified by the administration of antilymphocyte serum.[14] The underlying genetic vulnerability seems to reside in the manner in which the beta cell handles the environmental factor. The infective potential of viruses with pancreotropic properties appears to be genetically determined, and uptake and replication of viruses in beta cells may be influenced by recessive gene(s). Such inborn factors could account for the relative rarity of IDDM despite the seeming frequency of infections with the viruses which have been implicated. Genetic determinants could also influence the efficacy of repair processes once beta cell injury has been triggered by viruses, chemicals, and/or other, as yet unidentified, environmental agents.

Finally, genetic factors could determine the initiation of autoimmune processes spontaneously or in combination with the traumatizing variables cited above. Various disturbances of immune mechanisms are operative in most IDDM;[8-10] it remains to be established whether any or all are simple reflections of beta cell damage or components in a self-perpetuating cycle of auto-aggression.[15] The distinctions will be important in planning therapeutic strategies for possible intervention during the acute phase of islet insult.

Recognition of the interacting etiological variables in IDDM prompts certain hopes as well as reservations. Definition of appropriate genetic markers may make it possible to identify and categorize vulnerable populations on the basis of their heterogeneous susceptibilities. It should also facilitate eventual administration of appropriate preventatives (i.e., immunization, immune sera, etc.), where such subjects are exposed to identifiable risks. At the same time, it must be recognized that unique problems may arise with treatments, such as islet transplantation, in subjects in whom certain forms of autoimmune destruction are genetically programmed and etiologically contributory.

References

1. Craighead JE: Current views on the etiology of insulin-dependent diabetes mellitus. N Engl J Med 299:1439–45, 1978
2. Fajans SS: Diabetes mellitus. *In:* The Year in Metabolism, 1975–1976. Freinkel N, (ed) New York, Plenum Publishing Corp., 1976, p. 45–71
3. Fajans SS, Cloutier MC, and Crowther RL: Clinical and etiological heterogeneity of idiopathic diabetes mellitus. Diabetes 27:1112–25, 1978
4. Rotter JI, Rimoin DL:Heterogeneity in diabetes mellitus—Update, 1978. Diabetes 27:599–605, 1978
5. Friedman J, and Fialkow PJ: The genetics of diabetes mellitus. *In:* Progress in Medical Genetics. Steinberg, AG et al. (eds) Philadelphia, W. B. Saunders Co., 1980, In Press
6. Tattersall RB, and Pyke DA: Diabetes in identical twins, Lancet 2:1120–25, 1972
7. Nerup J, Platz P, Ortved Anderson O, et al: HL-A antigens and diabetes mellitus. Lancet 2:864–66, 1974
8. Irvine WJ, MacCuish AC, Campbell CJ, et al: Organ-specific cell-mediated autoimmunity in diabetes mellitus. Acta Endocrinol 83, Suppl 205:66–76, 1976
9. Lernmark A, Freedman AR, Hormann C, et al: Islet-cell-surface antibodies in juvenile diabetes mellitus. N Engl J Med 299:375–80, 1978
10. Lendrum R, Walker G, and Gamble DR: Islet-cell antibodies in juvenile diabetes mellitus of recent onset. Lancet 1:880–83, 1975
11. Tager H, Given B, Mako M, et al: Characterization of an abnormal insulin from a patient with diabetes. Clin Res 27:378A, 1979
12. Raum D, Stein R, Alper CA, et al: Genetic marker for insulin-dependent diabetes mellitus. Lancet 1:1208–10, 1979
13. Yoon JW, Austin M, Onodera T, et al: Virus-induced diabetes mellitus: Isolation of a virus from the pancreas of a child with diabetic ketoacidosis. N Engl J Med 300:1173–1213, 1979
14. Rossini AA, Like AA, Chick WL, et al: Studies of streptozotocin-induced insulinitis and diabetes. Proc Nat Acad Sci 74:2485–89, 1977
15. Huang SW, Maclaren NK: Insulin-dependent diabetes: A disease of autoaggression. Science 192:64–66, 1976

2

Morphologic View of the Islets in Diabetes Mellitus

Philip M. Lecompte, M.D.

NEW CONCEPTS

In recent years, the use of new methods, chiefly electron microscopy and immunocytochemistry, has shown that some of the same cell types found in the pancreatic islets also occur in the gastrointestinal tract and that interactions occur between these populations of cells. Such discoveries have led to a broadening of concepts, and it has become customary to use terms such as "gastro-entero-pancreatic (GEP) endocrine system,"[1] "gut hormones,"[2] and "entero-insular axis."[2]

With newer developments in neuroendocrinology, it has been demonstrated that most peptide hormones are produced by cells that may be considered to be "neuroendocrine programmed" (although not all of neural crest origin, as previously suggested) and that share certain cytochemical attributes summed up in the acronym APUD (amine precursor uptake, decarboxylation). It is customary now to speak of the APUD series of cells and even to use the term "apudoma" for tumors of such cells. The demonstration of neurohormones (e.g., somatostatin) in the islets as well as monoamine neurotransmitters has led to the term "paraneuron" applied to the cells of the GEP endocrine system.[3] Also, the revelation by electron microscopy of the rich innervation of the islets has resulted in a revival of interest in

7

what have been termed "neuro-insular complexes." Of special note is the recent demonstration of vasoactive intestinal peptide (VIP) and perhaps other peptides in the nerves of the islets and exocrine tissue, with the result that these nerves are being referred to as "peptidergic."

One of the most interesting modern concepts, especially as applied to the pancreas, represents a revival of that of Feyrter, who, some 40 years ago, began referring to the scattered cells that make up most of the GEP system as the "*diffuse (parakrine) endokrine*" system, and indicated that the secretion of such cells might influence adjacent cells, this being apparently at least in part what he meant by "*parakrine.*"[4] Recently, Unger and Orci have suggested that the D cells are strategically located in relation to the A and B cells and that a "paracrine" intercommunication among these three cell types may exist and may be important in noninsulin-dependent diabetes.

CELL TYPES AND HORMONES OF THE ISLETS

The classification of the cells of the GEP endocrine system, revised frequently by an International Commission, is based mainly on the size, shape, and density of secretory granules as seen with the electron microscope, combined with identification of hormones by immunocytochemistry. The following table is based on the Lausanne 1977 classification.[5]

The B cell is found only in the pancreas. The A cell is described in the stomach of various mammals, but so far in man only in the fetal stomach. D and D_1 cells are present in the stomach and small intestine. F cells storing pancreatic polypeptide are found throughout the gastrointestinal tract of dogs and other mammals, but, according to some workers, these differ from the human PP cell. The presence or absence of enterochromaffin (EC) cells, gastrin cells, and cells producing GIP (gastric inhibitory polypeptide) in the pancreas of man must be considered controversial at the present time. The production of more than one hormone by the same cell has been described but is not generally accepted.

Table 2-1. Cell Types in the Pancreatic Islets

Cell	Synonyms	Approximate frequency	Hormone produced
B	β, beta, insulin cell	60–80%	Insulin
A	α, alpha, A_2, glucagon cell	24–40%	Glucagon
D	δ, delta, A_1, somatostatin cell	6–15%	Somatostatin
PP*	Called F cell by some workers	1%	Pancreatic polypeptide
D_1	Type IV, "fourth cell type"	1%	Disputed (? VIP, ?PP)

*Varies in different parts of pancreas. Most abundant in certain lobes of head region.[5]

CONTRIBUTIONS OF MORPHOLOGY TO PHYSIOLOGY

These are beyond the scope of this article, but note should be taken of the contributions of electron microscopy (both by the usual section technique and by freeze-fracture) to the study of formation and migration of secretory granules, the role of micro-tubules, gap junctions and tight junctions between cells, and the nature and relation of nerve endings to the islet cells.[6] A recent outstanding contribution of immunocytochemistry is the demonstration of kallikrein (possibly essential to metabolism of proinsulin) in human islets.[7]

CHANGES IN THE PANCREAS AS A WHOLE IN DIABETES

For reasons that are not clear, the pancreas in insulin-dependent diabetes is often smaller than usual. It has been suggested that the pancreas of a child stops growing at the onset of diabetes, but this is not established. Destructive processes that involve the pancreas as a whole may injure the islets. Conditions of this type, which may or may not be associated with diabetes, include cancer (primary or secondary); hemochromatosis; fibrosis, inter- or intra-lobular; arterio- and arteriolosclerosis; pancreatitis, acute and chronic (including lithiasis). These are adequately discussed elsewhere.[6, 8]

CHANGES IN THE ISLETS IN IDIOPATHIC DIABETES MELLITUS [6, 8, 9, 10, 11]

Qualitative Changes

GENERAL APPEARANCE

Although the islets in noninsulin-dependent diabetes may *appear* normal with routine stains, there are usually obvious changes in insulin-dependent diabetes. The most common is shrinkage, with narrow cords of cells that, in the past, have been regarded as atrophic, but that are now known, with modern immunocytochemical methods, to be actively secreting hormones. Another major change, much less frequent and seen only in cases of recent onset, is hyperplasia, with occasional islets that appear large and are composed mainly of B cells showing signs of activity such as enlarged Golgi apparatus and large dark nuclei suggesting polyploidy.[11] This phenomenon of hyperplastic islets in the early onset insulin-dependent diabetic correlates with C-peptide excretion,[12] and may well explain the early remission or "honeymoon period" noted in so many young diabetics soon after treatment is begun. After some years of diabetes, B cells disappear almost entirely.

A striking hyperplasia, mainly of B cells, occurs in the infants of diabetic mothers, also in so-called "nesidioblastosis."

HYDROPIC CHANGE

The presence of cells with clear cytoplasm, now known to be B cells, was recognized frequently in juvenile diabetics dying in the pre-insulin era. It has been shown to be due to glycogen deposits and can be reproduced experimentally. The reason for such an accumulation in the same cell that makes insulin has never been established. It is rare today, probably because of the scarcity of untreated cases.

INSULITIS

Infiltration of the islets by lymphocytes was noted by early workers, often in association with hydropic change. It has since been shown to be a frequent finding in insulin-dependent diabetes, most often in children who die soon after onset of the disease.[8,9,10] It has also been found in two cases of noninsulin-dependent diabetes, both somewhat unstable. It is now generally accepted as representing an autoimmune reaction and perhaps of major importance in the pathogenesis of diabetes.

Another form of insulitis is the infiltration of eosinophile leukocytes often seen in and around the islets of infants of diabetic mothers.[6,8]

HYALINOSIS

Deposits of a hyaline substance, now considered to be a form of amyloid, are a common, but nonspecific, finding in noninsulin-dependent diabetes, as are insulinomas.[6,8]

FIBROSIS

Fibrosis of the islets occurs occasionally, usually in the juvenile, and often in the "atrophic" type of islet. Recently it has been described in the pancreas of infants of diabetic mothers.

REGENERATION

Signs of regeneration of islets, apparently from ducts and acini, are seen especially in the insulin-dependent diabetic.

QUANTITATIVE CHANGES[6,8,9,10]

Application of quantitative methods has been difficult because of the small volume and irregular shape of the islets, as well as the lack of appropriate techniques in the past. For these reasons, definitive conclusions are not yet possible.

In the insulin-dependent diabetic, the islets are definitely reduced in number and size, especially in cases of long duration. The same phenomenon seems to occur, but to a lesser extent, in the noninsulin-dependent type.

CHANGES IN CELLULAR COMPOSITION

Recent advances in immunocytochemical methods have led to entirely new concepts in this area. In particular, the "atrophic" islets of the insulin-dependent diabetic, previously considered inactive, have been shown to consist of actively secreting glucagon, somatostatin, and PP cells.[11] Of special interest is the finding that islets having a ribbon-like or serpentine pattern are often composed exclusively of PP cells.[11]

In general, it may be said that B cells are scarce or absent in insulin-dependent diabetes and reduced in number in noninsulin-dependent diabetes. It should be noted that the B cells are not all destroyed in early insulin-dependent diabetes, but persist in small numbers even for several years.[11]

ANIMAL MODELS OF DIABETES MELLITUS

Spontaneous

Useful spontaneous models of diabetes occur almost entirely in various rodents and can be divided into lethal or nonlethal, depending upon the species' ability to regenerate B cells (see A. A. Like in reference 3). Some forms are associated with obesity and hyperplasia of the islets. Perhaps the one most similar to the insulin-dependent human type is that of the recently discovered BBL strain of Wistar rat, which is nonobese and develops insulitis with destruction of B cells.[13]

Experimental

Most models involve: (a) chemical agents (alloxan, streptozotocin, diazoxide) which either visibly injure or else inhibit the B cells, or (b) hormones (glucagon, growth hormone, glucocorticoids, sex hormones) which seem to act by antagonizing insulin or by other poorly understood mechanisms. By far the most interesting and instructive animal model is the multiple-dose streptozotocin one, in which repeated small doses of the drug given to a suitable strain of mice lead to hyperglycemia with insulitis and the appearance ("induction") of C-type virus particles in the B cells. Most fascinating is the fact that prior treatment of susceptible mice with 3-O-methyl-D-glucose (which delays the streptozotocin effect) or anti-mouse-lymphocyte serum (which reduces the number of circulating lymphocytes) causes attenuation of the diabetic syndrome, and that both agents together prevent it.[14]

SUMMARY: RECENT CONTRIBUTIONS OF ISLET MORPHOLOGY TO UNDERSTANDING OF DIABETES MELLITUS IN MAN

Cellular Composition

The newer immunocytochemical methods have clarified the function of the various cells of the islets, established the presence of somatostatin and pancreatic polypeptide in addition to insulin and glucagon, and identified the cells producing all four hormones as well as revealing their topographical relation to one another. The latter, suggesting a "paracrine" relation, seems to be supported by studies of the isolated, perfused rat pancreas.

The small islets of insulin-dependent diabetes, formerly considered "atrophic," have been shown to be composed of cells actively secreting glucagon, somatostatin, and pancreatic polypeptide, the latter being the sole component of some islets. This finding has stimulated search for a possible role of PP in diabetes. Further, it has been shown that many B cells may be present at the onset of insulin-dependent diabetes and that they are not completely destroyed, but persist for at least several years in most cases;[11] this finding correlates with C-peptide excretion and with the clinical course of insulin-dependent diabetes.[12]

Insulitis

This phenomenon, known for many years, is now recognized as suggesting a possible autoimmune reaction as one of the components of B-cell injury in insulin-dependent diabetes, probably "triggered" by a virus or a toxin in a susceptible host. This hypothesis is seemingly confirmed by a recent case report,[15] and its validity is also strengthened by the multiple-dose streptozotocin experimental model described above. Further correlations are, of course, represented by the extensive literature on islet-cell antibodies, HLA subtypes, and epidemiologic evidence for virus infection preceding diabetes.

Regeneration

The dwindling number of B cells as insulin-dependent diabetes progresses, and the evidence of feeble attempts at regeneration, together with animal models, give morphologic support to the now widely held hypothesis that a fundamental factor in the pathogenesis of human diabetes mellitus may be a limited capacity of the B cell to replicate.

References

1. Fujita T (ed): Endocrine Gut and Pancreas. Proceedings of the International Symposium on the Gastro-Entero-Pancreatic (GEP) System, Kyoto, 1975. Amsterdam and New York, Elsevier Publishing Company, 1975
2. Bloom SR (ed): Gut Hormones. Edinburgh, London, New York, Churchill Livingstone, 1978
3. Coupland RE and Forssman WG (eds): Peripheral Neuroendocrine Interaction (Symposium). Berlin, Heidelberg, New York, Springer-Verlag, 1978
4. Feyrter F, in Handbuch der allgemeine Pathologie, F Büchner et al. (ed), Berlin and Heidelberg, Springer-Verlag, vol 8/2:344–423, 1966
5. Orci L, Malaisse-Lagae F, Baetens D, et al: Pancreatic-polypeptide-rich regions in human pancreas. Lancet ii, 1200–1201, 1978
6. Volk BW and Wellmann KF (eds): The Diabetic Pancreas, New York and London, Plenum Press, 1977
7. ole-MoiYoi O, Pinkus GS, Spragg J, et al: Identification of human glandular kallikrein in the beta cell of the pancreas. N Engl J Med 300:1289–94, 1979
8. Warren S, LeCompte PM, and Legg MA: The Pathology of Diabetes Mellitus. Philadelphia, Lea and Febiger, 1966

9. Gepts W: Pathologic anatomy of the pancreas in juvenile diabetes mellitus. Diabetes 14:619–33, 1965

10. Gepts W: Pathology of islet tissue in human diabetes, Chapter 17 in Handbook of Physiology, Section 7, Vol 1. Endocrine Pancreas, DF Steiner and N Freinkel (eds), Washington, American Physiological Society, 1972

11. Gepts W and DeMey J: Islet cell survival determined by morphology. Diabetes 27(suppl 1):251–61, 1978

12. Ludvigsson J and Heding LG: Beta-cell function in children with diabetes. Diabetes 27 (suppl 1):230–34, 1978

13. Nakhooda AF, Like AA, Chappel CI, et al: The spontaneously diabetic Wistar rat: metabolic and morphologic studies. Diabetes 26:100–12, 1977

14. Rossini A, Williams RM, Appel MC, et al: Complete protection from low-dose streptozotocin-induced diabetes in mice. Nature 276:182–84, 1978

15. Yoon JW, Austin M, Onodera T, et al: Virus-induced diabetes. Isolation of a virus from the pancreas of a child with diabetic ketoacidosis. N Engl J Med 300: 1173–79, 1979

3

Pathophysiology of Diabetes Mellitus

Robert S. Sherwin, M.D.
Philip Felig, M.D.

INSULIN SECRETION IN DIABETES

Current evidence favors the concept that a deficiency in the insulin secretory mechanism of the beta cell is the predominant or primary lesion in most forms of diabetes. This secretory abnormality may vary from complete failure to a partial defect apparent only in circumstances of increased demands such as obesity, pregnancy, or aging.

In insulin-dependent or juvenile-onset diabetes, insulin secretion is either totally defective or severely impaired. Endogenous insulin secretion, as determined by C-peptide measurements, is generally not detectable in juvenile-onset diabetics who have received insulin therapy for more than 5 years.[1] In noninsulin-dependent maturity-onset diabetic the secretory failure is less severe or insulin secretion may be intact. Basal insulin levels are generally normal or increased, whereas glucose-stimulated insulin secretion is generally diminished. In its mildest form, the beta-cell defect involves only the initial phase of insulin release; the later phase response remains intact. In such individuals the loss of responsiveness to glucose is demonstrable despite normal responsiveness to other insulin secretogogues.[2] These findings suggest a specific abnormality involving glucose recognition

17

and/or metabolism by the beta cell in the earliest stages of diabetes.

It should be noted that early reports of plasma insulin levels in maturity-onset diabetes emphasized the presence of hyperinsulinemia. This seeming paradox was subsequently shown to be more apparent than real if obesity and ambient blood glucose levels are considered. When comparison is made between obese maturity-onset diabetics and an appropriate weight-matched nondiabetic control group, insulin levels in most obese diabetics are lower than those observed in obese subjects with normal glucose tolerance. Furthermore, when the glucose tolerance curve of the mild diabetic is simulated in normal individuals, the insulin response is generally greater than that of the diabetic. Nevertheless, it is clear that insulin secretion in maturity-onset diabetes is heterogeneous, some patients demonstrating hyperinsulinemia even when obesity and hyperglycemia have been accounted for.

INSULIN RESISTANCE IN DIABETES

The importance of insulin resistance in the pathogenesis of maturity-onset diabetics is suggested by the usually high incidence (80%) of obesity in such patients. Obesity, per se, is associated with resistance on the part of target tissues (muscle, liver, and adipose tissue) to the action of insulin and a reduction in insulin receptors on these cells as well as circulating monocytes. On the basis of these studies and data demonstrating a remarkably close correlation between circulating monocytes and in vivo sensitivity to exogenous insulin in nonobese and obese humans, it has been suggested that decreased insulin binding to target tissues contributes to the insulin resistance of obesity.

With respect to insulin resistance in diabetes, reduced insulin binding to circulating monocytes has been observed in nonobese, as well as obese, maturity-onset diabetics. Furthermore, in vivo resistance to the action of exogenously infused insulin has been reported in some maturity-onset diabetics even in the absence of obesity.[3] Overall, the available data suggest the presence of heterogeneity with respect to insulin sensitivity as well as insulin secretion in maturity-onset diabetics. In most cases, maturity-onset diabetes is brought about by a failure of insulin secretion to keep pace with augmented demands for insulin engendered by obesity. However, in some patients, insulin resistance may be present even in the absence of obesity and may be an important factor in the development of the diabetic state. Again, there is a remarkably good correlation between insulin sensitivity and insulin binding to monocytes in maturity-onset diabetes.[3] In juvenile-onset diabetes and more severely hyperglycemic maturity-onset diabetics in whom there is absolute insulinopenia, insulin binding and responsiveness to insulin are comparable to normal subjects.

FUEL HOMEOSTASIS IN DIABETES

Insulin is the primary factor which controls the storage and metabolism of ingested nutrients. The action of insulin involves the three major metabolic fuels—carbohydrate, protein, and fat—and occurs in three principal tissues—liver, muscle, and adipose tissue. In each of these tissues there are anticatabolic, as well as anabolic, effects of insulin that act to reinforce each other (Table 3-1). The metabolic alterations observed in diabetes reflect the degree to which there is an absolute or relative deficiency of insulin. Viewed in the context of insulin as the major storage hormone, a minimal deficiency results in a diminished ability to increase effectively the storage reservoir of body fuels because of inadequate disposal of ingested food stuffs (e.g., glucose intolerance). With a major deficiency of insulin, not only is fuel accumulation hampered in the fed state, but excessive mobilization or production of endogenous metabolic fuels also occurs in the fasted condition (e.g., fasting hyperglycemia, hyperaminoacidemia, and elevated free fatty acids). In its most severe form (diabetic ketoacidosis), there is overproduction of glucose and marked acceleration of all catabolic processes (lipolysis, proteolysis) (Figure 3-1).

Carbohydrate

In the patient with glucose intolerance, fasting blood glucose levels are normal, but ingested glucose fails to elicit an adequate

Table 3-1. Metabolic Actions of Insulin.

	Liver	Adipose Tissue	Muscle
Anticatabolic effects	↓ Glycogenolysis ↓ Gluconeogenesis ↓ Ketogenesis	↓ Lipolysis	↓ Protein catabolism ↓ Amino acid output
Anabolic effects	↑ Glycogen synthesis ↑ Fatty acid synthesis	↑ Glycerol synthesis ↑ Fatty acid systhesis	↑ Amino acid uptake ↑ Protein synthesis ↑ Glycogen synthesis

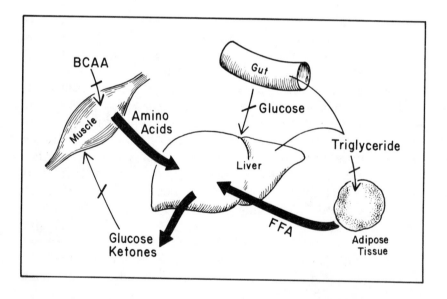

Figure 3-1. Alterations in carbohydrate, protein, and fat metabolism associated with severe insulin deficiency. Hyperglycemia results from reduced glucose uptake by liver and muscle and accelerated glucose production by the liver. Augmented amino acid release from muscle and hepatic uptake of these amino acids and the availability of energy-yielding equivalents derived from free fatty acid (FFA) oxidation account for hepatic glucose overproduction. Hypertriglyceridemia largely results from diminished triglyceride uptake by adipose tissue. Hyperketonemia is due to increased delivery of FFA to the liver, accelerated conversion of FFA to ketones, and reduced ketone uptake by muscle. Branched chain amino acid (BCAA) uptake by muscle is reduced, leading to decreased repletion of muscle nitrogen and hyperaminoacidemia.

early insulin release and, consequently, glucose is not taken up the liver in normal amounts (the liver is the primary site of glucose disposal after oral glucose ingestion) and is more slowly metabolized by peripheral tissues. The quantity of glucose that escapes uptake by the liver and enters the systemic circulation after oral glucose feeding is increased nearly twofold in the maturity-onset diabetic and is the major factor responsible for postprandial hyperglycemia in these patients.[4] A heretofore undefined factor, possibly emanating from the GI tract, has recently been reported to regulate insulin-mediated hepatic uptake of ingested glucose in normal humans.[5]

When absolute or relative insulin deficiency occurs in the basal state, an elevation in fasting blood glucose ensues. In this circumstance, normal basal levels of insulin may be maintained but only at the expense of fasting hyperglycemia. In such patients, hepatic glucose production is normal or only mildly increased, while fractional glucose turnover is reduced. Since only mild hyperglycemia in a normal individual is sufficient to inhibit hepatic glucose output, the diabetic with fasting hyperglycemia is always in a state of relative or absolute glucose overproduction.

In the extreme situation of total beta cell failure, an ever-increasing fasting blood glucose level fails to elicit an insulin secretory response. In the absence of the restraining influence exerted by insulin, the rate of glucose release by the liver may increase threefold or more, largely as a result of augmented gluconeogenesis. The clinical correlate of this sequence of events is severe hyperglycemia as observed in diabetic ketoacidosis or nonketotic hyperosmolar coma. The various gradations of disordered carbohydrate metabolism are shown in Table 3-2.

Protein

In the fasted state, plasma alanine is reduced and the hepatic uptake of this key glycogenic amino acid (as well as other glucose precursors) is increased twofold. Gluconeogenesis can account for over 30 to 40 percent of hepatic glucose production in the diabetic as compared to 15 to 20 percent in normal man.[6]

Table 3-2. *Relationship Between Insulin Secretion and Glucose Regulation in Diabetes.*

	Insulin Secretion		Glucose uptake		Glucose production
	Early	Late	Hepatic	Peripheral	
Abnormal glucose tolerance	↓	Normal	↓	Normal or ↓	Normal
Fasting hyperglycemia	↓	↓	↓	↓	Normal
Ketoacidosis	↓ ↓	↓ ↓	↓ ↓	↓ ↓	↑ ↑

Repletion of muscle nitrogen after protein feeding is reduced in the diabetic. In normal subjects, after a protein meal the branched chain amino acids (leucine, isoleucine, and valine) preferentially escape hepatic uptake and/or metabolism after intestinal absorption and account for most of the hyperaminoacidemia and amino acid uptake by muscle tissue.[6] In contrast, in the diabetic, the total uptake of these amino acids by muscle is decreased and the plasma levels of amino acids are consistently elevated following the ingestion of protein.[6] Diabetes thus may be viewed as a disorder of protein tolerance as well as glucose tolerance.

While the alterations in gluconeogenesis and the protein intolerance associated with mild to moderate insulin lack are not generally discernible clinically, the consequences of severe insulin deficiency on protein metabolism are readily apparent. The stunted growth of the juvenile diabetic observed in the preinsulin era and the negative nitrogen balance and protein wasting of the diabetic in ketoacidosis represent obvious clinical examples. In the latter case, augmented protein catabolism and accelerated output of amino acids from muscle also accentuate hepatic overproduction of glucose by increasing the availability of protein-derived gluconeogenic substrates.

Fat

With relatively mild or moderate insulin deficiency, circulating triglycerides may be increased, presumably as a result of a reduction in lipoprotein lipase activity which facilitates the disposal of both exogenous and endogenously derived triglycerides. Accelerated mobilization of body fat stores and ketone accumulation are generally observed only under conditions of more severe insulin deficiency. The failure to observe ketosis in many cases of diabetes with fasting hyperglycemia derives from the fact that lipolytic processes within the fat cell, ketogenesis in the liver, and ketone removal by muscle are exquisitely sensitive to small quantities of insulin. When insulin secretion is inadequate to suppress lipolysis, fatty acids are mobilized in increased quantities from adipose tissue. Hepatic metabolism of these fatty acids supplies energy for gluconeogenesis and substrate for the generation of ketone bodies. In addition, lack of insulin may account for the increased capacity of the diabetic liver to oxidize fatty acids irrespective of substrate availability ("ketogenic capacity") by increasing the activity of acylcarnitine transferase within the liver. Finally, decreased muscle ketone metabolism also contributes to ketone accumulation in the diabetic state. Diminished ketone disposal has, in fact, been observed in diabetics with normal ketone production, suggesting that the rate of ketone utilization may be a more sensitive index of insulin deficiency than ketone overproduction.[7] Hyperketonemia in diabetes is thus a consequence of changes in processes in adipose tissue, liver, and muscle.

ROLE OF INSULIN ANTAGONISTIC HORMONES

It has been suggested that the metabolic abnormalities associated with diabetes result not from the insulin lack by itself, but rather from a bihormonal disturbance of alpha and beta cell function.[8] The importance of glucagon in the development of the diabetic syndrome is suggested by the demonstration that suppression of glucagon by glucose is lost in diabetes and that protein-stimulated glucagon secretion is augmented. However, recent studies suggest that glucagon contributes to the diabetic state primarily in circumstances of insulin deficiency. Elevations of plasma glucagon (within the range observed in most hyperglucagonemic states) have no effect on glucose tolerance in normal man or in diabetic patients as long as insulin is available.[9]

On the other hand, glucagon excess contributes to endogenous hyperglycemia when insulin is deficient. In this circumstance, the glycemic effect of hyperglucagonemia is excessive because insulin lack precludes rapid disposal of glucose transiently released by the liver in response to glucagon. Similarly, hyperglucagonemia is insufficient to cause hyperketonemia in the face of a normal insulin secretory response (even if free fatty acid delivery is increased), but can accelerate the development of ketosis in circumstances of insulin lack. Thus, glucagon hypersecretion may exaggerate the metabolic alterations accompanying insulin deficiency. However, relative or absolute insulin lack is the essential factor necessary for the changes in fuel mobilization and utilization which characterize diabetes.

In contrast to glucagon, physiologic elevations of cortisol or epinephrine markedly accentuate hyperglycemia and hyperketonemia in diabetics even in the face of insulin treatment.[10] Hypersensitivity to cortisol- and epinephrine-induced hyperglycemia in diabetes is a consequence of increased hepatic responsiveness to the stimulatory effects of these hormones on glucose production. This hypersensitivity may account for the metabolic decompensation frequently observed during major stress despite usual insulin treatment.

EFFECT OF INSULIN TREATMENT

The primacy of insulin deficiency in the derangements of glucose, protein, and fat metabolism observed in diabetes is underscored by recent studies using mechanical insulin delivery systems which simulate the normal pattern of insulin release. The "closed-loop" glucose-monitored systems have been shown to normalize plasma glucose levels for 12–24 hours in insulin-dependent diabetics. Using an "open-loop" preprogrammed portable infusion system which delivers insulin by the subcutaneous route in basal amounts with pulse dose increments before meals, normalization of glucose, lipid, and amino acid metabolism has been achieved for periods of 2 weeks to 4 months.[11] Furthermore, exercise-induced secretion of catecholamines and growth hormone, which is exaggerated during conventional insulin treatment, is reduced to normal levels after 1–2 weeks of insulin pump treatment.[12] These findings thus provide additional evidence that inadequate insulin availability is the primary factor underlying the alterations in fuel homeostasis and counterregulatory hormone secretion which characterize the diabetic syndrome.

References

1. Block MB, Mako ME, Steinerer DF, et al: Circulating C-peptide immunoreactivity. Studies in normals and diabetic patients. Diabetes 21:1013–1018, 1972
2. Robertson RP, and Porte D, Jr: The glucose receptor. A defective mechanism in diabetes mellitus distinct from the beta adrenergic receptor. J Clin Invest 52:870–876, 1973
3. DeFronzo R, Deibert D, Hendler R, et al: Insulin sensitivity and insulin binding to monocytes in maturity-onset diabetes. J Clin Invest 63:939–946, 1979
4. Felig P, Wahren J, and Hendler R: Influence of maturity-onset diabetes on splanchnic glucose balance after oral glucose ingestion. Diabetes 27:121–126, 1978
5. DeFronzo RA, Ferrannini E, Hendler R, et al: Influence of hyperinsulinemia, hyperglycemia, and the route of glucose administration on splanchnic glucose exchange. Proc Natl Acad Sci USA 75:5173–5177, 1978
6. Felig P, Wahren J, Sherwin R, et al: Amino acid and protein metabolism in diabetes mellitus. Arch Intern Med 137:507–513, 1977
7. Sherwin RS, Hendler R, and Felig P: Effect of diabetes mellitus and insulin on the turnover and metabolic response to ketones in man. Diabetes 25:776–784, 1976
8. Unger RH: Diabetes and the alpha cell. Diabetes 25:136–151, 1976
9. Sherwin RS, Fisher M, Hendler R, et al: Hyperglucagonemia and blood glucose regulation in normal, obese and diabetic subjects. N Engl J Med 294:455–461, 1976
10. Shamoon H, Hendler R, and Sherwin RS: Hypersensitivity to cortisol and epinephrine in normoglycemic insulin-treated diabetics: A mechanism for diabetic instability. Diabetes 28 (Suppl 1):353, 1979
11. Tamborlane WV, Sherwin RS, Genel M, et al: Restoration of normal lipid and amino acid metabolism in diabetic patients treated with a portable insulin-infusion pump. Lancet 1:1258–1261, 1979
12. Tamborlane WV, Sherwin RS, Koivisto V, et al: Normalization of the growth hormone and catecholamine response to exercise in juvenile-onset diabetics treated with a portable insulin infusion pump. Diabetes 28:785–788, 1979

4

Biosynthesis of Insulin

Arthur H. Rubenstein, M.D.

PROINSULIN

Significant information has accumulated in recent years regarding the biochemical and morphological details of insulin biosynthesis and secretion. In 1967 Steiner and his coworkers discovered that insulin was synthesized in pancreatic beta cells by way of a single chain precursor, proinsulin, and demonstrated that intracellular proteolytic conversion of the precursor to the hormone takes place prior to its storage and secretion.[1]

Proinsulin consists of a single polypeptide chain ranging in length from 78 (dog) to 86 (human, horse, rat) amino acid residues. The variations in length in the mammalian proteins occur only in the connecting polypeptide portion, which links the carboxy-terminus of the insulin B chain to the amino-terminus of the A chain. The known mammalian proinsulins have pairs of basic residues at either end of the connecting peptide which link it to the insulin chains. These residues are excised during the conversion of proinsulin to insulin, giving rise to native insulin plus the remainder of the connecting polypeptide segment lacking amino- and carboxy-terminal basic residues. This peptide has been designated the C-peptide.

BIOSYNTHETIC ORGANIZATION OF THE BETA CELL

Proinsulin, in common with many other exportable proteins, is synthesized by ribosomes associated with the rough endoplasmic reticulum. After biosynthesis, peptide chain folding, and sulfhydryl oxidation to the native structure have occurred, newly synthesized proinsulin is transported by an energy requiring process to the Golgi apparatus. Conversion of proinsulin to insulin and the C-peptide is initiated in the Golgi apparatus or in the progranules as they leave the Golgi region, and continues for many additional hours within the secretory granules as they collect and mature in the cytosol.

The proteolytic enzymes responsible for the conversion of proinsulin to insulin have not been definitively identified. However, several lines of evidence indicate that the major types of proteolytic cleavage in this process involve the combination of a trypsin-like protease with another having specificity similar to that of carboxypeptidase B. The latter enzyme is necessary to remove the C-terminal basic residues left behind after tryptic cleavage, giving rise to the important naturally-occurring products, native insulin and the C-peptide. Approximate mixtures of pancreatic trypsin and carboxypeptidase B can quantitatively convert proinsulin to insulin in vitro. This model system can account for the known major intermediate forms and products that occur naturally in pancreatic extracts.

PREPROINSULIN

It has recently become clear that a precursor larger than proinsulin (preproinsulin) participates in the biosynthesis of insulin.[2] This form has been less readily detected because it turns over so rapidly in the cell. Preproinsulin and related precursors of many other secreted prohormones appear to provide the solution to a long-standing problem in the biosynthesis of secretory proteins, namely the mechanism by which the sequestration of peptide chains destined for secretion takes place within the cell. Thus, although it has been known that secretory proteins are synthesized in the rough endoplasmic reticulum by membrane-bound ribosomes, it has not been clear how the rough endoplasmic reticulum is formed or how the messenger RNA (mRNA) for secretory proteins is made available exclusively to membrane-bound ribosomes. The recent development of cell-free systems that efficiently translate mRNA in the absence of an appreciable background of endogenous protein synthesis has been of great importance in resolving this problem. One such system that has been widely used is the wheat-germ ribosomal system, which not only faithfully translates mRNA molecules in vitro, but also lacks proteolytic enzymes that might break down or alter the initial translation products as they are formed. Examination of the product obtained when nucleic acids, extracted from normal rat islets or rat islet cell tumors, were translated in a wheatgerm ribosomal system showed a major translation product, which was immunoprecipitable with insulin antibodies and had a molecular size of about 11,500 daltons. On the basis of these studies, it was concluded that preproinsulin consists of proinsulin with an amino-terminal extension of approximately 2,500 daltons.

INSULIN GENE

The identification of preproinsulin strongly suggests that the 51 residue insulin molecule is derived from a single gene which codes for a polypeptide containing 110 amino acids. Within the additional 49 amino acids of preproinsulin is the information required to direct its sequestration and storage within secretory granules, as well as the means to direct its efficient folding and the correct oxidation of its sulfhydryls. Several laboratories have now succeeded in using cloned cDNAs corresponding to insulin mRNA sequences as probes for the identification of the chromosomal genes for insulin. This approach will undoubtedly shed further light on questions regarding the structure, evolution, and possible defects in the genes for insulin.[3, 4]

On the basis of these new findings we can now summarize the flow of information in the beta cell. The gene or genes for insulin are located somewhere in the chromosomal DNA. The genes are transcribed by RNA polymerases in the nucleus, giving rise to the mRNA molecules, which encode the preregion as well as the B-, C-, and A-chain regions of proinsulin. The mRNA consists of a series of trinucleotide codons corresponding to these sequences and also contains a polyadenylic acid extension attached to its 3'-end. Translation of this mRNA leads initially to the synthesis of the preregion, which presumably aids in the binding of the appropriate ribosomes to the membranes of the endoplasmic reticulum, thus forming the rough endoplasmic reticulum of the beta cell. After the vectorial discharge of the proinsulin into the cisternal spaces, its subsequent processing and storage then proceed as detailed in the preceding sections.

SECRETION OF C-PEPTIDE

Insulin and C-peptide are derived from one molecule of proinsulin and are stored in equimolar quantities in beta cell granules prior to secretion. Thus, the serum levels of these peptides should correlate well and permit the use of the serum C-peptide concentration as a marker of beta cell function. This has proven to be particularly useful in insulin-treated diabetic patients in whom injected exogenous insulin and circulating insulin antibodies interfere with the measurement of endogenous insulin.[5, 6]

Circulating C-peptide levels are very low or undetectable in patients presenting in ketoacidosis. However, some two to ten weeks later, most subjects show partial recovery of beta cell secretory function as evidenced by a rise in peripheral C-peptide concentrations. This resumption of insulin secretion is associated with a decrease in exogenous insulin requirements and accounts for the "Brush effect" or honeymoon period. Following this recovery, sequential studies have shown that some diabetics retain the ability to secrete C-peptide over a number of years, albeit at a markedly reduced rate, while others become completely insulin deficient. An important question is whether there is any difference in the clinical course of patients with residual beta cell function compared to those who are entirely dependent on exogenous insulin for their metabolic control. The presently available results indicate that those patients with significant C-peptide secretion are more stable,[7] with fewer hypoglycemic reactions or episodes of ketoacidosis.

References

1. Steiner DF and Oyer PE: The biosynthesis of insulin and a probable precursor of insulin by a human islet cell tumor. Proc Nat Acad Sci USA 57:473–480, 1967
2. Steiner DF: Insulin today. Diabetes 26:322–340, 1977
3. Ullrich A, Shine J, Chirgivin J, et al: Rat insulin genes: construction of plasmids containing the coding sequences. Science 196:1313–1319, 1977
4. Villa-Komaroff L, Efstratiadis A, Broome S, et al: A bacterial clone synthesizing proinsulin. Proc Nat Acad Sci USA 75:3727–3733, 1978
5. Rubenstein AH, Steiner DF, Horwitz DL, et al: Clinical significance of circulating proinsulin and C-peptide. Recent Prog Hormone Res 33:435–468, 1977
6. Proceedings of an International C-peptide Symposium. Binder C and Rubenstein AH (eds). Diabetes 27 (Suppl 1):145–285, 1978
7. Gonen B, Goldman J, Baldwin D, et al: Metabolic control in diabetic patients. Diabetes 28:749–753, 1979

5

Current Concepts of Insulin Secretion in Diabetes Mellitus

Jeffrey B. Halter, M.D.
Daniel Porte, Jr., M.D.

INTRODUCTION

The importance of impaired insulin secretion in the pathogenesis of metabolic abnormalities of diabetes mellitus has been recognized for many years. This chapter will review the current state of knowledge about normal mechanisms and regulation of insulin release by the beta cells of the islets of Langerhans. In addition, alterations of beta cell function described in diabetic patients will be reviewed and updated.

NORMAL PHYSIOLOGY

The Role of Glucose

Glucose is the key physiological regulator of beta cell function. Glucose directly stimulates insulin release from the islets and regulates insulin responses to all other stimuli. Studies both in vitro and in vivo have documented that the insulin secretory response to direct glucose stimulation is multiphasic.[1] There is an early spike of insulin release (first phase) that occurs immediately after a glucose challenge and is over within 10–15 minutes despite continued hyperglycemia. Subsequently there is a gradual increase of insulin release (second phase) that continues as long as the stimulus of hyperglycemia persists. This latter response, especially if the stimulus is prolonged, is partially dependent upon the synthesis of insulin. The first phase response appears to be an important determinant of the glucose disappearance rate during a standard intravenous glucose tolerance test.

In addition to responding to glucose, the beta cell responds to a variety of other signals,[2,3] some of which are stimulatory while others are inhibitory (Table 5-1). It is now clear that the beta cell response to these other signals is modulated by the prevailing glucose level. We have used the term *potentiation* to describe this regulatory effect of glucose. For example, the insulin response to the beta adrenergic agent, isoproterenol, in man increases dramatically when plasma glucose levels are elevated, and falls when the glucose level is lowered.[4] Similarly, the gastrointestinal peptide, GIP, has no demonstrable effect on insulin release at basal levels of glucose, but GIP clearly stimulates insulin release when plasma glucose levels are elevated.[5] Glucose levels can also modulate effects of beta cell inhibitors. Although somatostatin is a potent inhibitor of insulin responses to a variety of beta cell secretagogues, such insulin responses can be at least partially restored when plasma glucose levels are increased.[6]

The Beta Cell as an Integrator

The beta cell may be best considered as an integrator of multiple stimulatory and inhibitory signals (Figure 5-1). There is evidence

Table 5-1. Signals Affecting Insulin Release.

Stimulators	Inhibitors
Glucose	Catecholamines (α-adrenergic)
Amino acids	Somatostatin
Fatty acids	Serotonin
Catecholamines (β-adrenergic)	Prostaglandin E
Acetylcholine	
Intestinal peptide hormones	

that insulin secretion in the basal state (i.e., after an overnight fast) is determined by this integrating function in response to endogenous signals.[7] When there is resistance to insulin action (e.g., obesity), beta cell stimulators such as glucose, amino acids, and fatty acids tend to increase, leading to an increase of basal insulin. Conversely, during starvation, plasma glucose declines, and meal-related signals are absent, resulting in a decrease of basal insulin levels. Following ingestion of a meal, an integrated insulin response occurs which is related to the increased glucose and amino acid levels, the release of gastrointestinal hormones, and the increase of visceral parasympathetic tone. The importance of these neuroendocrine stimulatory signals during a meal is demonstrated by the augmented insulin secretory response to orally ingested glucose or protein compared to the response to the same amount of nutrient given intravenously.

Cellular Mechanisms for Insulin Release

Exocytosis of intact granules is the major mechanism by which insulin is released from the beta cell. The process of exocytosis involves activation of the microtubular-microfilamentous system and appears to be dependent on shifts of intracellular calcium ions.[8] Therefore, the regulation of intracellular calcium may provide a signaling mechanism by which glucose and other stimulators and inhibitors modulate beta cell function. The second messenger cyclic AMP system is known to modulate insulin release rate, but regulation of intracellular calcium seems to be the prime mechanism for insulin secretion in a manner analogous to excitation-contraction coupling in muscle.[9, 10] Glucose and other beta cell modulators have been observed to cause striking changes of islet cell electrical activity,[11] suggesting that changes of membrane permeability and resulting ionic currents are an important component of an intracellular calcium signaling mechanism. Initiation of this signaling process appears to involve interaction of the beta cell regulator with specific membrane receptors. Although the existence of such receptors for neuroendocrine peptides and classical neurotransmitters is well

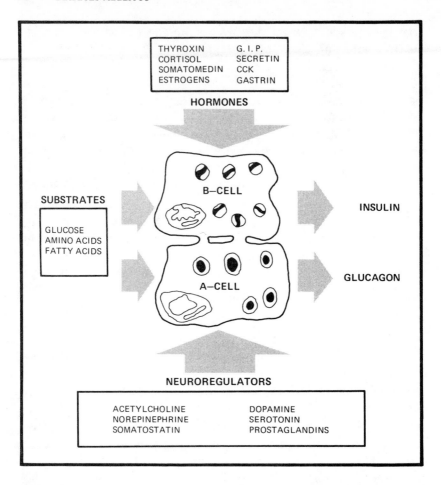

Figure 5-1. Pancreatic islet cells integrate signals due to substrates, extrapancreatic hormones, and neuroregulators to provide appropriate plasma levels of glucagon and insulin.

established, membrane receptors for nutrients such as glucose and amino acids have not yet been directly demonstrated. The possibility that intracellular metabolism of nutrient substrates is also involved in initiation of a signaling process for insulin release has been considered, but, at present, metabolic intermediates critical for such a process have not been identified.

INSULIN SECRETION IN DIABETES MELLITUS

Insulin-dependent Diabetes Mellitus

The beta cell function of patients with insulin-dependent diabetes can be characterized as uncompensated. Such patients are unable to maintain enough insulin secretion to meet their anticatabolic needs despite the presence of hyperglycemia, which would normally result in secretion of large amounts of insulin. They have subnormal basal insulin levels and inadequate insulin secretory responses to beta cell stimuli. In the absence of exogenous insulin administration, marked hyperglycemia, lipolysis, and proteolysis occur. Many patients with insulin-dependent diabetes, after an initial period of therapy, demonstrate a partial and temporary return of beta cell function (a "honeymoon" phase). During this period, endogenous insulin secretion occurs, as documented by measurement of C-peptide in plasma and urine.[12] This residual endogenous insulin release may increase the ease of diabetes control and may be of sufficient magnitude that exogenous insulin is not required to maintain a compensated metabolic state. However, recovery of beta cell function is temporary, and dependence on exogenous insulin therapy invariably recurs.

Noninsulin-dependent Diabetes Mellitus

Beta cell function of patients with noninsulin-dependent diabetes mellitus can be characterized as compensated. Such patients are able to secrete adequate amounts of insulin to meet anticatabolic needs. Thus, such patients are metabolically stable in the absence of a supervening illness. Lipolysis and proteolysis are normally inhibited, and basal plasma glucose levels, though elevated, are stable from day to day.[13]

The results of early studies of circulating insulin levels of noninsulin-dependent diabetics were somewhat surprising since the expectation of low levels was not confirmed. Plasma insulin levels of such patients were found to be of normal magnitude, or even elevated. However, these early studies did not take into account the insulin resistance of obesity, which leads to increased basal and stimulated insulin levels. Thus, when noninsulin-dependent diabetics, who are often overweight, are compared with weight-matched controls, the basal insulin levels of the diabetics are of normal magnitude but the insulin responses to an oral glucose challenge are impaired.[14] These findings are illustrated in Figure 5-2. Furthermore, studies of insulin secretory responses to an intravenous glucose challenge have demonstrated a more striking qualitative diabetic defect. Patients with fasting plasma glucose levels greater than 115 mg/dl do not have a measurable first-phase insulin response to glucose.[15]

In addition to having an impaired acute insulin response to glucose stimulation, patients with noninsulin-dependent diabetes demonstrate an impairment of glucose potentiation of nonglucose signals.[4] Patients with higher fasting plasma glucose levels have progressively greater impairment of glucose potentiation. These findings provide the basis for a new hypothesis to explain the remarkable consistency of basal hyperglycemia from day to day, the normal basal insulin levels, and the normal insulin responses to nonglucose stimuli of patients with noninsulin-dependent diabetes. As shown in Figure 5-3, this hypothesis suggests a feedback loop between the steady-state plasma glucose level and basal insulin secretion. Glucose is shown as the key regulator of beta cell output by both direct stimulation of insulin release and potentiation of the effects of other secretagogues to release insulin. The secreted insulin then regulates glucose production by the liver and glucose utilization by peripheral tissues. Through the operation of the feedback loop, a new, regulated, steady-state plasma glucose level is achieved.

In diabetics, the ability of the islet to respond to glucose, both as a direct stimulator of insulin release and as a potentiator of nonglucose stimuli, is impaired. Therefore, insulin secretion drops, resulting in increased production and decreased removal of glucose and an increase of the plasma glucose level. The resulting hyperglycemia increases the size of the glucose signal. The larger glucose signal remains ineffective in terms of a direct effect on the islet (hyperglycemic diabetics have markedly impaired first-phase insulin responses to a glucose challenge). However, this hyperglycemia results in augmentation of insulin

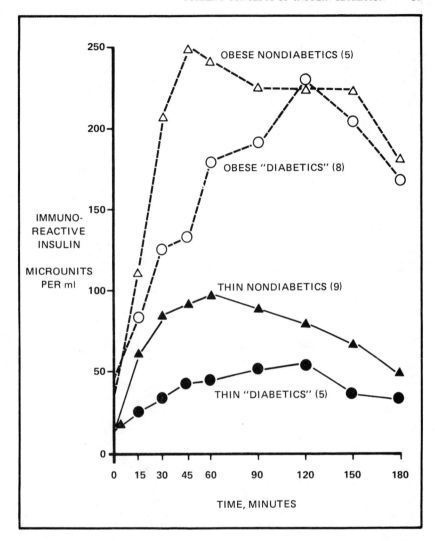

Figure 5-2. Mean insulin response of thin and obese nondiabetic and diabetic subjects during 3 hour (100 gram) oral glucose tolerance tests.[14]

responses to nonglucose signals.[4] When the basal glucose level has risen high enough to provide sufficient potentiation of nonglucose signals, a new steady-state is achieved in which basal insulin secretion is compensated. Under these circumstances, production and removal of glucose, basal insulin levels, and acute insulin responses to nonglucose stimuli are all normal.

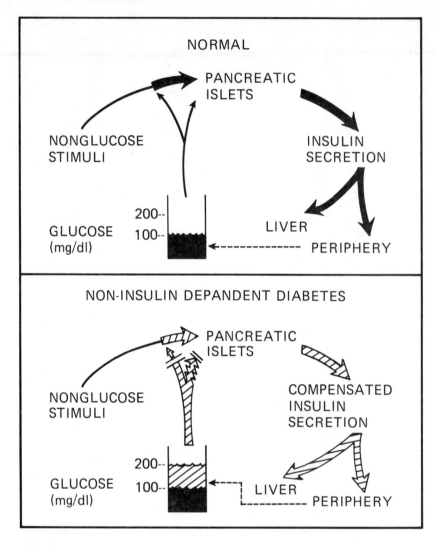

Figure 5-3. Schematic representation of an hypothesis about the relationship between steady state plasma glucose levels and insulin secretion in the normal state and in compensated diabetes mellitus (see text for explanation).

Due to renal excretion of glucose, the basal and postprandial glucose levels cannot rise indefinitely. Therefore, patients with more severe deterioration of islet function may not be able to maintain a high enough plasma glucose level to fully compensate for their impairment of glucose potentiation. These patients have low basal insulin levels and subnormal insulin responses both to glucose and nonglucose stimuli.[4] Such uncompensated patients may have accelerated basal glucose production and/or increased lipolysis, thereby falling into the category of insulin dependency.

In addition to decompensation of metabolic status due to a primary deterioration of islet function, it is apparent that a number of other factors could influence the delicate balance of compensation in diabetic subjects. Thus alpha-adrenergic inhibition of insulin release accompanying stress could lead to decompensated islet function in an otherwise compensated patient. Similarly, the development of insulin resistance due to obesity or the release of hormones which antagonize the effects of insulin (growth hormone, cortisol, glucagon, or catecholamines), such as might occur during a stressful illness, could lead to decompensation.[3] Reversal of the cause of insulin resistance or impaired insulin release would then be expected to result in return of the patient to a compensated state.

CONCLUSION

Studies of insulin secretion have helped to clarify the mechanisms by which regulation of beta cell function occurs in man. Such studies have identified glucose as a direct stimulator of the beta cells as well as an important potentiator of a variety of nonglucose signals. An understanding of beta cell regulation in the normal state has provided an explanation for a number of alterations of beta cell function in patients with diabetes mellitus. However, the molecular mechanisms involved in insulin secretion by the beta cell are not completely known. It is hoped that further understanding of these mechanisms will lead to better characterization of the causes of impaired beta cell function of patients with both insulin-dependent and noninsulin-dependent diabetes mellitus.

References

1. Porte D, Jr, and Bagdade JD: Human insulin secretion: an integrated approach. Ann Rev Med 21:219–240, 1970

2. Gerich JE, Charles MD, and Grodsky GM: Regulation of pancreatic insulin and glucagon secretion. Ann Rev Physiol 38:353–388, 1975
3. Porte D, Jr, Woods SC, and Smith PH: Neural control of the pancreatic islet and its relation to stress hyperglycemia. *In* Diabetes Mellitus: A Pathophysiologic Approach to Clinical Practice. Assan R, Girard JR, and Marliss EG, (eds), John Wiley & Sons, New York, In Press
4. Halter JB, Graf RJ, and Porte D, Jr: Potentiation of insulin secretory responses by plasma glucose levels in man: Evidence that hyperglycemia in diabetes compensates for impaired glucose potentiation. J Clin Endocrinol Metab 48:946–954, 1979
5. Andersen DK, Elahi D, Brown JC, et al: Oral glucose augmentation of insulin secretion. Interaction of gastric inhibitory polypeptide with ambient glucose and insulin levels. J Clin Invest 62:152–161, 1978
6. Taborsky GJ, Jr, Smith PH, Halter JB, et al: Glucose infusion potentiates the acute insulin response to non-glucose stimuli during the infusion of somatostatin. Endocrinology 105:1215–1220, 1979
7. Goodner CJ and Porte D, Jr: Determinants of basal islet secretion in man. *In* Handbook of Physiology. Greep RO, (ed), Williams and Wilkins Co., Baltimore, 1973, pp. 597–609
8. Malaisse WJ, Malaisse-Lagae F, Van Obberghen E, et al: Role of microtubules in the phasic pattern of insulin release. Ann NY Acad Sci 253:630–652, 1975
9. Charles MA, Lawecki J, Pictet R, et al: Insulin secretion. Interrelationships of glucose, cyclic adenosine 3′:5′ - monophosphate, and calcium. J Biol Chem 250:6134–6140, 1975
10. Wollheim CB, Kikuchi M, Renold AE, et al: The roles of intracellular and extracellular Ca^{++} in glucose-stimulated biphasic insulin release by rat islets. J Clin Invest 62:451–458, 1978
11. Meissner HP and Atwater IJ: The kinetics of electrical activity of beta cells in response to a "square wave" stimulation with glucose or glibenclamide. Horm Metab Res 8:11–16, 1976
12. Block MB, Rosenfield RL, Mako ME, et al: Sequential changes in beta-cell function in insulin-treated diabetic patients assessed by C-peptide immunoreactivity. N Engl J Med:1144–1148, 1973
13. Holman RR and Turner RC: Maintenance of basal plasma glucose and insulin concentrations in maturity-onset diabetes. Diabetes 28:227–230, 1979
14. Bagdade JD, Bierman EL, and Porte D, Jr: The significance of basal insulin levels in the evaluation of the insulin response to glucose in diabetic and nondiabetic subjects. J Clin Invest 46:1549–1557, 1967
15. Brunzell JD, Robertson RP, Lerner RK, et al: Relationship between fasting plasma glucose levels and insulin secretion during intravenous glucose tolerance tests. J Clin Endocrinol Metab 42:222–229, 1976

6

Insulin-Glucagon-Somatostatin Interactions

Roger H. Unger, M.D.

Recent advances in our understanding of the physiology and pathophysiology of glucagon, together with the discovery of somatostatin in the islets of Langerhans, have forced major conceptual modifications concerning islet cell function in health and disease. These changes warrant the attention of clinicians with an interest in diabetes mellitus and related diseases. Some of the material contained in this chapter is still unconfirmed and may require revision by the time of the next edition in this series. Nevertheless, the fundamental issues of the normal relationships between the islet cells, the hormones they secrete, and the aberrations of diabetes seem likely to stand the test of time.

THE MICROANATOMY OF THE ISLET AND INTERCELLULAR RELATIONSHIPS

The islets of Langerhans, the vital regulators of fuel homeostasis, constitute unique endocrine microorgans dispersed in a well-protected solid retroperitoneal structure, the pancreas. Each of the many hundreds of thousands of microorgans has a constant nonrandom topographical arrangement of its cells[1] (Figure 6-1). In man, the outer rim of each islet is made up principally of glucagon-containing A-cells. In one segment of the pancreas A-cells are largely replaced by F-cells containing pancreatic polypeptide, the function of which is yet to be elucidated. The A-cells make up approximately 25 percent of the islet cell population. Under this outer shell of A-cells is a sparser layer of somatostatin-containing D-cells comprising about 10 percent of the normal endocrine population. The central portion of the islet consists largely of B-cells, which make up at least 60 percent of the islet. All of the islet cells are connected to one another by the intercellular channels called "gap junctions," through which small molecules can flow from the interior of one cell to the interior of another cell without entering the intercellular space. Thus, each islet is, in the functional sense, a syncytium, and the intercellular connections may provide a means by which the individual cells of a single islet coordinate their respective secretory activities (see Reference 1 for a review).

CONTROL OF ISLET CELL SECRETION

The output of islet hormones is controlled by means of signals from various sources inside and outside the islets. These are depicted schematically in Figure 6-2.

Signals Originating Within the Islets: Inside the islet, locally produced prostaglandins may influence the behavior of the islet cells. But the islet hormones themselves may exert profound local effect upon the secretory activities of nearby cells. For example, somatostatin released from D-cells located between A- and B-cells may locally inhibit both insulin and glucagon secretion, while glucagon may stimulate both insulin and somatostatin, and insulin may inhibit both glucagon and somatostatin secretion. An interlocking "paracrine" or local system may, thus, govern islet cell function[2] (Figure 6-3), although definitive proof of this is not yet available. Perhaps the hyperglucagonemia of diabetes is the result of a loss of the inhibitory influence of local somatostatin and insulin upon A-cell secretion as a consequence of profound distortion of islet microanatomy and cell-to-cell relationships (Figure 6-3).

Signals Originating Outside the Islets: The islets of Langerhans are obviously under the tight control of influences

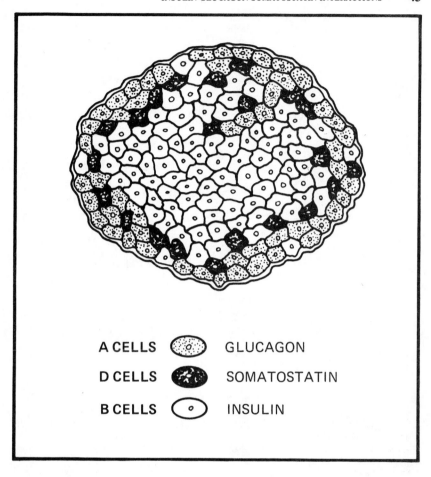

A CELLS   GLUCAGON

D CELLS   SOMATOSTATIN

B CELLS   INSULIN

Figure 6-1. Schematic representation of an islet of Langerhans, showing distribution of glucagon, somatostatin, and insulin-containing cells based on immunofluorescent studies for these hormones. Islet cell types for which no positive function has yet been established are omitted from this scheme, as are the afferent blood vessels and nerves which enter in the tricellular zone. (Reprinted courtesy of Arch Int Med).

arising from outside the islets. Inasmuch as their function is to regulate the homeostasis of many fuels, of which glucose is of a particular importance, it is not surprising that the level of circulating glucose and other fuels exerts an important influence on the secretion of insulin and glucagon. Similarly, in view of the dependence of the central nervous system on the delivery of glucose (or ketones) through proper islet cell responses, it is not

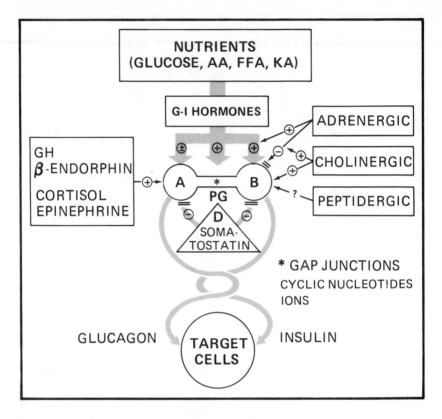

Figure 6-2. Hypothetical scheme depicting the islets of Langerhans as a multihormonal unit in which coordinated function of the component cells makes possible precise regulation of the homeostasis of glucose and other nutrients. In the case of glucose, the most tightly controlled of the nutrients, coordinated secretion of insulin and glucagon appropriately matches insulin-mediated glucose utilization with glucagon-mediated glucose production by the liver, thereby maintaining normal glucose levels irrespective of change in flux rates. Somatostatin may serve as a regulator of the entry of ingested nutrients into the circulation (still unproven), in which case, coordinated secretion of somatostatin and insulin would balance somatostatin-regulated entry of ingested nutrients with their insulin-mediated utilization. (Reprinted courtesy of Life Sciences.)

surprising that neurotransmitters play an important role in shaping the islet hormone response to stress, famine, or physical danger (fight or flight situations), when survival depends upon the maintenance of optimal function of the central nervous system. To maintain a high rate of hepatic fuel production (glucose and ketones) insulin levels must be low and glucagon levels relatively high; this islet response can be produced by adrenergic

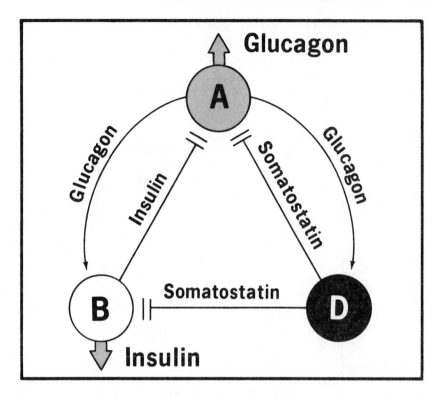

Figure 6-3. Schematic representation of the postulated paracrine or within-islet function of insulin, glucagon, and somatostatin. (Reprinted courtesy of Ann Rev Physiol)

input, hormones of stress (epinephrine, cortisol, and β-endorphin), and perhaps other factors not as yet identified.

On the other hand, the optimal storage of ingested fuels requires an appropriate rise in insulin; while the nutrients themselves influence the islet cell response to meals, the gastrointestinal hormones released during the processing of a meal, together with cholinergic signals, probably exert the most profound influence in determining both the timing, form, and magnitude of insulin secretion in response to a meal.

Actions of Insulin and Glucagon: Figure 6-4 reviews the antagonistic actions of these two islet hormones. By varying the relative concentrations of these two peptides, fuels can be moved to and from various tissues according to moment-to-moment needs. However, insulin-mediated utilization of glucose is maintained at relative equality with glucose production by the liver, mediated by glucagon, and glucose absorption from the gut, thereby restricting glucose concentrations to the normal range. Put differently, insulin prevents hyperglycemia during increased glucose entry, and glucagon prevents hypoglycemia during increased glucose utilization (see Reference 3 for a review).

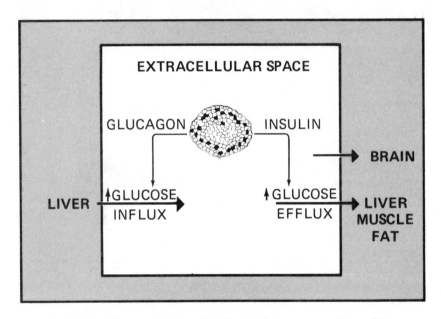

Figure 6-4. Schematic representation of insulin and glucagon as regulators of the movement of nutrients such as glucose through the extracellular space. The brain is depicted as consuming glucose at a constant rate independent of insulin concentration. The islet produces insulin in increased amounts whenever blood glucose levels rise, as after a meal, and enhances glucose efflux into liver, muscle, and perhaps, fat tissue. Glucagon, by contrast, enhances glucose production by the liver whenever glucose concentration in the extracellular space begins to fall. Thus, during increased glucose efflux—in exercise, for example—enhanced glucagon secretion would replace the utilized glucose, thereby maintaining extracellular glucose concentration constant. Thus, the coordinated secretion of insulin and glucagon makes it possible to change flux rates through the extracellular space without permitting glucose concentration to exceed the upper or lower limits of normal.

IS SOMATOSTATIN A HORMONE?

As already mentioned, many have assumed that the somatostatin in the islets exerts a local inhibitory action on its neighboring islet cells, although incontrovertible proof of this is lacking. The hormonal status of somatostatin remains similarly uncertain.

However, it has been hypothesized (Figure 6-5) that somatostatin of the islets is a third hormone with a regulatory role in the homeostasis of ingested nutrients.[4] Teleologically, it seems reasonable that the islets of Langerhans, which control the main pathways of nutrient flux (endogenous fuel production by the liver through glucagon and the rate of fuel disposal into insulin-responsive tissues such as liver, fat, and muscle via insulin), should also have an influence on the major route of nutrient flow, i.e., influx of ingested nutrients from the gastrointestinal tract. It has long been known that somatostatin, at least in pharmacologic doses, can inhibit virtually all important post-prandial gastrointestinal and digestive events, and now it appears that even small physiological increments of exogenous somatostatin retard the rate at which ingested nutrients enter the circulation. It has, therefore, been hypothesized that islet somatostatin controls the rate at which ingested nutrients enter the circulation, thereby making possible coordination between the rate at which ingested nutrients enter the circulation and the rates at which they are utilized by insulin-responsive tissues (Figure 6-5). While this concept is far from proven, it appears to fit with all presently available facts. For example, gastrointestinal hormones released during meals stimulate the release of pancreatic somatostatin in parallel with the release of insulin, and somatostatin, in turn, inhibits the release of these gut hormones in a positive-negative gut-islet-gut axis. Moreover, in the dog, endogenous somatostatin-like immunoreactivity rises in plasma after meals,[5] and its neutralization by somatostatin antibodies is associated with an exaggerated postprandial rise of plasma triglyceride levels.

THE PATHOPHYSIOLOGY OF THE ISLETS IN DIABETES MELLITUS

Juvenile Diabetes: In addition to the well-known disturbances in B-cell function, diabetes mellitus of all types is associated with glucagon levels which are high relative to both the insulin levels and the glucose levels.[6] This abnormal A-cell function is expressed in at least two ways: (1) the normal reciprocal relationship between glycemia and glucagonemia is lost; glucagon is no longer suppressed by hyperglycemia nor increased by

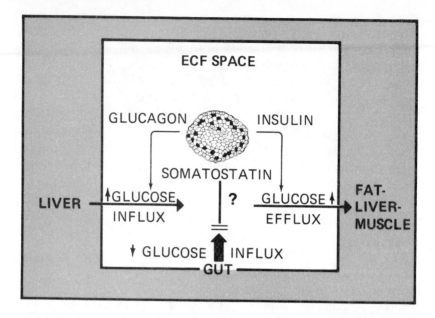

Figure 6-5. This diagram is identical to Figure 4 except that somatostatin has been added as a third hormone of nutrient homeostasis. The current concept is that somatostatin may regulate the rate at which nutrients enter the extracellular fluid space from the gut. Coordination between the somatostatin-secreting D-cells, depicted as black cells, and the insulin-secreting B-cells, depicted as white cells, would make possible relative equality between the influx of nutrients such as glucose from the gut and their insulin-mediated efflux to tissues, thereby giving the islets control of the rate at which ingested nutrients move through the extracellular space, while maintaining their concentrations in that space within relatively narrow limits.

hypoglycemia; and (2) the response of the A-cell to stimuli such as arginine and other A-cell secretogogues is exaggerated, and is not diminished by hyperglycemia, as is the case in nondiabetics.

In the juvenile-type diabetic, these A-cell abnormalities are believed to be the result of the lack of a normal insulin pattern appropriate for the circulating glucose concentration. Insulin can restore to normal the A-cell response to changes in glucose.[7] A constant rate of insulin delivery will not achieve this; rather, insulin delivery must simulate the nondiabetic pattern if the A-cell response is to be made entirely normal, something which conventional treatment with insulin obviously cannot achieve.

The islets of the juvenile-type diabetic are grossly deformed. They are small because of the loss of the central mass of B-cells, and they consist of about 75 percent A-cells and 25 percent D-cells. It is not surprising that, in addition to hyperglucagonemia, hypersomatostatinemia has been reported.[5] Why doesn't the increase in islet somatostatin restrain the A-cell in the juvenile diabetic? Perhaps in the absence of the restraining influence of insulin, the relatively small quantities of somatostatin in the islets are insufficient to produce a normal level of suppression, particularly with the extensive disruption of the intimate anatomical contiguity between A- and D-cells that characterizes normal islets.

Adult-Onset Diabetes: Abnormal A-cell function is also present in the maturity-onset diabetic, but seems to vary with the degree of B-cell dysfunction.[8] Loss of glucose suppressibility is less marked, particularly in the obese hyperinsulinemic type of diabetic, than in the juvenile-type diabetic, but hyperresponsiveness to A-cell secretogogues is just as marked. The most striking difference between the normal A-cell function of the adult-onset diabetic and that of the juvenile-type diabetic is that, whereas, in the latter, insulin corrects the A-cell hyperresponsiveness to a protein meal and to arginine, in the adult-onset diabetic even very high doses of insulin fail to diminish the A-cell hyperresponsiveness.[9] Since insulin is often present in abundance in the latter form of diabetes, this observation is not surprising and suggests that the etiology of the A-cell dysfunction in this form of diabetes cannot be ascribed to insulin lack as in juvenile diabetes.

THE DELETERIOUS ROLE OF ABNORMAL A-CELL FUNCTION IN DIABETES

The presence of glucagon, a powerful glycogenolytic, gluconeogenic, ketogenic antagonist of insulin, produces the severe endogenous hyperglycemia and ketosis that characterizes the insulin-deficient state. Insulin deficiency alone, in the absence of glucagon, does not cause the overproduction of glucose or ketones that otherwise occurs.[10-12] Even when insulin is present in normal quantities but its effective concentration is fixed by secretory malfunction or resistance to its action on target cells, a rise of glucagon contributes to the hyperglycemia.[13] Only a normal capacity of insulin to respond to glycemic change can prevent glucagon from adding to diabetic hyperglycemia. This should be obvious—after all, stimulation of glucagon in a normal person by a protein meal does not raise blood sugar, but in a diabetic, receiving a constant intravenous insulin infusion, ingestion of a carbohydrate-free protein meal raises the plasma glucose by 50 mg/dl within an hour.[14]

THERAPEUTIC IMPLICATIONS

This deleterious action of glucagon can obviously be prevented by a normal increase in insulin. Islet transplants, the artificial B-cell, or open-loop insulin pumps can achieve this and thus overcome the effects of glucagon. However, when insulin delivery cannot be made to match insulin need, then suppression of glucagon and glucagon-mediated glucose production may be useful in blood glucose control.

Pharmacologic doses of somatostatin inhibit glucagon secretion in the juvenile diabetic.[11] This action, together with a retarding effect on the rate of nutrient entry from the gut,[15] makes possible better glycemic control than with insulin delivered at a constant rate. While the usefulness of somatostatin as an adjunct to conventional therapy remains to be established, this new approach appears sufficiently promising to warrant thorough exploration.[16]

References

1. Orci L and Unger RH: Hypothesis: Functional subdivisions of islets of Langerhans and possible role of D-cells. Lancet ii:1243–44, 1975
2. Unger RH and Orci L: Hypothesis: The possible role of the pancreatic D-cell in the normal and diabetic states. Diabetes 26:241–44, 1977
3. Unger RH and Orci L: Physiology and pathophysiology of glucagon. Physiological Reviews 56:778–826, 1976
4. Unger, RH, Ipp E, Schusdziarra V, et al: Hypothesis: Physiologic role of pancreatic somatostatin and the contribution of D-cell disorders to diabetes mellitus. Life Sci 20:2081–86, 1977
5. Schusdziarra V, Rouiller D, Harris V, et al: The response of plasma somatostatin-like immunoreactivity to nutrients in normal and alloxan diabetic dogs. Endocrinology 103:2264–73, 1978
6. Unger RH and Orci L: Hypothesis: The essential role of glucagon in the pathogenesis of diabetes mellitus. Lancet i:14–16, 1975
7. Shichiri M, Kawamori R, and Abe H: Normalization of the paradoxic secretion of glucagon in diabetics who were controlled by the artificial beta cell. Diabetes 28:272–75, 1979

8. Hatfield HH, Banasiak MF, Driscoll T, et al: Glucose suppression of glucagon: Relationship to pancreatic beta cell function? J Clin Endocrinol Metab 44:1080–87, 1977
9. Raskin P and Unger RH: Effect of insulin therapy on the profiles of plasma immunoreactive glucagon in juvenile-type and adult-type diabetics. Diabetes 27:411–19, 1978
10. Dobbs RE, Sakurai H, Sasaki H, et al: Glucagon: Role in the hyperglycemia of diabetes mellitus. Science 187:544–47, 1975
11. Gerich JE, Lorenzi M, Bier DM, et al: Prevention of human diabetic ketoacidosis by somatostatin: Evidence for an essential role of glucagon. N Engl J Med 292:985–89, 1975
12. Cherrington AD, Lacy WW, and Chiasson JL: Effect of glucagon on glucose production during insulin deficiency in the dog. J Clin Invest 62:664–77, 1978
13. Raskin P and Unger RH: Effects of exogenous hyperglucagonemia in insulin-treated diabetics. Diabetes 26:1034–39, 1977
14. Raskin P, Aydin I, Yamamoto T, et al: Abnormal alpha cell function in human diabetes: The response of oral protein. Amer J Med 64:988–97, 1978
15. Wahren J and Felig P: Influence of somatostatin on carbohydrate disposal and absorption in diabetes mellitus. Lancet ii:1213–16, 1976
16. Raskin P and Unger RH: Hyperglucagonemia and its suppression. Importance in the metabolic control of diabetes. N Engl J Med 299:433–36, 1978

7

Glucoregulatory Effects of Neurogastrointestinal Peptides: The Diffuse Neuroendocrine System

Marvin R. Brown, M.D.
Wylie W. Vale, Ph.D.

A large number of biologically active small peptides (molecular weight < 3500) have been demonstrated to be present within brain, gut, and pancreas. Some of these peptides, e.g., somatostatin, luteinizing hormone releasing factor, and thyrotropin releasing factor, have established physiological roles as regulators of anterior pituitary functions.[1] These peptides and others (Table 7-1) have pharmacologic actions on the brain, gut, and/or pancreas as well as other tissues. Evidence now supports the concept that some of these neurogastrointestinal peptides are messengers of a diffusely distributed intercellular communication system. The widespread distribution and multiple actions of these small peptides in mammalian tissues leads to the consideration of the teleologic significance of this peptide messenger system. Neurogastrointestinal peptides, members of the diffuse neuroendocrine system, may play a variety of roles in various tissues as transsynaptic (neurotransmitter or neuromodulator), paracrine, or endocrine mediators. The proposed common neuroectodermal origin of cells containing various secretory peptides is an appealing unifying concept.[2] Unfortunately, considerable reservations have been expressed recently concerning this hypothesis, particularly with regard to the derivation of the endocrine cells of the gut and pancreas.[3] Refinement of the APUD (amine precursor uptake decarboxylation) concept by

Pearse suggests that these peptides are from a neuroendocrine programmed epiblast.[4] Alternatively, it can be proposed that the nervous, endocrine, and gastrointestinal systems evolved a variety of extracellular peptide regulatory agents, and that it was advantageous to the organism for those systems to communicate with one another by means of such peptides. According to this hypothesis, a mutation allowing one system to detect and appropriately respond to signals from other systems would be selected for. Mutations permitting local expression (production) of that peptide signal could have occurred subsequently.[5] A consequence of this evolutionary expansion of a peptide's roles would be the potential for the peptides to coordinate the actions of various physiologic systems. Coordination of several actions by a single peptide is perhaps characteristic of oligopeptides as extracellular transmitter substances; there may be an advantage to the organism to have a single extracellular messenger that regulates and organizes qualitatively and temporally the activities of systems.[6] For example, insulin modifies the entry or exit of fat, carbohydrate, and protein into a variety of cell types. Likewise, neurogastrointestinal peptides may act at a variety of sites to regulate and synchronize various cellular functions.

Table 7-1. Neurogastrointestinal Peptides: Members of The Diffuse Neuroendocrine System.

Somatostatin
Thyrotropin Releasing Factor (TRF)
Luteinizing Hormone Releasing Factor (LRF)
Neurotensin (NT)
Substance P (SP)
Cholecystokinin (CCK)
Bombesin
β-Endorphin/enkephalins
Glucagon
Insulin

Small peptides may participate in varied morphologically arranged systems. That is, peptides may act as specific endocrine messengers in addition to being transsynaptic or paracrine mediators. Endocrine specificity may result from the apparent highly restricted receptor distribution, a characteristic that probably is related to the size and greater complexity of peptides as compared with the smaller non-peptide chemical messenger substances. As transsynaptic or paracrine mediators, an additional level of specificity is conferred by virtue of the restriction of anatomic distribution of such messengers.

It is probable that the secretory oligopeptides are produced by post-translational modification of larger precursor peptides which were biosynthesized by ribosomal mechanisms. In the nervous system, the parakaryia, rather than axon terminals, are the sites of biosynthesis; the secretory capacity of peptidergic neurons is dependent upon axonal transport and the presence of sizable pools near release sites rather than on local synthesis, as in the case for monoamines. Another potential distinguishing feature of peptides or their post-translational products is the biosynthetic proximity of these substances to genomic control. Whether primary genomic products versus cytoplasmic products offer an operational advantage in the system's control remains an unanswered question.

Somatostatin represents an excellent example of a neurogastrointestinal peptide. Indeed, the plethora of somatostatin actions on the brain, gastrointestinal tract, and pancreas led to the initial conclusion by one endocrinologist that this peptide was the endocrine cyanide.[7] More careful inspection of the various actions that somatostatin exerts may indicate that this peptide, like many others, exerts actions on multifocal sites, which, in a general sense, can be viewed as coordinated to reach a common physiological goal. Perhaps the most common action of somatostatin is to influence nutrient metabolism.[1, 8, 9] Somatostatin may alter hepatic glucose production by a direct effect on the liver[10, 11, 12] or by altering pancreatic insulin or glucagon secretion, which, in turn, affects hepatic glucose output.[8] Somatostatin alters the pituitary secretion of growth hormone that secondarily might affect carbohydrate metabolism.[13] Unger and co-workers have also suggested that somatostatin may play a role in controlling nutrient entry from the gut.[14] In addition, somatostatin has recently been demonstrated to influence those mechanisms by which the brain may control nutrient metabolism and appetite.[9, 15] In doses that are ineffective when given systemically, somatostatin and somatostatin analogs, given intracisternally or into the lateral ventricle of rats, reduce hyperglycemia and hyperglucagonemia produced by a variety of CNS active glucogenic substances, e.g., bombesin, 2-deoxyglucose, β-endorphin, carbachol, neurotensin, and stress. Recent studies have demonstrated that the mechanisms by which somatostatin produces these CNS effects on glucoregulation are via alteration of plasma catecholamine levels.[15,16] The various actions of somatostatin to inhibit gastrointestinal hormone secretion, produce pancreatic exocrine secretions, and inhibit gallbladder contraction are all consistent with somatostatin's coordinated actions to influence nutrient mobilization.[1,8]

Another neurogastrointestinal peptide, bombesin, is similar to somatostatin in that it possesses a variety of intriguing pharmacologic or physiologic actions.[6] However, in contrast to somatostatin, bombesin, a tetradecapeptide isolated from anuran skin, has not been chemically characterized in mammalian tissues. Highly purified extracts of mammalian brain and gastrointestinal tract do, however, contain an immunologically and biologically active bombesin-like peptide.[6,17,18] Bombesin placed into the various brain regions produces a prompt adrenal-dependent hyperglycemia in animals which lasts for several hours, an effect which is independent of hypothermia produced by this peptide.[19,20] This hyperglycemia is associated with elevation of plasma epinephrine and glucagon and decrease in plasma insulin.[16,20]

The action of bombesin to affect the brain to influence adrenal epinephrine secretion while apparently having little, if any, effect on levels of norepinephrine, suggests that the sympathetic nervous system may be subdivided functionally.[20] Thus, adrenal secretion of epinephrine may occur in the absence of generalized increase of sympathetic activity. Similar selective activation of a branch of the sympathetic nervous system occurs following insulin-induced hypoglycemia,[21] i.e., rise in plasma epinephrine greater than norepinephrine. The possibility exists that there is a metabolic advantage of only epinephrine secretion following some physiologic stimuli; that is, hypoglycemia or CNS nutrient deprivation would best be served by activation of nutrient-mobilizing systems and not by generalized sympathetic activity. Generalized sympathetic activity would result in utilizing substrates possibly critical for CNS function. We have suggested that a parallel response to the activation of the nutrient-mobilizing component of the sympathetic nervous system is activation of adaptive hypothermia. Lowering of body temperature would reduce cellular utilization substrates that would be of adaptive value in states of nutrient deprivation. The neural pathways stimulated by bombesin are capable of increasing nutrient mobilization and lowering body temperature to provide a mechanism to ensure adequate substrate for tissues such as the brain during periods of nutrient deprivation. Bombesin given to rats intracisternally or intracerebroventricularly reversibly lowers body temperature and activates the adrenomedullary sympathetic nervous system,[19, 20, 22] thus showing that a single putative neurochemical messenger can produce these two effects. These observations further demonstrate the concept of a single messenger exerting coordinated actions.

Similar to bombesin, neurotensin, at high doses, when placed into the central nervous system, produces a rise in plasma catecholamines, glucagon, and glucose, with a decrease in plasma insulin. Neurotensin and substance P, given systemically to animals, result in an increase in plasma glucagon and glucose, an effect which appears to be secondary to direct effects of these peptides on the endocrine pancreas and, subsequently, glucagon effect on hepatic glucose production.[23, 24, 25] Neither substance P nor neurotensin has been demonstrated to have any direct effect on hepatic glucose production.[1] The possibility that the actions of substance P and neurotensin to elevate glucagon might be secondary to release of endogenous histamine is supported by the observation that these effects are reversed by H_1 antihistamine blockers.[26, 27] Although histamine has extremely potent effects to alter the secretion of insulin and glucagon from the endocrine pancreas,[26] little attention has been given to what role this biogenic amine might have in the physiologic regulation of endocrine pancreatic secretions. Animals given streptozotocin have been demonstrated to have increased pancreatic levels of neurotensin and increased gastric levels of substance P.[28] Whether these increased tissue levels of neurotensin and/or substance P may contribute to the diabetic state of these animals has not been determined. It would be of interest to determine if antihistamines would improve the glucose intolerance of these animals.

The morphinomimetic peptides, including β-endorphin, have been reported to influence the CNS to produce hyperglycemia in animals.[9, 29, 30] We have found that development of hyperglycemia is dependent on intact adrenal gland and occurs only in animals whose motor activity is severely impaired. We have so far been unable to demonstrate any CNS hyperglycemic action of the enkephalins.

Ipp et al.[31] have recently demonstrated that β-endorphin stimulates the secretion of insulin and glucagon from the perfused dog pancreas. Systemic administration of β-endorphin does not alter blood glucose concentrations or modify the dose response of epinephrine to produce hyperglycemia (Brown, unpublished observation). What role, if any, β-endorphin might have in influencing normal carbohydrate metabolism remains to be determined.

TRF (thyrotropin releasing factor) has recently been demonstrated to be distributed throughout the rat gastrointestinal tract and the pancreas.[32, 33] TRF secretion from the perfused rat pancreas may be induced by arginine. In addition, it has been demonstrated that TRF enhances arginine-induced glucagon secretion from the isolated perfused rat pancreas.[34] While we were unable to demonstrate enhancement of arginine-induced glucagon secretion by TRF, the potent TRF analog, 3-methyl-his-2-TRF, significantly enhances arginine-induced glucagon secretion (Brown, unpublished data). Neither TRF nor 3-methyl-his-2-TRF significantly influenced arginine-induced insulin secretion.

This short summary of some of the effects of neurogastrointestinal peptides on the neuroendocrine regulation of carbohydrate metabolism serves to point out the diverse possible sites of action of these peptides to potentially influence carbohydrate metabolism. As pointed out above, these peptides may potentially influence carbohydrate metabolism by neurocrine, paracrine, or endocrine actions, or a combination of the above. Whether any of these substances are physiologic participants in the regulation of carbohydrate metabolism remains to be determined. However, each may be used as a tool to pharmacologically explore the regulation of those systems which influence carbohydrate metabolism. Models which can be derived from the effects of bombesin and somatostatin to influence brain control of the sympathetic nervous system allow exploration into possible mechanisms in the importance of stress-induced changes in carbohydrate metabolism.

References

1. Vale W, Rivier C, and Brown M: Regulatory peptides of the hypothalamus. Ann Rev Physiol 29:473–527, 1977
2. Pearse AGE and Polak JM: The diffuse neuroendocrine system and the APUD concept. *In* Gut Hormones. Bloom SR, (ed), London, Churchill Livingston, 1978, pp. 33–39
3. Le Douarin NM: The embryological origin of the endocrine cells associated with the digestive tract. *In* Gut Hormones. Bloom SR, (ed), London, Churchill Livingston, 1978, pp. 49–56.
4. Pearse AGE: The common peptides and the APUD concept. In International Society of Psychoneuroendocrinology, Xth International Congress, August 8–11, 1979, Park City, Utah, p. 33 (Abstract).
5. Vale WW: Distribution, metabolism, and pharmacology of peptides. Neurosci Res Prog Bull 16:521–533, 1978
6. Brown M and Vale W: Bombesin—a putative mammalian neurogastrointestinal peptide. Trends in Neurosci 2:95–97, 1979
7. Besser GM: Hypothalamus as an endocrine organ—II. Br Med Jour 3:613–615, 1974
8. Brown M and Vale W: Somatostatin: Five years of progress. Biomedicine 28:93–96, 1978
9. Brown M, Rivier J, and Vale W: Somatostatin: Central nervous system actions on glucoregulation. Endocrinol 105:1709–1715, 1979
10. Oliver JR and Wagle SR: Studies on the inhibition of insulin release, glycogenolysis and gluconeogenesis by somatostatin in the rat islet of Langerhans in isolated hepatocytes. Biochem Biophys Res Commun 62:772, 1975
11. Sacks H, Waligora K, Matthews J, et al: Inhibition by somatostatin of glucagon induced glucose release from the isolated perfused rat liver. Diabetes 26:22, 1977 (Abstract)
12. Sacca L and Sherwin R: Somatostatin (SRIF) alters sensitivity to glucagon and epinephrine independent of insulin and glucagon availability. Diabetes 26:23, 1977 (Abstract)
13. Pfeiffer EF, Missner C, Beischer W, et al: The anti-diabetic action of somatostatin assessed by the artificial β-cell. Metabolism (suppl 1) 27: 1415, 1978
14. Unger RH, Ipp E, Schusdziarra V, et al: Hypothesis: physiologic role of pancreatic somatostatin and the contribution of D-cell disorders to diabetes mellitus. Life Sci 20:2081, 1977
15. Fisher DA and Brown M: Somatostatin: Plasma catecholamine suppression mediated by the central nervous system. Science, submitted 1979
16. Brown M and Fisher DA: Plasma catecholamines: regulation by brain peptidergic and cholinergic systems. 61st Ann Endocrine Soc Meeting, June, 1979, Anaheim, A211, p. 125 (Abstract)

17. Brown M, Allen R, Villarreal J, et al: Bombesin-like activity: radioimmunologic assessment in biological tissues. Life Sci 23:2721–2728, 1978
18. Villarreal J and Brown M: Bombesin-like peptide in hypothalamus: chemical and immunological characterization. Life Sci 23:2729–2734, 1978
19. Brown M, Rivier J, and Vale W: Bombesin affects the central nervous system to produce hyperglycemia in rats. Life Sci 21:1729–1734, 1977
20. Brown M, Tache Y and Fisher D: Central nervous system action of bombesin: Mechanisms to induce hyperglycemia. Endocrinol, In Press, 1979
21. Lewis GP: Physiological mechanisms controlling secretory activity of adrenal medulla. In Handbook of Physiology and Endocrinology. Geiger SR, (ed), Washington, D.C., Amer Physiological Soc, 1975, Vol 6, pp. 309–319
22. Brown M, Rivier J, and Vale W: Bombesin: potent effects on thermoregulation in the rat. Science 196:998–1000, 1977
23. Brown M and Vale W: Effects of neurotensin and substance P on plasma insulin, glucagon and glucose levels. Endocrinol 98:819–822, 1976
24. Carraway RE, Demers LM, and Leeman SE: Hyperglycemic effect of neurotensin, a hypothalamic peptide. Endocrinol 99:1452–1462, 1976
25. Nagai K and Frohman LA: Hyperglycemia and hyperglucagonemia following neurotensin administration. Life Sci 19:273–280, 1976
26. Brown M, Villarreal J, and Vale W: Neurotensin and substance P: Effects on plasma insulin and glucagon levels. Metabolism 25:1459–1461, 1976
27. Nagai K and Frohman LA: Neurotensin hyperglycemia: evidence for histamine mediation and the assessment of a possible physiologic role. Diabetes 27:577–582, 1978
28. Fernstrom MH, Mirski MA, Carraway RE, et al: Effect of streptozotocin-induced diabetes on tissue levels of substance P and neurotensin. Endocrinol 104:A448, 1979 (Abstract)
29. Feldberg W: Pharmacology of the central actions of endorphins. In Gut Hormones. Bloom SR, (ed), London, Churchill Livingston, 1978, pp. 495–500
30. Brown M and Vale W: Somatostatin (SS): Central nervous system (CNS) actions on glucose and temperature regulations. Endocrinol 102:A770, 1978
31. Ipp E, Dobbs RE, and Unger R: Morphine and β-endorphin influence the secretion of the endocrine pancreas. Nature 276:190–191, 1978
32. Morley JE, Garvin TJ, Pekary AE, et al: Thyrotropin-releasing hormone in the gastrointestinal trace. Biochem and Biophys Res Commun 79:314–318, 1977
33. Leppäluoto J, Koivusalo F, and Kraama R: Thyrotropin-releasing factor: Distribution in neural and gastrointestinal tissues. Acta Physiol Scand 104:175–179, 1978
34. Morley JE, Steinbach JH, Feldman EJ, et al: The effects of thryotropin releasing hormone (TRH) on the gastrointestinal tract. Life Sci 24:1059–1066, 1979

8

Insulin Receptors and Hyperglycemia

Jesse Roth, M.D.
Michele Muggeo, M.D.

Background: Historically, diabetes has been viewed as a disorder due to insulin deficiency. In fact, only a minority of patients with hyperglycemia are absolutely insulin-deficient and absolutely require insulin regularly. These patients have been designated Type I, or insulin-dependent, ketosis-prone diabetics.

The large majority of patients with hyperglycemia have normal or supernormal amounts of insulin in the circulation. This insulin is biologically intact insulin (Note 1), but the cells of the hyperglycemic patient do not respond to it as well as do the normal cells. Not only are the cells less responsive to the endogenous insulin, but they are less responsive to exogenously administered insulin as well. Thus, in the majority of hyperglycemic patients, the major defect is at the level of the target cell.[1]

The Target Cell and its Receptors: The first step in the action of insulin at the target cell is binding of hormone to specific receptors at the cell surface (Table 8-1, Figure 8-1). The receptors for insulin and for most hormones are complex proteins that reside in the plasma membrane of the cell; each hormone or other bioactive ligand has a unique set of receptors which serves to recognize that particular bioactive species. The binding of hormone to receptor serves two fundamental functions, recognition and activation. The receptor allows the cell to recognize insulin, although the hormone represents only one out of every few million molecules to which the cell is exposed. Further, the combination of hormone with receptor initiates, at the cell surface, the series of biochemical events within the target cell that lead ultimately to the characteristic action of the hormone, e.g., with insulin, glucose storage, or utilization (Figure 8-1). If the responsiveness of the target cell is subnormal, the defect could lie at any site with the target cell.[1-3] With the introduction of methods by which receptor binding can be measured specifically and quantitatively,[1,4] it is now clear that many patients with hyperglycemia and/or insulin resistance (Note 2) have defects at the level of the receptor.[1-10] Either the receptor for insulin is deficient in number or its affinity for insulin is reduced, and these alterations at the level of the receptor appear to be important in the manifestation of the disease.

Modulators of the Insulin Receptor: The receptors on the cell surface are being turned over rapidly with half-lives in the order of a few hours. A steady-state level of receptors indicates that

Table 8-1. The Interaction of Hormone With Receptor.

1. The primary interaction:

$$H + R \leftrightharpoons HR$$

H = free hormone
R = free receptor
HR = hormone-receptor complexes
R_o = total receptor $(R + HR)$

2. The equilibrium constant (K_a) for this reaction:

$$K_a = \frac{[HR]}{[H][R]}$$

3. The biological effect (E) is some function (f) of the strength of the signal to the cell; the signal strength is directly related to [HR].

$$E = f([HR])$$
$$= (K[H][R])$$

Thus, the signal strength to the cell depends equally on K, H, and R (or R_o).

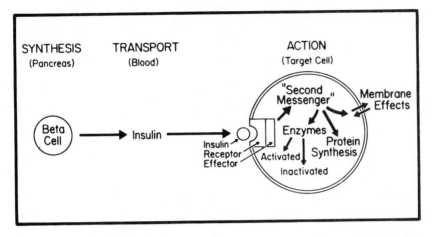

Figure 8-1. Schematic representation of insulin synthesis, transport, and action at its target cell. The part of the receptor molecule that recognizes insulin is labeled "receptor" while that portion of the receptor molecule that initiates the activation of the target cell is designated "effector." (Bar RS, Harrison LC, Muggeo M, et al. Advances in Intern Med Vol 24, 1979:23, Year Book Med Pub, Chicago.)

the synthetic rate is equal to the degradation rate. Both the concentration and the affinity of receptor for hormone are highly regulated by a wide range of signals from inside and outside the cell. For example, the chronic ambient insulin concentration to which the cell is being exposed (i.e., basal insulin) regulates the receptor concentration and affinity. Diet can have major effects. High-calorie, high-fat, or high-carbohydrate diets lower insulin binding. High-fiber diets, as well as exercise (both acute and systematic training), elevate binding of hormone to receptor and increase sensitivity to insulin. In addition, one or more hormones, by any of several mechanisms, can affect hormone binding to receptor. Thus, the receptor, like the hormone, has as a major feature of its biology a propensity to respond quickly and widely to changes in the internal and external environment of the cell.[1-3, 6]

Methods: To measure receptors, carefully prepared ^{125}I-insulin is incubated for a few hours with whole cells or the components of broken cells that are rich in plasma membrane, both in the absence and presence of unlabeled insulin. The amount of hormone bound to receptor is expressed as a function of the total insulin concentration (Figure 8-2). The specificity of binding has been verified by comparing the receptor binding to the biological properties of dozens of insulins and related substances.[1,4]

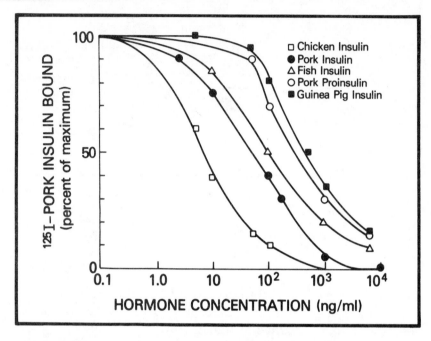

Figure 8-2. Specificity of the insulin receptor. The binding *in vitro* of ^{125}I-pork insulin to receptor on cells or membranes of cells is plotted as a function of the hormone concentration. In competing for ^{125}I-insulin binding, chicken insulin > pork > fish > proinsulin > guinea pig insulin, which parallels the relative biological potencies of these insulins. Receptors in all species of vertebrates and all cell types show this same specificity. (Muggeo M, Ginsberg BH, Roth J, et al. Endocrinology, 104:1393, 1979.)

The insulin receptor is extremely similar functionally in all vertebrates and in all tissues (Figure 8-2). In animals, essentially all tissues are accessible, whereas in humans, tissue is limited. Human blood cells (monocytes, erythrocytes, and granulocytes), placenta, and adipocytes can be obtained fresh for study. What we really wish to know most in humans is the state of insulin receptors on liver and secondarily on muscle. The insulin receptors on other cells are most useful when they mirror accurately the state of their counterparts in liver and muscle. The current favorites for study in humans are monocytes and erythrocytes. How can we extrapolate from receptors on blood cells to liver and muscle? If the receptor in either erythrocytes or monocytes changes in the same way as liver and muscle in the analogous state in animals, or if both of these cell types in people give the same pattern of binding, or if the binding changes correlate with the severity of the problem and to therapeutic responses, then it may be surmised that this pattern of receptor binding may be widepread in the individual and include liver and/or muscle. To distinguish effects on receptors due to the in vivo environment, the insulin receptors on cultured fibroblasts and B-lymphocyte cell lines have been used. More methods are now being introduced to study receptors, including morphological, chemical, and immunological tools and a technique to measure receptor binding in vivo in the whole animal or person.

Obesity in Rodents: The first studies to relate a disease state to a defect in a cell surface receptor were those with insulin receptors in obese insulin-resistant mice.[5] In obese mice, irrespective of whether the obesity is genetic or acquired, hyperinsulinemia and insulin resistance are associated with a deficiency of insulin receptors in liver and all other cells examined including muscle, fat, heart, and lymphocytes (but not brain). Among the obese mice, the severity of the insulin resistance correlates with the severity of the receptor defect. Treatments that improve cellular responsiveness to insulin (and glucose tolerance) markedly improve binding to receptors.

Obesity in Humans and Dieting: The majority of adult diabetics are obese. In fact, obesity and diabetes are commonly associated in individuals as well as in populations worldwide. In most obese diabetics, plasma insulin levels in the basal state, as well as in the postprandial state, are above normal, and measurements of sensitivity to insulin in vivo (and in vitro) show subnormal responsiveness, i.e., resistance to insulin at the level of the target cell. In obese humans, as in the mice, there is an excellent correlation between the magnitude of the insulin resistance and the severity of the receptor defect, even to the extent that, in those obese patients who are not hyperinsulinemic or insulin-resistant, receptor concentrations are normal. Furthermore, calorie-restricted diets lead to a prompt improvement in glucose tolerance, amelioration of the hyperinsulinemia, and restoration of receptors to normal (Figure 8-3A). It should be emphasized that calorie-restricted diets show their beneficial effects very quickly (even within a week or two) long before the patient has been restored to normal weight.[2, 3, 6–8]

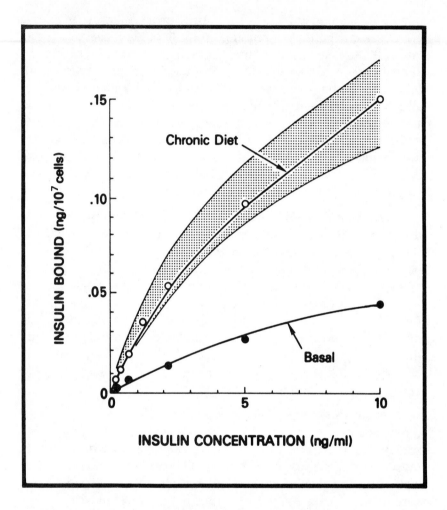

Figure 8-3. Insulin binding to circulating monocytes. Blood was drawn and mononuclear cells were isolated and interacted with ^{125}I-insulin and unlabeled insulin. Insulin bound to receptor (vertical axis) is plotted as function of the insulin concentration to which the cell is exposed in the assay. (A.) An obese patient in the "basal" state is compared to the same patient after a calorie-restricted diet ("chronic diet") and to normal subjects (shaded area). Note that insulin binding in the basal state is reduced uniformly at all concentrations of insulin. (Bar RS and Roth J: Arch Intern Med 137:474, 1977.) (B.) Four acromegalic patients (individual lines) are compared to normal subjects (shaded area). Patient 1 is most insulin resistant and patient 4 is least resistant. Note that insulin binding is less impaired at low insulin concentrations (< 1 mg/ml), equivalent to basal insulin *in vivo* then at high concentrations (> 2 mg/ml) equivalent to stimulated levels *in vivo*. (Muggeo M, Bar RS, Roth J et al. Journal of Clinical Endocrinology and Metabolism 48:17, 1979.) (C.) Patients with Type A and Type B extreme insulin resistance are compared to an obese subject and to normal volunteers. (Kahn CR, Flier JS, Bar RS, et al. Journal of Medicine, 294:739, 1976.) (For (B) and (C) see pp. 69 and 70.)

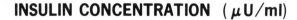

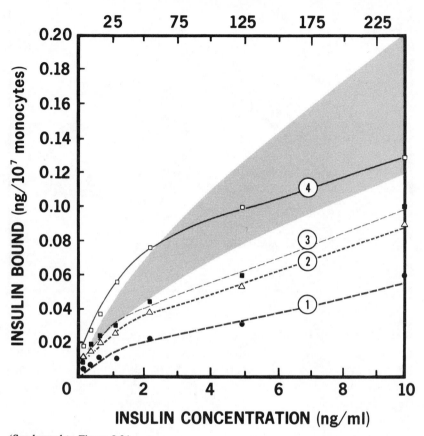

(See legend to **Figure 8-3.**)

Thin Diabetics: Although most are obese, some of the adult-type Type II, noninsulin-dependent diabetics are not over-weight. Some of these thin diabetics have normal insulin sensitivity, while others show hyperinsulinemia and insulin resistance. Those with insulin resistance have a decrease in the number of receptor sites per cell, whereas those with normal insulin sensitivity have normal concentrations of receptor (Figure 8-4A).[6]

Sulfonylureas: When thin adult diabetics with decreased receptors were treated with sulfonylureas, receptor concentrations increased, along with substantial improvement in the blood glucose levels (Figure 8-4B).[6] In a few of the patients, sulfonylureas

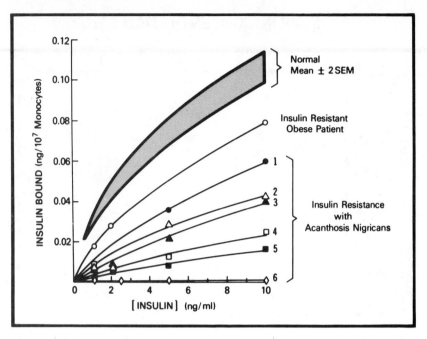

(See legend to **Figure 8-3.**)

caused no change or a decrease in receptors, and these patients failed to respond clinically to the drug. The effect of sulfonylureas, to elevate receptor concentrations, has also been shown in rodents. Thus, contrary to long-held theories, sulfonylureas, when they work, appear to operate at the level of the receptor rather than at the level of the hormone. (The largely ignored paradox had been that sulfonylureas do act acutely to stimulate hormone release in vivo and in vitro, but, curiously, with chronic treatment of diabetics with sulfonylureas, circulating hormone concentrations failed to increase.)

Caution: While sulfonylureas do appear to act to increase receptors in receptor-deficient patients, I am not prepared, on that basis, to recommend the use of these agents in the treatment of diabetes. The mechanism of their action is a pharmacological question; their clinical usefulness is a therapeutics question, the answer to which depends on their safety and long-term efficacy, which have been in some doubt.

Other Forms of Insulin Resistance: With growth hormone excess, commonly encountered in patients with acromegaly (and,

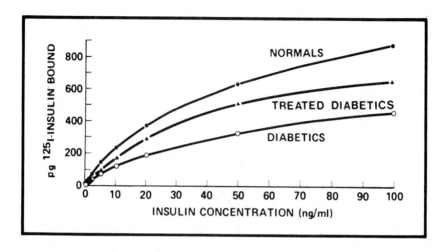

Figure 8-4. Thin patients with noninsulin-dependent (Type II) diabetes as a group are compared before and after treatment with sulfonylurea (4A and 4B) versus normal subjects (4A) (see Figure 3 legend for general methods). The three patients who failed to increase insulin binding on sulfonylurea treatment (broken lines, open circles, and crosses) failed to respond clinically. (Olefsky JM and Reaven GM, Am J Med 60:89, 1976.) (For (4B) see next page.)

very rarely, in growth hormone deficient patients who are being overzealously treated with growth hormone replacement), hyperinsulinemia and insulin resistance are associated with a decrease in insulin binding to its specific receptor sites. In acromegaly, as in obesity, among individual patients, there is excellent correlation between the severity of the insulin resistance and the severity of the receptor defect (Figure 8-3B).

Receptors are just starting to be characterized in other forms of moderate insulin resistance. Glucocorticoid excess produces insulin resistance similar to that encountered in obesity and acromegaly, and a decrease in hormone binding at the receptor has likewise been observed. However, the effects of glucocorticoids appear to be quite complex since acute and chronic therapy in humans and rodents, in vivo and in vitro, each appear to give somewhat different results. Similarly, in one form of experimental uremia, the insulin resistance is accounted for by the receptor defect, whereas chronic renal failure in humans appears to be more complicated, involving receptor and

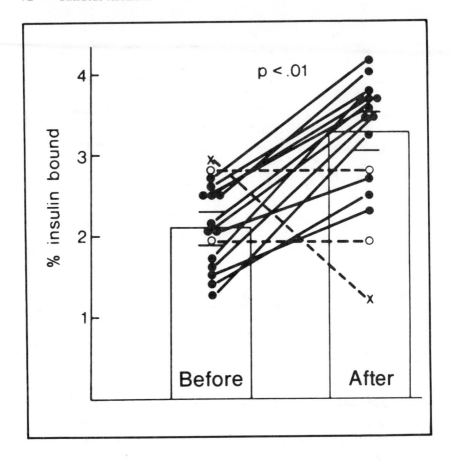

postreceptor sites. Pregnancy, myotonic dystrophy, and Werner's syndrome have likewise been studied, but the relative role of receptor and postreceptor events is as yet uncertain.[1,2]

Extreme Insulin Resistance: In contrast to the patients described above, who have moderate insulin resistance, are several groups of patients with extreme insulin resistance (Tables 8.2 and 8.3).[2,3,10] They are substantially more hyperinsulinemic in both the basal and stimulated states, and their response to exogenous insulin is distinctly more impaired than that found in obese or other patients with moderate insulin resistance. Acanthosis nigricans (Figure 8-3C), which may be quite marked, is found in many of these patients, irrespective of the cause of the extreme insulin resistance, and the severity of this skin lesion waxes and wanes in phase with the hyperinsulinemia. The relationship at the biochemical or cellular level of the skin lesion to the glucose and insulin problems is obscure. Finally, it should be pointed out that anti-insulin antibodies, due to treatment with insulin, can be of unusually high titer and thereby cause insulin resistance that may be quite severe. In all patients with insulin resistance that we ascribe to defects at the target cell, we have shown that anti-insulin antibodies are absent or that the titer is not high enough to account for the insulin resistance.

Table 8-2. Extreme Insulin Resistance at the Target Cell.

Antireceptor Antibodies	Prevalence of Antibodies	
Type B	All, by definition	
Ataxia telangiectasia	Few?	
IgA, IgE deficiency	Few?	
NZO mice	All obese diabetic ones?	
Lacking Antibodies to Receptor	**Receptor or Postreceptor Defect**	
Type A	Receptor ⎫	by definition
Type C	Postreceptor ⎭	
Lipoatrophic diabetes	Either—or both	
Leprechaunism	Either—or both	

Antireceptor Antibodies: This group of patients with extreme insulin resistance, in addition to insulin-resistant diabetes, has clinical and laboratory findings that we associate with autoimmune phenomena (Table 8-3). A minority of these patients fulfill the diagnostic criteria for one of the well-characterized autoimmune diseases (e.g., lupus), but the majority do not. Insulin binding to their cells is markedly decreased, and they have in their circulation antibodies directed against the receptor for insulin. These antibodies bind to the receptor and impair the ability of the receptor to bind insulin. The severity of the insulin resistance correlates well with the severity of the hyperinsulinemia, the severity of the defect in insulin binding to their own cells, and to the titer of antireceptor antibody in their circulation.

Table 8-3. Patients with Acanthosis Nigricans and Insulin Resistance.

Type A and Type B	Type A	Type B
Hyperglycemia—usually	Young, 12–24 yr	Older, 30–60 yr
Hyperinsulinemia—may	Hirsutism, virilization	Autoimmune features
be extreme	Polycystic ovaries	+ antinuclear antibodies
Insulin resistance—may	No autoimmune	+ anti-DNA
be extreme	features	↑ erythrocyte
Acanthosis nigricans		sedimentation rate
		↑ γ-globulins
		↓ WBC
		Alopecia, proteinuria
		Anti-receptor antibodies

Spontaneous or drug-induced remissions of the disease are associated with coordinate improvement or complete disappearance of all of these abnormalities (and of the acanthosis nigricans). In addition to the patients who fulfill the criteria for Type B insulin resistance with acanthosis nigricans, antireceptor antibodies have been detected in two patients with insulin-resistant diabetes associated with ataxia telangiectasia; in New Zealand obese mice with autoimmunity and insulin-resistant diabetes; and in occasional patients with isolated deficiencies of IgA or IgE.[2, 3, 10]

Extreme Insulin Resistance Without Antibodies: Another group of patients with extreme insulin resistance associated with acanthosis nigricans are those designated Type A (Table 8-3). Insulin binding to their receptors is markedly diminished, but they have no circulating antibodies or autoimmunity. All of these patients are thin females who have difficulties with sexual maturation and often have polycystic ovaries. In one patient, we observed the characteristic Type A syndrome, but the patient had normal binding of insulin to her receptors, indicating that a postbinding defect was the sole cause of her insulin resistance. This patient, designated Type C, and the patients with typical Type A show many similarities with a broad group of patients who have long been described under the rubric of lipoatrophic diabetes. The latter group of patients, in addition to their lipoatrophy, often show marked hyperinsulinemia and severe insulin resistance. Insulin binding to receptors in these patients has been subnormal, normal, or elevated, suggesting a heterogeneity of mechanism.[1–3,10]

Leprechaunism: Of a mixed group of young infants with leprechaunism (failure to thrive; facies thought to resemble the mythical leprechauns), some have been found who have severe hyperinsulinemia and insulin resistance. With cultured fibroblasts from two of these patients, insulin binding to receptor was normal, implicating a postreceptor site, whereas in two cases, severe binding defects were detected in cultured cells, suggesting major congenital or genetic defects at the level of the receptor.

Insulin Deficiency: Up to here we have covered situations where changes in the receptor dominated the clinical picture; hormone levels were opposite to the clinical. However, even in hyperglycemic states where hormone deficiency is the dominant influence by far, receptor binding may change and these changes may be quite considerable, even if subordinate in the ultimate to the insulin deficiency. The most striking example, though incompletely worked out, is diabetic ketoacidosis. Insulin deficiency is the major problem. Poor control (i.e., hyperglycemia), ketones, and acidosis all have major effects on the receptor. Lowering pH from 7.4 to 6.8, as can occur in this disorder, can markedly depress the affinity of the receptor for insulin. Of potentially greater importance, recent studies showed that moderate acidosis itself can depress receptor levels, and severe acidosis (pH $\leq$ 7.0) can cause complete disappearance of receptor from the cell surface. This may account for the observation that occasional diabetics with severe ketacidosis do not respond to insulin until fluid and electrolyte corrections have started. We interpret it as follows: insulin deficiency leads to severe acidosis which leads to receptor disappearance and refractoriness to insulin via a receptor mechanism.

Conclusions: In patients with hyperglycemia, only a minority are absolutely insulin deficient. In a majority, insulin is being delivered to the target cell at normal or supernormal concentrations, but the target cell responds inadequately to the signal. In many of these patients, defects in the first step at the target cell, hormone binding to receptor, play an important role in the observed abnormalities. The receptor abnormality in each disorder is characteristic; typically the severity of the receptor defect in individual patients is correlated with the severity of the insulin resistance; and often successful therapy is associated with marked improvement in insulin resistance and in hormone binding to receptor. Steps beyond the receptor have not been as well characterized but may be involved as well.

Practical Considerations: Insulin receptors on erythrocytes can be studied on 5–10 ml of blood,[9] but reticulocytes or transfused cells at high concentrations may affect results. Studies on monocytes require 60–100 ml of blood; a better alternative is to remove 500 ml of blood, use the buffy coat for testing, and return most of the red cells and plasma to the patient, which allows a full monocyte and erythrocyte study with minimal net blood loss.

Many research laboratories in North America, Europe, Japan, and Australia do these types of studies regularly and are interested in patients with potential receptor disorders. Studies with monocytes are always done on the same day that the blood is drawn, whereas erythrocytes, if prepared properly, can be stored for later testing.

Receptor evaluation should be considered at least in the following situations: (a) any patient (even if blood glucose is normal) with an unexplained elevation of the basal insulin; (b) any patient with unexplained hyperglycemia with normal or supernormal insulin following oral glucose (especially if blood glucose response to intravenous insulin, 0.1 U/Kg body weight, is borderline or subnormal); or (c) any patient with acanthosis nigricans or autoimmunity (clinical and/or laboratory) associated with disordered blood glucose or insulin.

Notes

1. Very rare groups of patients make insulin molecules that are biologically defective.
2. The term, i.e., "insulin resistance" is often misinterpreted by the clinician. It does not indicate absolute refractoriness to insulin;

rather, a higher than normal concentration of insulin is needed to achieve any given level of response.

References

1. Roth J, Lesniak MA, Bar RS, et al: An introduction to receptors and receptor disorders. Proc Soc Exp Biol Med 162:3, 1979
2. Kahn CR: The role of insulin receptors and receptor antibodies in states of altered insulin action. Proc Soc Exp Biol Med 162:13, 1979
3. Bar RS and Roth J: Insulin receptor status in disease states of man. Arch Intern Med 137:474, 1977
4. Freychet P, Roth J, and Neville DM, Jr: Insulin receptors in the liver: Specific binding of [^{125}I]-insulin to the plasma membrane and its relation to insulin bioactivity. Proc Natl Acad Sci USA 68:1833, 1971
5. Kahn CR, Neville DM, Jr, Gorden P, et al: Insulin receptor defect in insulin resistance: Studies in obese-hyperglycemic mouse. Biochem Biophys Res Commun 48:135, 1972
6. Olefsky JM: The insulin receptor: Its role in insulin resistance of obesity and diabetes. Diabetes 25:1154, 1976
7. Beck-Nielsen H, Pedersen O, and Swartz-Sorensen N: Effects of diet on the cellular insulin binding and insulin sensitivity in young healthy subjects. Diabetologia 15:289, 1978
8. Felig P and Soman V: Insulin receptors in diabetics and other conditions. Amer J Med 67:913, 1979
9. Gambhir KK, Archer JA, and Carter L: Insulin radio-receptor assay for human erythrocytes. Clin Chem 23:1590, 1977
10. Kasuga M, Akanuma Y, Tsushima T, et al: Effect of anti-insulin receptor autoantibodies on the metabolism of human adipocytes. Diabetes 27:938, 1978

9

Genetics of Diabetes Mellitus

Carol E. Anderson, M.D.
Jerome I. Rotter, M.D.
David L. Rimoin, M.D., Ph.D.

INTRODUCTION

Although diabetes mellitus (DM) has often been termed the "geneticist's nightmare,"[1] current research efforts are giving clues into the genetics of the many disease entities that constitute DM. In this chapter we will briefly review the background for genetic heterogeneity, the implications of population and family HLA studies, as well as the current status of genetic counseling of families with a member affected with DM.

EVIDENCE FOR HETEROGENEITY

The increased prevalence of DM amongst the families of diabetics, as compared to the general population, suggested that genetic factors may be important in the etiology of the disease. Despite this familial aggregation, however, studies of large numbers of families were not consistent with any single mode of inheritance; and all of the different Mendelian modes of inheritance (autosomal dominant, sex linked and, most popularly, autosomal recessive), as well as polygenic inheritance, have been postulated.[2] One of the major difficulties in finding a single mode of inheritance to explain all DM was the lack of appreciation of genetic heterogeneity. This concept implies that DM is really a symptom complex, which is the result of many different genetic mechanisms; and, thus, different types of DM may be inherited in different ways.

One of the earliest pieces of evidence for genetic etiologic heterogeneity in DM in man was the recognition that glucose intolerance is a feature of many different genetic syndromes, due to mutations at different genetic loci.[3] These syndromes are listed in Table 9-1, classified according to the probable pathogenetic mechanisms.

Table 9-1.* Genetic Syndromes Associated With Glucose Intolerance or Clinical Diabetes.

Syndromes Associated with Pancreatic Degeneration	
Hereditary relapsing pancreatitis	AD
Cystic fibrosis	AR
Polyendocrine deficiency disease	AR
Hemochromatosis	AR
Hereditary Endocrine Disorders with Glucose Intolerance	
Isolated growth hormone deficiency	AR, AD
Hereditary panhypopituitary dwarfism	sporadic, AR, X-linked
Pheochromocytoma	AD
Multiple endocrine adenomatosis	AD
Inborn Errors of Metabolism with Glucose Intolerance	
Glycogen storage disease type 1	AR
Acute intermittent porphyria	AD
Hyperlipidemias	AD, AR
Syndromes with Nonketotic, Insulin-resistant, Early-onset Diabetes	
Ataxia telangiectasia	AR
Myotonic dystrophy	AD
Lipoatrophic diabetes syndromes	AR
Hereditary Neuromuscular Disorders with Glucose Intolerance	
Muscular dystrophy	AD, X-linked
Late-onset proximal myopathy	AR
Huntington chorea	AD
Machado disease	AD
Herrmann syndrome	AD

Optic atrophy-diabetes mellitus syndrome	AR
Friedreich's ataxia	AR
Alstrom syndrome	AR
Laurence-Moon-Biedl syndrome	AR
Pseudo-Refsum syndrome	AD

Progeroid Syndromes with Glucose Intolerance
Cockayne syndrome	AR
Werner syndrome	AR

Syndromes with Glucose Intolerance Secondary to Obesity
Prader-Willi syndrome	AR, sporadic
Achondroplasia	AD

Miscellaneous Syndromes with Glucose Intolerance
Steroid-induced ocular hypertension	Multifactorial
Mendenhall syndrome	AR
Epiphyseal dysplasia and infantile-onset diabetes	AR

AD=autosomal dominant
AR=autosomal recessive
NB: These indications of mode of inheritance are not meant to indicate that every case is inherited in this fashion. They are simply to indicate the suspected or proven modes of inheritance where they exist.
*After Rimoin[2]

Physicians have long appreciated clinical heterogeneity in DM; e.g., the different clinical characteristics of juvenile-onset and adult-onset types of diabetes. Family and twin studies have provided direct evidence for genetic heterogeneity between these two clinical disorders. For example, MacDonald found no greater prevalence of the adult-onset type of disease amongst families ascertained through a proband with a juvenile-onset type disease than would be expected in the general population.[4] This indicated that the two disorders were genetically independent. In monozygotic twins, Tattersall and Pyke found a 93 percent concordance for the adult-onset disease (onset at greater than 40 years) and a 50 percent concordance for the juvenile-onset disease (onset at less than 40 years), again indicating genetic differences between these two entities.[5] However, insulin-dependent (IDDM) and noninsulin-dependent (NIDDM) diabetes have now been accepted as more useful criteria for purposes of genetic studies than age of onset in distinguishing between these two major syndromes.[6]

There is now evidence for possible heterogeneity even within IDDM and NIDDM. For example, Tattersall and Fajans described families with the characteristics of maturity-onset DM, where the onset of the disease was in young people (less than 25 years of age).[7] Pedigree analysis showed that this maturity-onset disease of the young (MODY) was vertically transmitted from generation to generation, with approximately half the offspring of each affected person being affected, consistent with autosomal dominant inheritance. In addition, Leslie and Pyke have now found that chlorpropamide primed, alcohol-induced flushing may serve as a genetic marker for certain forms of NIDDM.[8]

HLA ASSOCIATIONS WITH INSULIN-DEPENDENT DIABETES MELLITUS (IDDM)

Studies utilizing the human leukocyte antigen (HLA) system have also provided significant new information on the genetic heterogeneity of DM, with positive HLA associations with IDDM and no association with NIDDM. By the way of explanation, the human leukocyte antigen system is a group of tightly linked genes on human chromosome number 6. Each of the three loci, A, B, and C, code for a number of antigens which can be serologically defined, using white cells. The D locus codes for antigens present only on lymphocytes and are determined by a mixed lymphocyte culture (MLC) reaction. Each individual inherits one set of antigens, a haplotype, from one parent, and the other set of alleles, or haplotype, from the other parent. The prevalence of each antigen varies from population to population. When a particular antigen is found in persons with a given disorder more often than is seen in the general population from which that person comes, there is said to be a positive association between the antigen and the disorder. The strength of the association is indicated by relative risk, e.g., the increase in risk for the disease of the group with the marker antigen as compared to the risk in the general population for developing the disorder.

Population studies in Caucasians in Western Europe have revealed positive associations on the order of 2-fold increased risk for IDDM with HLA-B8, B15, and B18 antigens. Even stronger associations on the order of a 5-fold increase were found with Dw3 and Dw4.[9] It is worth pointing out that many persons with B8 or the B8/Dw3 combination have no problems at all. These antigens, however, do occur in increased frequency in several autoimmune disorders, such as Grave's disease, Addison's disease, Sicca syndrome, myasthenia gravis, dermatitis herpetiformis with coeliac disease, and SLE.[10] The observation that antiadrenal antibodies are seen significantly more often in Dw3-positive Addison's patients than Dw3-negative patients is comparable to the increased persistence of islet cell antibodies that have been found in B8-positive IDDM patients. Persistence of islet cell antibodies has not been found, however, in the B15-positive IDDM group, suggesting heterogeneity even within typical IDDM.[2]

The way in which these markers may be related to specific entities within IDDM may be clarified by family studies. In a family where more than one sibling is affected with IDDM, the affected siblings are identical for both haplotypes approximately 60 percent of the time instead of the 25 percent expected on the basis of Mendelian inheritance.[11] Ultimately, the mechanism for increased susceptibility in the haplotype identical sibling as well as more exact estimation of the risk of disease associated with haplotype identity may be delineated for IDDM subgroups.

GENETIC COUNSELING

At this time, HLA typing of families with members affected with IDDM is still a research tool. The practicing physician's approach to questions the family might have about genetic risks must be based on empiric risk figures, which have been derived from retrospective surveys of large numbers of families with diabetes; however, these did not separate out individual disease entities. Thus, after a careful family history and physical examination, to help rule out any of the complex inherited syndromes listed in Table 9-1, the following figures can be offered so as to give the family the best possible estimate of risk of recurrence. It is important to distinguish between IDDM (requiring insulin in order to prevent ketosis) and NIDDM (possibly controlled by diet). In a given family, the risk would only be for the specific disease seen in that family. If a child had IDDM, the risk of his siblings developing IDDM is in the range of 5 to 10 percent. If a parent has IDDM, the risk that their offspring would develop IDDM is in the range of 1 to 5 percent. As with most empiric risk figures, the risk increases slightly when more than one person in a family is affected. Reports of offspring where both parents had IDDM are too rare to develop exact recurrence figures.

The risk to siblings of a NIDDM is influenced by environmental factors such as degree of overweight and life-style. The risk is greater with increasing age and, taking this into account, may be as high as 25 percent for NIDDM to occur sometime before 85 years. If both parents have NIDDM, the observed risk to their offspring (not adjusting for age of onset) is observed to be approximately 10 percent.[12] Thus the WHO advice against two diabetics marrying each other and having children must be seriously reevaluated.

Since MODY is an autosomal dominant trait, if one parent has MODY, then the risk to his or her offspring is 50 percent. With the exception of the risk figures for MODY, which are based on the laws of Mendelian inheritance, the physician at this time must rely on these rough estimates, which may not necessarily be accurate for the specific family. However, these figures may be reassuring, since families frequently have unrealistic fears about how high their risks are. The precision of the genetic counseling available should improve substantially as the full extent of the genetic heterogeneity of diabetes is uncovered and biochemical markers for the individual disease entities are found.

References

1. Neel JV: The genetics of diabetes, *In* The Genetics of Diabetes Mellitus. W Creutzfeldt, J Kobberling, and JV Neel (eds), Berlin, Springer Verlag, 1976, pp. 1–11
2. Rimoin DL: Inheritance in diabetes mellitus. *In* Medical Clinics of North America 55:806–819, 1971

3. Rotter JI and Rimoin DL: Genetic heterogeneity in diabetes mellitus and peptic ulcer. *In* Genetic Epidemiology. Morton NE and Chung CS (eds), New York, Academic Press, 1978, pp. 381–414
4. MacDonald MJ: Equal incidence of adult onset diabetes among ancestors of juvenile diabetics and non-diabetics. Diabetologia 10:767–73, 1974
5. Tattersall RB and Pyke DA: Diabetes in identical twins. Lancet 2:1120–25, 1972
6. Irvine WJ, Toft AD, Holton DE, et al: Familial studies of type I and type II idiopathic diabetes mellitus. Lancet 2:325–28, 1977
7. Fajans SS, Cloutier MC and Crowther RL: Clinical and etiologic heterogeneity of idiopathic diabetes mellitus. Diabetes 27:1112–25, 1978
8. Leslie RDG and Pyke DA: Chlorpropamide alcohol flushing: a dominantly inherited trait associated with diabetes. British Medical Journal 2:1521–22, 1978
9. Christy M, Green A, Christau B, et al: Studies of the HLA system and insulin-dependent diabetes mellitus. Diabetes Care 2:209–14, 1979
10. Nerup J, Cathelineau CR, Seignalet J, et al: HLA and endocrine diseases. *In* HLA and Disease. Copenhagen, Munksgard, 1977, pp. 148–67
11. Barbosa J, King R, Noreen H, et al: The histo-compatibility (HLA) system in juvenile insulin dependent diabetes in multiplex families. Journal of Clinical Investigation 60:989–98, 1977
12. Ganada OP, Soeldner JS: Genetic, acquired, and related factors in the etiology of diabetes mellitus. Arch Int Med 137:461–69, 1977

10

The Epidemiology of Diabetes Mellitus

Peter H. Bennett, M.B., F.R.C.P., F.F.C.M.

INTRODUCTION

Epidemiology is the study of the distribution and determinants of disease and its complications, through which hypotheses concerning the etiology and cause are generated, and upon which measures for treatment, control, and prevention are based. As much information on etiology and the complications of diabetes is reviewed elsewhere, the present chapter will be restricted to the distribution and determinants of diabetes itself, with particular reference to populations in the United States.

In 1975, there were an estimated 4.8 million persons, or 2.3 percent of the noninstitutionalized civilian population of the United States, who reported diabetes[1] (Table 10-1). In addition, there were an unknown number of persons with undiagnosed diabetes. The proportions reporting diabetes increased from 0.6 percent in those under 45 years of age to 8.3 percent in those age 65 and over, with the rates in females higher at all ages. Age-specific rates in Black Americans were 1.4 to 1.9 times greater than among Whites. The prevalence of diabetes varies enormously among native Americans, ranging from very low rates among Eskimos to rates of about 50 percent among those aged 45 and over in some tribes, such as the Pima Indians of Arizona.[2]

87

Table 10-1. Prevalence of Diabetes in the United States, 1975[1]

(Self reported diabetes during the U.S. Health Interview Survey)

Age Group (years)	Rates/1000 Population		
	Males	Females	Both Sexes
<17	1.2	0.9	1.1
17–44	8.1	10.7	9.4
45–64	47.9	52.4	50.3
65 and over	77.9	86.6	83.0
All ages	20.1	25.4	22.9

INSULIN-DEPENDENT DIABETES MELLITUS (IDDM)

IDDM characteristically has an onset before 40 years of age and appears to be a disease found predominantly in Europe and North America, whereas in people of Asian, African, Oriental, and American Indian origin without Caucasian admixture it appears to be rare. The occurrence of the disease correlates with the distribution of certain HLA antigens (especially B8 and Bw15) which are found characteristically and in relatively high frequency in certain Caucasoid populations. In the Japanese, however, while IDDM is infrequent compared to Caucasians, its occurrence is associated with another HLA antigen, Bw22.

In the United States and Europe, known diabetes occurs in approximately 1 in 800 persons below 17 years of age, with similar frequencies in males and females (Table 10-2). The majority of these probably have insulin-dependent diabetes mellitus. It is estimated that there were approximately 86,000 diabetics below 20 years of age in the United States in 1973.[3] While the disease undoubtedly sometimes begins at older ages, the incidence and prevalence of the disorder in the older age groups is not known, largely because of the difficulties of distinguishing satisfactorily for epidemiologic purposes between IDDM and noninsulin-dependent diabetes, which is severe enough to require treatment with insulin. In spite of these difficulties, there is no doubt that IDDM constitutes a minority of the total diabetes in the United States, as only 22 percent of persons reporting diabetes take insulin. This proportion falls progressively with age, from 62% below age 20 to 18 percent in those aged 60 years and over.[1]

Table 10-2. Prevalence of Diabetes in Selected Populations in Persons Below 30 Years of Age.

		Age group	Rate/1000
National Center for Health Statistics (US, 1973)	Interviews	0–16	1.3
Michigan School Children Gorwitz (1976)	Questionnaire	5–18	1.6
Minnesota School Children Kyllo and Nutall (1978)	Questionnaire to schools	5–18	1.9
Rochester, Minnesota Palumbo and LaBarthe (1978)	Survey of clinical records	0–14 15–29	0.6 2.9
British Children (cohort) Wadsworth and Jarrett (1974)	Medical records	17 25	0.6 3.0

(See Reference 7 for further details.)

Even in young persons, not all diabetics are of the insulin-dependent type. A number of those with onset in childhood and adolescence do not require insulin to sustain life and prevent the development of ketosis. These children and adolescents may conform to the recently described and characterized Maturity-Onset-type Diabetes of the Young (MODY). Thus, even in children and young persons, the prevalence of truly insulin-dependent diabetes is uncertain, as an unknown proportion of those who do take insulin are probably not ketosis prone. The proportion of children and adolescents with undiagnosed diabetes in the population is unknown, but is generally believed to be very small.

Etiology

The rates of concordance for diabetes in identical twins are extremely high when the onset of diabetes is at 40 years of age and over (Table 10-3), whereas a much lower rate is found when the age of onset is before 40 years and in the age range where insulin-dependent diabetes occurs proportionately more frequently. Nevertheless, there is now overwhelming evidence that genetic factors do alter the likelihood of the development of IDDM, since a variety of markers in the HLA region of chromosome 6 show associations with the disease, e.g., HLA-B8, B15, Dw3, but the mode of inheritance of the predisposition to IDDM and whether genetic predisposition to the disease is a prerequisite to its development remain unknown.

Table 10-3. Concordance Rates for Diabetes in Identical Twins.

Age of onset of diabetes in index twin	Concordant	Discordant	Percent of pairs concordant for diabetes
≤40	31	28	53%
>40	34	3	92%

(From Tattersall RB and Pyke DA, Lancet 2, 1120–1125, 1972.)

Environmental factors currently believed to precipitate IDDM include several viruses such as mumps, Coxsackie B4, and rubella infection. The disease is also found in association with a variety of autoimmune disorders, such as Hashimoto's thyroiditis and Addison's disease. A number of immunological disturbances, including islet cell (cytoplasmic) antibodies and pancreatic beta cell surface antibodies, are found very commonly in those who have recently developed the disease.[5] The extent to which genetic, immunologic, and/or environment factors interact in causing insulin-dependent diabetes is an area of active investigation at this time.

NONINSULIN-DEPENDENT DIABETES MELLITUS (NIDDM)

The majority of persons with diabetes in the United States have insulin-independent diabetes. Approximately 70% develop diabetes after 45 years of age (Table 10-4). Although greater numbers of persons developed the disorder between 45 and 64 years of age, the incidence in those aged 65 and over is higher than in those aged 45–64 years, because of the greater numbers of persons in the population at risk in the 45–64 year age range. The risk of developing the disease increases with increasing age and is somewhat greater in women of all ages.

Table 10-4. Annual Incidence of Reported Diabetes: Number of Persons and Rates/1000 Persons Reporting the Diagnosis of Diabetes Within the Past 12 Months.

(1973 Health Interview Survey.)

Age	Males		Females		Total	
<17	8,000	0.3	12,000	0.4	20,000	0.3
17–44	57,000	1.5	113,000	2.8	70,000	2.1
45–64	109,000	5.4	137,000	6.1	246,000	5.6
65+	41,000	4.9	134,000	11.3	176,000	6.7
All ages	215,000	2.2	396,000	3.7	612,000	3.0

NIDDM occurs in all races, but some groups, such as American Indians, Micronesians, and Polynesians, appear to be particularly susceptible when in suitable environments. These groups, under the influence of increased acculturation and with the adoption of western foods, reduced levels of physical activity, and increasing degrees of obesity, have higher prevalence rates of NIDDM than found in Caucasians. The extent to which these differences are due to genetic factors is uncertain, but environmental factors undoubtedly play an important role in the emergence of the disease, as demonstrated by migrant studies of the East Indians and Japanese.

As with IDDM, the mode of inheritance of NIDDM is unknown, but the concordance rates in identical twins suggest that genetic factors are extremely important (and perhaps a prerequisite) for the development of the disease, but evidence of linkage or association with defined genetic loci has not yet been obtained. Although it has been suggested that NIDDM in young persons (MODY) may show a dominant form of transmission, it is quite likely that NIDDM is a heterogeneous disease, with the predisposition inherited in different ways resulting from the action of different genes.

Obesity and NIDDM

The evidence that obesity is related to the development of NIDDM is extensive and compelling: the majority of subjects (perhaps 80%) with NIDDM are obese at the time of diagnosis; NIDDM is more prevalent in persons who are overweight; the disorder is more prevalent in populations that are more obese; and the risk of developing diabetes in subgroups of a population is strongly related to preceding degree of obesity. The incidence of NIDDM over a ten-year period in middle-aged men in Scandinavia varied 10-fold among those who were of normal weight compared to those who were 40 percent or more overweight,[6] and similar results have been reported among the Pima Indians.[2]

The degree of obesity is also related to the age of onset of diabetes such that the most obese show the highest incidence in earlier decades, whereas those with moderate obesity show a later age of onset. This suggests that obesity may precipitate diabetes at an earlier age in susceptible persons, whereas those who are inherently predisposed to the disorder but who do not become obese may have the onset delayed until later in life or may perhaps never develop it.

SPECIFIC TYPES OF DIABETES MELLITUS

Diabetes secondary to pancreatic calcification and fibrosis constitutes an important, and in some populations the predominant, form of diabetes mellitus, but is not endemic in the United States.[7] This disease has a distinctive geography and epidemiology. Diabetes due to other specific causes, such as hemochromatosis and that associated with a number of dintinctive, but relatively unusual, genetic syndromes, are all relatively uncommon and fall outside the scope of the present chapter.[7]

IMPAIRED GLUCOSE TOLERANCE

In the United States population, the frequency distribution of glucose levels, fasting and following a carbohydrate load, is unimodal and skewed without any clear separation between those with and without diabetes. Consequently, criteria for diabetes based solely on glucose tolerance and statistical limits were arbitrary. In some populations with a very high prevalence of diabetes, the frequency distributions of glucose levels in the population are bimodal, allowing a more logical separation of those without diabetes and those who fall into the more hyperglycemic mode, whose fasting glucose levels are 140 mg/dl and over and two hour glucose levels ≥ 200 mg/dl, and who develop the specific complications of diabetes.[8] Similar glucose levels are associated with the development of these complications in studies from Great Britain.[9]

On the other hand, subjects with glucose levels above the conventional norms, but below the levels which are clearly indicative of diabetes, do have an increased risk of worsening (2–3 percent per year) to diabetes, but the majority either revert to normal or remain unchanged. Such subjects do not develop specific complications over prolonged follow-up[9] and consequently cannot be considered to have diabetes mellitus. Such persons with impaired glucose tolerance may have an increased risk of developing atherosclerotic vascular disease and, if pregnant, may have increased perinatal morbidity, but do not appear to have any appreciable risk of developing specific complications of diabetes unless glucose tolerance subsequently worsens.

MORTALITY

Diabetes is the sixth leading cause of death in the United States. In 1977, 33,000 deaths occurred in which diabetes is stated as the underlying cause. These data, however, seriously underestimate the contribution of diabetes to mortality as the majority of persons with diabetes die as a result of vascular complications, about half of them the result of heart disease, which may be directly or indirectly related to diabetes, but which are often described as the underlying cause of death. Those with diabetes described as the underlying cause of death constitute only about 25 percent of the total deaths among diabetics.

The impact of diabetes on mortality is more easily judged by comparing age-specific mortality rates among diabetics and nondiabetics. These rates are many fold higher for diabetics below 45 years of age, but overall, the rates are approximately twice those of nondiabetics.

References

1. Sayetta RF and Murphy RS: Summary of current diabetes-related data from the National Center for Health Statistics. Diabetes Care 2:105–119, 1979
2. Bennett PH, Rushforth NB, Miller M, and LeCompte PM: Epidemiological studies of diabetes in the Pima Indians. Recent Progress in Hormone Research 32:333–374, 1976
3. Diabetes Data compiled 1977. Bennett PH, Entmacher PS, Habicht J-P, et al, (eds): US Dept. of Health Education and Welfare, DHEW Publication No. (NIH) 78-1468. US Government Printing Office, Washington, 1978, pp. 119
4. Tattersall RB and Pyke DA: Diabetes in identical twins. Lancet 2:1120–1124, 1972
5. Irvine WJ, McCullum CJ, Gray RS, et al: Pancreatic islet-cell antibodies in diabetes mellitus correlated with the duration and type of diabetes, co-existent autoimmune disease, and HLA type. Diabetes 26:138–147, 1977
6. Westlund K, Nicholaysen R: Ten year mortality and morbidity related to serum cholesterol. Scand J Clin Lab Invest 30, Suppl 127, 3–24, 1972
7. West KM (1978): The Epidemiology of Diabetes and its Vascular Lesions. Elsevier, New York, pp. 579
8. Rushforth NB, Miller M, and Bennett PH: Fasting and two-hour postload glucose levels for the diagnosis of diabetes: the relationship between glucose levels and complications of diabetes in the Pima Indians. Diabetologia 16:373–379, 1979
9. Keen H, Jarrett RJ, and Alberti KGMM: Diabetes mellitus: a new look at diagnostic criteria. Diabetologia 16:283–285, 1979

11

Classification of Diabetes Mellitus

Stefan S. Fajans, M.D.

During recent years, newer knowledge of the etiology and pathogenesis of diabetes, although still very incomplete, has indicated that the disease is heterogeneous in nature. Thus, diabetes is not a single disease but a syndrome. Ideally a classification should be based on etiology and pathogenesis only. To be useful; (a) for the clinician in categorizing patients and (b) to serve as a framework for collection of clinical and epidemiological data in diverse population groups, it is convenient presently to include other considerations into a classification, such as factors recognizing the natural history of the disease. Since April 1978, an international work group, sponsored by the National Diabetes Data Group of the National Institute of Health, has been working on a "Classification of Diabetes Mellitus and Other Categories of Glucose Intolerance," a final version of which will probably be accepted internationally. The classification to be used in this chapter has been adopted essentially from the work and proceedings of the work group.[1] Indices by which other classifications could be devised have been reviewed and discussed by West.[2] At the present time, any classification is still arbitrary, sometimes inconsistent, and a compromise to accommodate different points of view.

The present classification (Table 11-1) includes both diabetes (characterized either by fasting hyperglycemia or levels of plasma glucose during a glucose tolerance test above defined limits) as well as "impaired glucose tolerance" (plasma glucose levels during a glucose tolerance test which lie above normal but below those defined as diabetes). The levels of plasma glucose in the fasting state or during a glucose tolerance test which are defined as normal, impaired, or diabetic are also compromises and not subscribed to as ideal by all investigators.[3,4] In addition, the classification includes gestational diabetes and stages in the natural history of diabetes in which there is an absence of abnormalities of carbohydrate metabolism, such as previous abnormality of glucose tolerance and potential abnormality of glucose tolerance.

Table 11-1. Classification of Diabetes Mellitus and Other Categories of Glucose Intolerance.

Class	Former terminology
A. *Diabetes Mellitus (DM)*	
I. Type I. Insulin-dependent type (IDDM)	juvenile diabetes juvenile-onset diabetes juvenile-onset type diabetes JOD ketosis-prone diabetes unstable or brittle diabetes
II. Type II. Noninsulin-dependent types (NIDDM) a. NIDDM in Nonobese b. NIDDM in Obese (includes families with autosomal dominant inheritance)	adult-onset diabetes maturity-onset diabetes maturity-onset type diabetes (MOD) ketosis-resistant diabetes maturity-onset type diabetes of the young (MODY) stable diabetes
III. Other types, including diabetes mellitus associated with certain conditions and syndromes: (1) Pancreatic disease (2) Hormonal (3) Drug or chemical induced (4) Certain genetic syndromes (5) Insulin receptor abnormalities (6) Other types	secondary diabetes

Table 11-1. continued

Class	Former terminology
B. Impaired Glucose Tolerance (IGT)	
a. IGT in Nonobese	asymptomatic diabetes
b. IGT in Obese	chemical diabetes
c. IGT associated with certain	latent diabetes
conditions and syndromes:	borderline diabetes
(1) Pancreatic disease, (2) Hormonal, (3)	subclinical diabetes
Drug or chemical induced, (4) Insulin	
receptor abnormalities, (5) Certain	
genetic syndromes.	
C. Gestational Diabetes (GDM)	gestational diabetes
D. Previous Abnormality of Glucose	subclinical diabetes
Tolerance (PrevAGT)	prediabetes
	latent diabetes
E. Potential Abnormality of Glucose	prediabetes
Tolerance (PotAGT)	potential diabetes

DIABETES MELLITUS

Type I. Insulin-Dependent Diabetes Mellitus (IDDM)

Diabetes mellitus is subdivided into three different types, which appear to differ in etiology and pathogenesis. The first is Type I or insulin-dependent diabetes mellitus (IDDM). Genetic factors are thought to be of importance in the majority of patients, as expressed by the associated increased or decreased frequency of certain histocompatibility antigens (HLA) on chromosome number 6. Environmental (acquired) factors, such as certain viral infections superimposed on genetic factors, may either destroy islet cells[5] or lead to autoimmune destruction of beta cells. Thus, genetically determined abnormal immune responses (postulated because of HLA associations) and autoimmunity are thought to play an etiological role. Frequently, islet cell antibodies are present at diagnosis. IDDM appears to be heterogeneous in terms of genetics and environmental factors which precipitate the disease. Classically, this type of disease occurs in juveniles; however, it can be recognized and may become symptomatic for the first time at any age. Usually there is an abrupt symptomatic onset, ketosis-proneness, and the patient is dependent upon insulin treatment for survival. In addition to the ketosis-prone stage, this type of disease can also be recognized in a symptomatic preketosis-prone stage. By prospective testing in asymptomatic siblings of insulin-dependent diabetics, one can discover patients with abnormal glucose tolerance and with normal fasting plasma glucose levels.[6] Their diabetes progresses rapidly to the ketotic form, usually within two years after recognition and occasionally after longer periods of time. IDDM is characterized by severe insulinopenia.

Type II. Noninsulin-Dependent Diabetes Mellitus (NIDDM)

The second type of diabetes, Type II or noninsulin-dependent diabetes mellitus (NIDDM) also has a genetic basis which is commonly expressed by a more frequent familial pattern of occurrence than is seen in IDDM. In this type, aggregation of HLA types and islet cell antibodies characteristic of Type I are not found. Within NIDDM are included families in whom diabetes presents in children, adolescents, and young adults (formerly referred to as maturity-onset type diabetes of the young, or MODY,[6]) and in which autosomal dominant inheritance of diabetes has been established. Autosomal dominant pattern of inheritance may be seen in as many as 20% of all NIDDM.[7] Environmental factors superimposed on genetic susceptibility are undoubtedly involved in the onset of NIDDM. Intake of excessive calories leading to weight gain and obesity are probably important factors in its pathogenesis. Although small changes in weight may be important, NIDDM has been subdivided according to the absence or presence of obesity, since in Western societies 60 percent to 90 percent of all NIDDM patients are obese. Hyperglycemia and glucose intolerance are usually improved by weight loss. Patients with NIDDM are noninsulin-dependent for prevention of ketosis (i.e., they are ketosis-resistant and not ketosis-prone), but they may require insulin for correction of symptomatic or persistent fasting hyperglycemia, if this cannot be achieved with the use of diet or oral agents. Occasionally it is difficult to distinguish nonobese NDDM patients treated with insulin from truly insulin-dependent (ketosis-prone) patients (IDDM). Patients with NIDDM may even develop ketosis under such circumstances as severe stress precipitated by infections or trauma. In Type II patients, insulinopenia may be mild or only relative, while insulin resistance may be of greater importance in the pathogenesis of hyperglycemia. The spectrum of insulin responses to glucose from low to supernormal has been found in patients of this group, many of whom do not have fasting hyperglycemia. Patients with NIDDM may be asymptomatic for years or decades and show very slow progression of the metabolic and morphologic aberrations of the disease. However, the typical chronic associations or complications of diabetes, namely macroangiopathy, microangiopathy, neuropathy, and cataracts, seen in IDDM may be seen in NIDDM as well. NIDDM undoubtedly is also heterogeneous.[6]

Other Types of Diabetes

Included are entities secondary to or associated with certain conditions or syndromes. This subclass can be divided according to the known or suspected etiologic relationships. Diabetes may be secondary to pancreatic disease or removal of pancreatic tissue, secondary to endocrine disease such as acromegaly, Cushing's syndrome, pheochromocytoma, glucagonoma, somatostatinoma, primary aldosteronism, etc., secondary to the administration of hormones causing hyperglycemia, and secondary to the administration of certain drugs.[1] Diabetes (or carbohydrate intolerance) may be associated with a large number of genetic syndromes.[1] Finally, diabetes may be associated with defects of insulin receptors, which may be due either to abnormalities in number or affinity of insulin receptors or due to antibodies to insulin receptors with or without associated immune disorders.

IMPAIRED GLUCOSE TOLERANCE (IGT)

The work group recommends that a category be established for individuals who have nondiagnostic fasting plasma glucose levels and levels during the glucose tolerance test which lie between normal and diabetic. It is well recognized that, in some subjects, IGT may represent a stage in the natural history of IDDM and may do so much more frequently in NIDDM. In such patients, conversion of IGT to NIDDM, and particularly to NIDDM with fasting hyperglycemia, has taken years or decades.[6] It has been found to occur in 10–50 percent of patients with IGT followed for 7–10 years. Thus, in the majority of various population groups, impaired glucose tolerance either does not progress or reverts to normal glucose tolerance. To avoid the psychological and socioeconomic stigma of a diagnosis of diabetes in these individuals, the category of impaired glucose tolerance has been established. Although clinically significant renal and retinal complications of diabetes (microangiopathy) are absent in patients with IGT, many studies have shown in such groups an increased death rate and increased prevalence of arterial disease, electrocardiographic abnormalities, or increased susceptibility to atherosclerotic disease associated with other known risk factors including hypertension, hyperlipidemia, and adiposity. Thus, impaired glucose tolerance, particularly in otherwise healthy and ambulatory individuals under the age of 50 (conditions appropriate for using the oral glucose tolerance test), may have prognostic implications and should not be ignored or taken lightly. In the obese, impaired glucose tolerance almost invariably reverts to normal glucose tolerance with weight reduction. Impaired glucose tolerance may be associated with the conditions and syndromes listed under *Other Types of Diabetes.*

GESTATIONAL DIABETES (GDM)

Impaired glucose tolerance may have its onset or may be first recognized during pregnancy. From a biochemical point of view (levels of plasma glucose), impaired glucose tolerance during pregnancy is similar to IGT, described in the previous section.

Impaired glucose tolerance during pregnancy is associated with increased perinatal morbidity and mortality and increased frequency of loss of viable fetuses. Therapy of this mild degree of glucose intolerance can prevent much of this. For these reasons, impaired glucose tolerance in this particular group of patients is termed gestational diabetes. Gestational diabetes usually returns to a state of normal glucose tolerance after parturition; even so, 30 percent to 40 percent of such women develop diabetes within 5–10 years after parturition. Thus, after termination of pregnancy, patients with gestational diabetes should be reclassified as patients with impaired glucose tolerance, diabetes mellitus, or previous abnormality of glucose tolerance.

PREVIOUS ABNORMALITY OF GLUCOSE TOLERANCE (PrevAGT)

This classification is restricted to individuals who previously had diabetic hyperglycemia or impaired glucose tolerance but who presently have normal glucose tolerance. Individuals who have had gestational diabetes but have returned to normal glucose tolerance after parturition are examples, as are individuals who were overweight or obese and whose diabetes or impaired glucose tolerance returned to normal glucose tolerance after loss of weight. Patients with impaired glucose tolerance or mild diabetes of the NIDDM form, particularly among pedigrees of four generations of diabetes inherited in an autosomal dominant fashion (MODY), may fluctuate between normal, impaired glucose tolerance and diabetes, with their having little or no change in weight.

POTENTIAL ABNORMALITY OF GLUCOSE TOLERANCE (PotAGT)

Individuals in this class have never exhibited abnormal glucose tolerance but have increased risk for the development of diabetes or impaired glucose tolerance. Factors associated with increased risk for IDDM include being a sibling or twin of an IDDM; having histocompatible haplotypes identical to those of an

IDDM first-degree relative, particularly a sibling; and having islet cell antibodies. Factors associated with increased risk for NIDDM include being a first-degree relative of an NIDDM diabetic, particularly in a family of several generations of NIDDM; giving birth to a neonate weighing more than 9 pounds; obesity associated with a family history of diabetes; and being a member of a racial or ethnic group with a high prevalence of diabetes, e.g., a number of American Indian tribes.

The terms *prediabetes* and *potential diabetes* have been used for individuals in this class in the past. If used at all, the term prediabetes should only be used retrospectively to refer to the period prior to the diagnosis of diabetes. It cannot be used prospectively since it is now known that diabetes occurs primarily in those in whom a precipitating environmental factor becomes superimposed upon a genetic predisposition.

PotAGT should never be applied as a diagnosis to an individual. It is included in this classification to identify groups of individuals for prospective research studies.

References

1. National Diabetes Data Group: Classification and diagnosis of diabetes mellitus and other categories of glucose intolerance. Diabetes 28: 1039–1057, 1979
2. West KM: Standardization of definition, classification, and reporting in diabetes-related epidemiologic studies. Diabetes Care 2:65–76, 1979
3. Mackenthun AV, Lehman AE, Bradford RH, et al: What is the normal range for the fasting plasma glucose (FPB)? Diabetes 28:361, 1979
4. O'Sullivan JB: Prevalence and course of diabetes modified by fasting blood glucose levels: implications for diagnostic criteria. Diabetes Care 2:85–90, 1979
5. Yoon J-W, Austin M, Onodera T, et al: Virus-induced diabetes mellitus. N Engl J Med 300:1173–79, 1979
6. Fajans SS, Cloutier MC, and Crowther RL: Clinical and etiologic heterogeneity of idiopathic diabetes mellitus. (Banting Memorial Lecture) Diabetes 27:1112–25, 1978
7. Pyke DA, and Leslie RDG: Chlorpropamide-alcohol flushing: a definition of its relation to non-insulin-dependent diabetes. Br Med J 2:1521–22, 1978

DIAGNOSIS AND TREATMENT

12

Diagnosis of Diabetes Mellitus

Kelly M. West, M.D.

There is now considerable support for the view that diabetes is simply "too much glucose in the blood." Some uncertainties remain, however, on how much glucose is too much, and on the relationship of diagnostic levels to factors such as age and to the size of the glucose load.

Roughly half of the patients with untreated diabetes have classical symptoms of diabetes. Weight loss occurs only with severe insulin insufficiency and is much less specific for diabetes. Pruritus vulvae is a very frequent early sign of diabetes. Other less specific symptoms suggesting the possibility of diabetes include blurring of vision, weakness, and a sense of fatigue. Diagnostic or screening tests are indicated in those with conditions strongly associated with diabetes. These may include obesity, coronary disease, gangrene, neuropathy, tuberculosis, and carbuncle.

BLOOD GLUCOSE METHODS

Several methods are available for determining with accuracy the concentration of glucose in blood. These methods include the Autoanalyzer ferricyanide and neocuprine methods, the glucose oxidase and hexokinase methods, and the ortho-toluidine and

Somogyi-Nelson methods. For clinical purposes, results with these six methods are interchangeable.

TYPES OF DIAGNOSTIC TESTS

Urine Tests and Random and Fasting Blood Glucose Values

Persons with gross hyperglycemia usually have glycosuria and symptoms of diabetes such as polyuria. These persons do *not* need, and should not have, glucose tolerance tests. In these cases, the diagnosis can be confirmed by determination of the fasting blood glucose or sometimes by a random blood glucose determination. Except in the immediate postprandial period, random glucose values above 200 mg/100 ml can usually be considered diagnostic. Values above this level are usually present in persons with typical symptoms of diabetes and in those with heavy glycosuria. Most persons with occult fasting hyperglycemia have glycosuria in specimens obtained 2 hours after a large meal, and most people with fasting glycosuria have diabetes.

Because of increasing conservatism in the interpretation of glucose tolerance tests, the fasting blood glucose is now being used more widely as a screening and diagnostic instrument. More data are needed, but it appears that the upper limit of the normal range in individuals who have fasted for three hours or more is approximately the same in those who have fasted overnight. For this reason, it is sometimes possible to perform this test in late morning or afternoon at an hour that is often more convenient to patients and their attendants than the traditional prebreakfast hour.

Oral Carbohydrate Loading Tests

The test most widely used in the diagnosis of diabetes is the oral glucose tolerance test. Opinion varies considerably about the clinical utility and the design and interpretation of such tests.[1,2] In general, this test is overused.[2]

Most authorities limit postload collections to blood specimens at 1 and 2 hours, but some advise that sampling be done at more frequent intervals and/or extended to 3 hours.

In interpreting glucose tolerance tests the following considerations apply:

Compared to venous values, capillary values are higher (about 5 percent, not mg %) for the fasting, approximately 20 percent for the 1-hour, and roughly 10% for the 2-hour value. Capillary values reflect arterial levels. The a-v difference at 2 hours is a bit smaller after 50 gm loads and somewhat larger after 100 gm.

In order to promote simplification and avoid age adjustment, the NIH Diabetes Data Group[1] and the World Health Organization recommend that, in adults of all ages, a 2-hour value of 200 mg/100 ml be required for the diagnosis of diabetes. By their criteria, 2-hour values between 140 and 200 indicate "impaired glucose tolerance," but not diabetes. Others, including the author, favor adjusting the diagnostic cut-off point with age (e.g., 180 mg/100 ml in those less than 40 years and 220 mg/100 ml in those over 60 years old). In elderly subjects, some authorities reserve the diagnosis for those with fasting hyperglycemia. In persons over 60 years of age, 2-hour values in the range of 140-199 mg/100 ml probably ought to be considered normal. The Diabetes Data Group suggests that fasting values above 140 are abnormal. However, values from 120 to 139 may be treated with suspicion (120–129) or considered diagnostic (130–139), if confirmed.

One- and 2-hour values are about 20 mg/100 ml higher with afternoon tests than with morning tests. These values are, on the average, about 20 mg/100 ml lower when the test is performed 2–4 hours after eating. Whole blood values are lower (by 15 percent, not mg percent) than plasma levels. With glucose loads of 100 gm, 1-hour values are about 5 mg/100 ml higher and 2-hour values about 15 mg/100 ml higher than with 75 gm. With 50 gm loads, these values are lower by a comparable degree. Postload values, particularly the 1-hour value, are affected by the relationship of the size of the load to the size of the subject. To adjust for body size, one may administer 1 gm per kg or 40 gm per sq. m; or one may use 75 gm except in adults who are very small or very large (e.g., 50 gm for those weighing less than 50 kg and 100 gm for those weighing more than 100 kg).

Many factors can induce falsely elevated values. These include: recent sharp restrictions of dietary carbohydrate, acute illness, and many medications, particularly contraceptive steroids and glucocorticosteroids. The 1-hour value tends to be high in patients who have had a gastrectomy. Subjects with impaired gastrointestinal absorption may have false negative tests.

In the presence of slightly elevated values, the diagnosis should require confirmation with at least one additional test. Day-to-day variations in the 1- and 2-hour values as great as 30 mg/100 ml are common.

With increasing frequency, nonglucose loading nutrients are being used to screen or test for diabetes. Typical of these is "Glucola" (Ames Co.). This is a mixture of simple carbohydrates that is somewhat more palatable than glucose. The carbohydrates in this solution produce increments of blood glucose and insulin that are very similar to those after equivalent amounts of glucose. Because of its lesser osmotic effect in the small bowel, unpleasant gastrointestinal effects are less with Glucola than with glucose.

Theoretically, measured loads containing nutrient mixtures (e.g., candy, rice meals, standard breakfasts, etc.) should be just as effective as glucose in testing for diabetes. The advantage of using glucose is the greater amount of data on ranges of normal response in subjects with varying characteristics. On the average, 2-hour values after 75 gm of oral glucose are about 20 mg/100 ml higher than after a typical breakfast containing 75 gm of carbohydrates.

Intravenous Tests

The advantages of intravenous testing include an avoidance of the vagaries of gastrointestinal absorption that affect oral tests. When properly performed, intravenous tests yield results that are more reproducible than do oral tests. Most of the intravenous tests require less than an hour. But these tests are not used frequently in clinical practice because of several disadvantages. If any of the injected high-concentration glucose escapes the vein at the site of injection, it is quite irritating. Intravenous challenges are in some respects unphysiologic. Consumption of food is attended by release of gut hormones that aid in its disposition, and ingested sugar normally enters through the portal circulation. The timing and configuration of the hyperglycemic bolus are quite different with typical intravenous challenge tests than with oral tests or normal meals. Another disadvantage is that only a small fraction of physicians know how to interpret results of such tests. Finally, as ordinarily performed, intravenous tests require several blood specimens. This usually entails several venipunctures or placing a catheter, although capillary blood may be used.

The test most commonly employed is one in which a rapid bolus of glucose is given (e.g., 25 gm in 2 minutes as 50 ml of a 50% solution). After about 15 minutes to allow for equilibration in the extracellular space, samples are drawn at intervals of approximately 5 minutes for 30 to 45 more minutes. Results are plotted on semi-log paper and a line of best fit drawn through the series of values. The rate of decline of the blood glucose can then be determined, using a standard formula. The K value, thus ascertained, reflects the rate of fall in percent per minute. Some have based calculations on incremental rather than absolute values. The incremental value is the absolute value minus the fasting value. These two approaches yield very similar information, although ranges of normal are different. When absolute values are used, K values below 1.0 are abnormal except in the elderly. Values above 1.2 are normal for all ages.

Other Tests

These include tolbutamide response tests and tests of response to glucagon, glucocorticosteroids, and amino acids. These are seldom useful in clinical practice, although capable of measuring beta-cell responsiveness. These and other diagnostic tests have been reviewed in detail.[2]

References

1. Bennett PH: Recommendations on the standardization methods and reporting of tests for diabetes and its microvascular complications in epidemiologic studies. Diabetes Care, Vol 2, No 2, 98–104, 1979
2. West KM: Diagnostic methods. *In* Epidemiology of Diabetes and Its Vascular Lesions. Elsevier North-Holland, 67–126, 1978

13

Diet and Diabetes

Ronald A. Arky, M.D.

Recent advances in genetics, immunochemistry, and cytophysiology establish that diabetes mellitus is not a single entity but a series of disease complexes characterized by hyperglycemia.[1] A corollary of this conclusion is that there is not a single dietary formula that suffices to treat satisfactorily all individuals with diabetes. Diabetics require no special foods—merely the same nutrients, vitamins, and minerals as nondiabetics.[2] The fundamental principles of nutrition that apply to diabetics are applicable to nondiabetics as well (Table 13-1). This review considers those general principles and their application to the insulin-dependent (Type I) and noninsulin-dependent (Type II) diabetic.[3] The principles are discussed with reference to the current concepts of the pathophysiology of the heterogeneous syndromes that comprise diabetes mellitus.

Calories Count

This most important dietary concept concerns total caloric intake. For the youth with hyperglycemia, caloric intake must be sufficient to assure normal growth, development, and maturation. For adults with the hyperglycemic syndrome and obesity, total caloric intake must be reduced. Obesity is diabetogenic and should be prevented. If present, obesity must be treated; even small amounts of weight loss improve the receptivity of tissue for insulin and lower glucose levels.[4] Alterations in caloric intake may be necessary during pregnancy or when the diabetics suffer from such complications as renal or cardiac disease.[5]

Table 13-1. Principles of Nutrition Applicable to the Hyperglycemic Syndromes.

---

1. There is no single "diabetic diet": the syndromes are heterogeneous.
2. Calories count
3. Carbohydrates.
    (a) Glucose-containing simple carbohydrates elevate blood glucose.
    (b) Equal amounts of complex carbohydrates do not induce equal
         increments in blood glucose.
    (c) Disproportionate restriction of carbohydrate is not warranted.
4. Fats.
    (a) Total intake should not exceed 30 percent of total calories.
    (b) Limit the ingestion of animal fats.
5. Instruction.
    (a) All individuals with hyperglycemic syndromes require counseling.
    (b) A single encounter with a diet counselor is ineffective—diet instruction
         demands time and repetition.
    (c) Instruction begins immediately after diagnosis.

Exercise

While diet therapy is the cornerstone in the treatment of the hyperglycemic syndromes, such therapy must be integrated with scheduled physical activity and exercise. Exercise augments the effectiveness of diet and facilitates the action of the hypoglycemic agents used in the treatment of diabetics.[6]

Carbohydrates

Ingestion of concentrated, simple carbohydrates (mono- and disaccharides) by diabetics aggravates hyperglycemia and causes wide fluctuations in blood glucose. Sucrose and sucrose-containing foods are to be avoided or consumed in moderation.* Insulin-dependent diabetics whose beta cells are unresponsive to fluxes in circulating glucose experience marked hyperglycemia after consuming foods that contain simple carbohydrates.

Glycemic responses to food containing complex carbohydrates (e.g., potatoes, rice) differ—equivalent quantities of complex carbohydrates do *not* induce equivalent increments in plasma glucose or insulin.[7] The reasons for this variation are unknown at this time.

Total carbohydrate intake should not be disproportionately restricted in diabetics.[8] Increases of dietary carbohydrate without increases in total caloric intake do not increase insulin requirements in insulin-dependent diabetics. In noninsulin-dependent diabetics (Type II), glucose tolerance may improve with substantial intake of carbohydrate. The carbohydrate content of the diet should comprise 55–60 percent of total calories; rarely, such an intake may induce or aggravate an underlying state of hypertriglyceridemia (hyper pre-beta lipoproteinemia).

Fats

Fat intake should supply no more than 35 percent of the total calories ingested by the diabetic (and the nondiabetic as well). Debate continues about the preventive value of polyunsaturated fats on the pathogenesis of atherosclerosis. Prudent clinicians urge the reduction in consumption of animal fats in efforts to avoid obesity and maintain normal plasma lipid levels.

Instruction[3]

Every individual with diabetes requires instruction in the basic principles of nutrition. A single educational session will not

---

*This does not preclude the insulin-dependent diabetic from always carrying an available source of simple carbohydrate to relieve or alleviate a hypoglycemic episode or to counteract the effects of strenuous exercise. Often, during periods of illness, simple carbohydrates are the best sources of calories.

achieve the behavioral changes that are essential if results are to be expected from educational experiences.* Nutrition counseling is an art, and few physicians have the know-how or time to devote to this important therapeutic measure. Whenever possible, the physician should utilize the services of a diet counselor and refer the patient for follow-up instruction periodically. Use of standard diets or "handouts" is discouraged.

SPECIFIC PRINCIPLES

Type I (Insulin-Dependent) Diabetics

Diabetics who require insulin must eat regularly and time their caloric intake with the temporal action of their insulin. Insulin-dependent diabetics should never miss a meal and always carry with them a "quick" source of simple carbohydrate. To facilitate meal planning, daily total caloric intake may be divided into tenths, so that 2/10ths to 4/10ths of calories are taken at meal time and 1/10th at snack time.† Dietary patterns must be tailored to fit the individual's activity and exercise schedule. Extra calories (concentrated carbohydrate) are required before strenuous exercise.

These simple concepts must be conveyed to the insulin-dependent diabetic and his/her family immediately after the diagnosis is made. Youngsters with diabetes must appreciate the need for balanced meals eaten at regular intervals early in the course of their disease. Pediatricians and other physicians must emphasize these principles lest the individual patient become recalcitrant to a reasonable approach and reject general self-care measures.

---

*Physicians treating diabetics must be able to determine the caloric need of patients and design a meal plan (Table 13-2).[5]

†As an example for the active youth going to school: 2/10ths of total calories are given for breakfast, 2/10ths at lunch, 1/10th as afternoon snack, 4/10ths at dinner, and 1/10th for bedtime snack.

Type II (Noninsulin-Dependent Diabetes

Most individuals with this form of diabetes are overweight, and frequently the loss of 7–10 pounds is accompanied by marked improvement in both fasting and postprandial hyperglycemia. Short-term fasts (7–10 days)[9] represent one approach, but should be undertaken only in persons who are: (1) under constant medical surveillance; (2) appreciative of the complications that might result from starvation; and (3) capable of measuring urine "ketones" and of seeking medical attention when symptomatic. Protein-sparing modified diets may be useful, but offer little benefit over hypocaloric mixed diets. The method of weight reduction in obese diabetics is much less important than the maintenance of that weight loss; efforts to achieve desired body weight (Table 13-2) should be continuous and patients urged to lose 1.5 to 2.0 pounds per week.

Noninsulin-dependent diabetics with normal weight should adhere to a caloric intake that assures maintenance of that weight and should consume a nutritious diet the composition of which should not differ from that of nondiabetics. Oral hypoglycemic agents should not be used until the patient appreciates the principles of nutrition that apply to his or her disease state.

SPECIAL PRINCIPLES

Fiber

Dietary fibers represent the skeletal remains of plant cells that resist digestion by human enzymes. Most dietary fibers are undigestible carbohydrates (cellulose, hemicellulose, pectin, and plant gums such as guar), while lignins are phenylpropane polymers.[10] Certain plant fibers, when ingested with glucose, improve glucose tolerance in both normal and mild diabetics. When diabetics are given fiber-enriched meals (bran is used as source of fiber), postprandial hyperglycemia is blunted.[11,12] These preliminary observations, which include both diabetics on insulin and on oral hypoglycemic agents, do not afford a definition of the mechanism(s) whereby the fiber content of a diet

Table 13-2. Determining Caloric Needs.

Estimate Desirable Body Weight

Build	Women	Men
Medium Frame:	100 lb for first 5 ft of height, plus 5 lbs for each additional inch	106 lb for first 5 ft of height, plus 6 lbs for each additional inch
Small Frame:	Subtract 10%	Subtract 10%
Large Frame:	Add 10%	Add 10%

Determine Caloric Needs

A. Basal Calories: Desired body weight × 10 = basal kilocalories
B. Add Activity Calories:

$$\text{Sedentary} = \text{Basal} + (\text{Desired body weight} \times 3)$$
$$\text{Moderate} = \text{Basal} + (\text{Desired body weight} \times 5)$$
$$\text{Strenuous} = \text{Basal} + (\text{Desired body weight} \times 10)$$

C. Weight gain situations = growth, pregnancy, and lactation; add 300–500 kilocalories daily.
D. Weight losing situations = OBESITY; subtract 750–1000 kilocalories to lose 2–2½ lbs/week.

alters glycemic excursions nor do they indicate the potential side effects of such diets on mineral (calcium, magnesium) balance. Nevertheless, there are indications that the addition of bran or guar gum to meals may blunt postprandial hyperglycemia of diabetics.

Sweeteners[13]

Since the governmental ban on cyclamates, saccharin and its salts are the most extensively used artificial sweeteners in the United States. Diabetics are among the principal users of saccharin and were concerned about the alleged relationship between saccharin and urinary bladder cancer. At the time of this writing, the available scientific data do not justify the complete restriction of the use of saccharin by diabetics. However, as with any food additive, "use in moderation" is a safe principle.

The nutritive sweeteners[14] fructose, xylitol, and sorbitol have the same caloric density as glucose and sucrose. Fructose is approximately 80 percent sweeter than sucrose and twice as sweet as sorbitol. In controlled diabetics, fructose does not adversely affect glucose metabolism and has been used as a "sweetener" for diabetics in several European centers. Extensive studies of the long-term effects of modest quantities of fructose, xylitol, and sorbitol used as a sweetener in diabetes are not available. Until such time as they are, the use of these sweeteners by the large population afflicted with the hyperglycemic syndromes cannot be advocated.

SUMMARY

The basic principles of nutrition are readily applicable to the treatment of the hyperglycemic syndromes, provided that an understanding of the pathophysiological changes that account for these states are appreciated. Total caloric intake has relevance in all forms of the hyperglycemic syndromes. While the guidelines for nutrition are simple, a number of questions remain unanswered. Among these are: (1) Why do equal amounts of different complex carbohydrates produce various excursions in plasma glucose? (2) Is the accelerated atherogenesis of diabetes influenced by a reduced fat intake? (3) Does the long-term usage of nutrient sweeteners such as fructose affect the course of diabetes?

A further challenge to the physician and other professionals involved in the care of diabetics relates to the communication of the basic nutrition principles to the patient. To assure success in this educational endeavor, better methods and tools are needed. Diet therapy is important—a fact that must be acknowledged by patient, physician, and all the others involved in the care process.

References

1. Rotter JI and Rimoin DL: Heterogeneity in diabetic mellitus—Update 1978. Diabetes 27:599–605, 1978

2. Talbot JM and Fischer KD: The need for special foods and sugar substitutes by individuals with diabetes mellitus. Diabetes Care 1:231–240, 1978
3. Arky RA: Current principles of dietary therapy of diabetes mellitus. Med Clinics of N America 62:655–662, 1978
4. De Fronzo RA, Soman V, Sherwin RS, et al: Insulin binding to monocytes and insulin action in human obesity, starvation and refeeding. J. Clin Invest. 62:204–213, 1978
5. A Guide for Professionals: The effective application of "Exchange Lists for Meal Planning," American Diabetes Association, Inc. and The American Dietetic Association, 1977
6. Murray FT, et al.: The metabolic response to moderate exercise in diabetic men receiving intravenous and subcutaneous insulin. J Clin Endocrinol Metab 44:708–720, 1977
7. Crapo PA, Reaven G, and Olefsky J: Postprandial glucose and insulin responses to different complex carbohydrates. Diabetes 26:1178–1183, 1977
8. Brunzell JD, Nuttall F et al: Principles of nutrition and dietary recommendations for patient with diabetes mellitus. Update 1979. Diabetes 28:1027–1030, 1979
9. Davidson JK: Controlling diabetes mellitus with diet therapy. Postgraduate Medicine 59:114–122, 1976
10. Kritchevsky D: Dietary fiber: what it is and what it does. Ann New York Academy of Sciences 300:283–289, 1977
11. Kiehm TG, Anderson JW, and Ward K: Beneficial effects of high carbohydrate, high fiber diet on hyperglycemic diabetic men. Am J Clin Nutr 29:895–899, 1976
12. Goulder TJ, Alberti KGMM, and Jenkins DA: Effects of added fiber on the glucose and metabolic response to a mixed meal in normal and diabetic subjects. Diabetes Care 1:351–355, 1978
13. Kalkhoff RK and Levin ME: The saccharin controversy. Diabetes Care 1:211–222, 1978
14. Brunzell JD, Use of fructose, xylitol or sorbitol as a sweetener in diabetes mellitus. Diabetes Care 1:223–230, 1978

14

Clinical Use of Insulin

John A. Galloway, M.D.
John K. Davidson, M.D., Ph.D.

The goal of insulin therapy is to normalize plasma glucose levels while minimizing or avoiding the complications of insulin therapy: significant hypoglycemia, allergy, immunologic resistance, lipoatrophy, hypertrophy, and edema. Available forms of insulin, their pharmacology and time action, and typical insulin treatment programs are reviewed in this chapter, and complications of insulin therapy and their treatment are noted.

Insulin therapy is indicated in: (1) persistently hyperglycemic individuals (fasting plasma glucose $\geq$130 mg/dl on appropriate diet and exercise therapy) who are at or below ideal body weight; (2) hyperglycemic pregnant women regardless of body weight; and (3) individuals in diabetic ketoacidosis or a hyperglycemic hyperosmolar state regardless of body weight.

The insulin preparations that are frequently used in the United States,[1] with their time actions and chemical characteristics, are listed in Table 14-1. An appreciation of factors known to affect insulin action is helpful in the proper use of these insulin preparations (Table 14-2). Since many Type I (insulin-dependent) diabetics require mixtures of intermediate and short-acting insulin, it is useful to know that Regular insulin may be mixed with NPH or with Lente insulin in the same syringe with the distinct effects of the two insulin preparations generally preserved. It should be pointed out, however, that recent

Table 14-1. Insulin Preparations.

Type of insulin	Appearance	Action	Peak activity (hours)	Duration (hours)	Zinc content (mg/100 units)	Buffer pH	Type of modifying protein	Amount of modifying proteins mg/100 units
Regular Crystalline	Clear	Rapid	2–4	5–7	0.01–0.04	None Neutral	None	—
NPH	Turbid	Intermediate	6–12	24–28	0.01–0.04	Phosphate Neutral	Protamine	0.03–0.06
Protamine Zinc	Turbid	Prolonged	14–24	36+	0.15–0.25	Phosphate Neutral	Protamine	1.25
Semilente	Turbid	Rapid	2–8	12–16	0.12–0.25	Acetate Neutral	None	—
Lente	Turbid	Intermediate	6–12	24–28	0.12–0.25	Acetate Neutral	None	—
Ultralente	Turbid	Prolonged	18–24	36+	0.12–0.25	Acetate Neutral	None	—

bioavailability studies in normal fasted subjects suggest that some binding of the added Regular insulin to the Lente may occur. However, the clinical significance of this finding may be minimal.

Table 14-2. Factors that Affect the Bioavailability of Insulin.

1. Site of Injection: Following a dose of Regular insulin, peak concentrations are most quickly achieved with abdominal injection and are slowest to occur with injection in the anterior thigh. Peak concentrations are highest in the deltoid area and lowest following buttock injection. Exercise increases insulin absorption from a given extremity.[2]
2. Depth of Injection: The deeper insulin is injected, the quicker its onset and the higher its peak.[3,4] However, the clinical significance of these differences may be minimal.
3. Concentration of insulin in the range of 40 to 100 U/ml is not a significant factor in insulin bioavailability.[5]
4. There is significant day-to-day variation in serum insulin and/or blood glucose response of normals and diabetics given the same dose of insulin twice or more.[3,6]
5. Insulin antibodies attract and hold injected insulin for variable periods of time, thereby delaying its onset and duration of effect.[7-9]
6. The most important factor(s) in insulin effect may be the dynamics of its interaction with insulin receptors, quantitative data on which are scant at the present time.[3]

INSULIN TREATMENT PROGRAMS

For patients in diabetic ketoacidosis or a hyperglycemic hyperosmolar state, Regular insulin should be used.[10] It may be administered in intravenous solutions, or by bolus intravenously, intramuscularly, or subcutaneously.

For chronic insulin treatment, NPH or Lente alone, or combined with Regular insulin, is preferred.[1,11,12] The precise insulin treatment program depends upon the plasma glucose profile obtained from sampling at various times while the patient is on a stable diet and exercise pattern. Some diabetologists prefer to measure 8 a.m. (fasting) and 4 p.m. plasma glucoses and, occasionally, 2- to 3-hour postbreakfast plasma glucoses. Others prefer to measure plasma glucose fasting and three hours after each meal, or fasting and 180 minutes postbreakfast.[6] Several days of monitoring in a hospital setting will provide adequate data on which to design initial insulin therapy or to change existing treatment programs. About two-thirds of insulin-dependent patients can be controlled on one dose daily of Lente or NPH insulin. The dose may range from as little as 2 units to as much as 100 units per day, with most individuals requiring from 20 to 40 units per day. Most in the remaining one-third will respond to one of the strategies outlined in Table 14-3. Rarely, a patient may benefit from Regular insulin before breakfast and lunch plus NPH and Regular before supper, or from an 8 a.m. and 8 p.m. dose of Ultralente each day.

Table 14-3.[1,12] *Common Problems in Response to Single Daily Injections of Intermediate-acting (NPH and Lente) Insulin and Their Remedies.*

Present treatment method	A.M. NPH or Lente	A.M. NPH or Lente	A.M. and P.M. NPH or Lente
Problem	Postbreakfast and/or early afternoon hyperglycemia	Prebreakfast hyperglycemia	Postbreakfast hyperglycemia
Approximate frequency*	20	10	3
Indicated therapy	Add a.m. Regular insulin	a.m. and p.m. NPH or Lente	Add a.m. Regular insulin**

*As percent of patients receiving NPH or Lente Insulin.
**Occasionally, the a.m. insulin dose (including the Regular) is given as much as two hours before breakfast so that the action of the Regular insulin matches the postbreakfast hyperglycemia.

Regardless of the insulin treatment program used, patients should be questioned at each visit for evidence of hypoglycemia, particularly at the time of peak action of the insulin they are using. Hospital and home monitoring techniques for determining plasma or blood glucose[13] make it possible to document suspected hypoglycemia and to rearrange the diet and/or exercise pattern in an appropriate fashion.

COMPLICATIONS OF INSULIN THERAPY[1]

The various complications of insulin therapy are listed in Table 14-4. Since all but insulin edema are related in varying degrees to the purity of insulin, information on the purity of insulin preparations available in North America is pertinent to the management of the complications of insulin therapy.

Table 14-4. Complications of Insulin Therapy and Their Currently Estimated Frequency[1]

1. Formation of antibodies in the serum to insulin—almost 100 percent
   Resulting in immunologic resistance—varies from 0.1 percent to 1.0 percent in different populations. (Intermittent insulin therapy increases its prevalence.)
2. Allergy to insulin
   Local—10 percent
   Systemic—less than 1 percent
3. Insulin lipodystrophy (atrophy and/or hypertrophy)—less than 5 percent
4. Insulin edema—100 percent of patients whose poor control is abruptly improved.

About 10 years ago, gel-filtration chromatography was added to the manufacturing process by Eli Lilly and Company, resulting in insulin which unofficially has been called "single peak" because of its chromatographic profile. Additional purification by ion-exchange chromatography results in insulin of even greater purity. Presently, the proinsulin content is being used to monitor insulin purity. It is expected that other substances will eventually be measured also as a part of the quality standards for insulin production. The proinsulin contents of insulins presently available and about to be introduced in the U.S. marketplace are listed in Table 14-5.

Table 14-5. Proinsulin Contents of Insulins Commercially Available in the United States in 1980.

(Parts per Million, ppm)

Conventional U.S.P.	>10,000
Single Peak*	<3,000
Improved Single Peak**	<50
Purified***	<10

*All Lilly beef-pork insulin manufactured between 1972–1979.
**All Lilly beef-pork insulin marketed after April 1980.
***Lilly Iletin II, Novo "Monocomponent," and Nordisk "Rarely Immunogenic."

Serum Antibodies To Insulin

Virtually all patients treated with insulin develop antibodies. Insulin immunogenicity is a function of the species source of the insulin (beef, being dissimilar to human insulin at two important parts of the molecule, is substantially more immunogenic than pork, which is identical to human insulin at those sites), purity, pharmaceutical form (Regular is less immunogenic than Lente), and the inherent immunologic make-up of the patient. Intermittent insulin therapy increases the prevalence of immunologic resistance.[9] The least immunogenic insulin available is purified pork insulin.

Insulin antibodies in high titer will reduce the promptness of response to a dose of insulin. Insulin antibodies may delay the onset and prolong the time action of Regular insulin[7, 8] and in some patients may reduce the amplitude of the blood glucose excursion which would result from the sudden action of absorbed Regular insulin were it not first intercepted by insulin antibody.[14] A study in animals has implicated insulin antibodies in the development of nodular glomerulosclerosis.[15] The significance of this finding is not known since the lesion also occurs in patients who have not received insulin.[16] A report correlating preservation of endogenous insulin secretion with reduced antibody formation suggests a deleterious effect of serum insulin antibodies.[17] Antibodies to exogenous insulin (beef, pork) cross-react with and neutralize endogenous human insulin.[18]

Immunologic Resistance[1,9]

Immunologic resistance is due to the development of high titers of IgG and IgA insulin-neutralizing antibodies (≥ 30 U/ml serum). Treatment consists in the use of purified pork insulin alone or with a short course of steroids.[19] Some patients need sulfated insulin.[9]

Insulin Allergy[1]

Allergy to insulin occurs in two forms, local and systemic. Local allergy consists of a hard, red, pruritic knot or indurated area appearing at the injection site from minutes to hours after injection. This may be due to impurities in the insulin, previous sensitization to beef or pork protein, or the insulin molecule proper.

The treatment of local allergy to insulin usually consists in switching the patient from beef-pork insulin to purified pork insulin. About 80 percent of patients with local allergy will improve on purified pork insulin. Of the remaining 20 percent, about one-third will respond to beef insulin, one-third can be desensitized, and one-third will continue to have allergy for at least a year. In this latter group, spontaneous improvement over time is the rule.

The treatment of patients with systemic allergy to insulin is desensitization. These patients usually have increased titers of IgE insulin antibodies. Since a high percentage of patients with systemic allergy to insulin also have elevated titers of IgG antibody to beef insulin, desensitization to pork insulin is preferable. For several years, Eli Lilly and Company has provided special kits which contain dilutions of Regular insulin for this purpose. In the Lilly series of 296 patients with systemic allergy to insulin, 17 could not be desensitized. If insulin therapy is essential, oral antihistamine drugs and/or steroid therapy may be of value.

Feinglos and Jegasothy[20] have demonstrated allergy to zinc and favorable responses to zinc-free insulin (obtainable from Eli Lilly and Company) in patients with insulin allergy who do not respond to the desensitization and species source change.

Lipoatrophy[1]

Lipoatrophy most commonly occurs in children and in young women, usually within the first few months of insulin therapy. It consists in loss of fat at the injection site and, in some cases, at sites other than those where insulin is administered. Clinical experience demonstrates that local allergy and atrophy frequently co-exist and that atrophy usually will not improve until the allergy has been adequately treated. Although the cause has not been definitely established, most workers feel that it is due to the presence of a lipolytic substance in the insulin. Thus, Wright et al.[21] found the frequency of lipoatrophy in patients receiving unchromatographed beef-pork or beef insulin to be 10 percent. In our experience,[22] 90 percent of patients on unchromatographed insulin with insulin lipoatrophy responded to single peak beef-pork insulin. Virtually all patients with lipoatrophy which occurs with single peak beef-pork insulin will respond if treated with purified pork insulin. The insulin should be injected into the affected areas until filling in occurs, which usually requires three to four months, at which time injection sites are rotated. Kumar et al.[23] have reported prompt resolution of insulin lipoatrophy with unchromatographed insulin to which dexmethasone 4 μg/unit has been added.

Insulin Hypertrophy[1]

This complication of insulin therapy consists in areas of adipose tissue accumulation where insulin has been administered. The cause of insulin hypertrophy is not known. However, since one of the chief actions of insulin is lipogenesis and since atrophy which has resolved may proceed to hypertrophy, insulin hypertrophy may well be due to the insulin molecule proper. Over half of the patients with insulin hypertrophy improve on the purified pork insulins. An essential part of the treatment of insulin hypertrophy is avoidance of the hypertrophied areas by rotation of injection sites. While the purified pork insulins are apparently less efficacious in insulin hypertrophy than in lipoatrophy, the data being accumulated currently clearly suggest that patients with hypertrophy should receive the purified pork insulins if they fail to respond to the other insulins in Table 14-5.

In view of the foregoing and in consideration of the commercial availability of purified pork insulins (Iletin II, Lilly; Monocomponent, Novo; Rarely Immunogenic, Nordisk),* attention is necessarily focused on when these insulins should be used. The current indications are listed in Table 14-6. Because the availability of purified insulins may lead to their use in situations where therapeutic advantages over other insulins have not been established, physicians may be tempted to prescribe purified pork insulins for patients with labile brittle diabetes or for patients using insulin for the first time. The decision to use purified pork insulin in this manner at the present time should be tempered by two important facts. First, we wish to mention our concern that patients will be treated with the purified pork insulins for reasons which are not substantiated by existing clinical data and that disappointment with the results will ensue. Second, in terms of the long-term survival of the patient, more important than the species source and purity of the insulin is the degree of control of the plasma glucose achieved with it. Conventional subcutaneous insulin administration rarely normalizes the blood glucose over the long term. Skillful use of diet, exercise, and insulin can improve plasma glucose control in the majority of patients. Nonetheless, until methods of delivery of insulin are improved so that the plasma glucose can be kept normal at all times, no insulin, regardless of its purity or similarity to human insulin, will completely prevent the complications of diabetes and the premature deaths that result therefrom.

Insulin Edema[24]

Finally, a frequently unrecognized complication of insulin therapy is fluid retention. This most commonly occurs in patients at the time blood glucose control is established following a

---

*These insulins will be identified officially in the United States as purified insulins, although they are, in fact, highly purified insulins that have been purified by multiple gel-filtration and ion-exchange chromatography processes to remove nearly all of the currently recognized contaminants, such as proinsulin and proinsulin-like substances, glucagon, somatostatin, pancreatic polypeptide, and other identifiable noninsulin materials.

Table 14-6. Suggested Indications for Chromatographically Purified Pork Insulin*

1. Patients who are now taking pork insulin.
2. Patients with persistent local or systemic allergy to beef-pork or beef insulin.
3. Patients who develop insulin lipoatrophy or hypertrophy now taking beef-pork or beef insulin.
4. In patients with immunologic resistance to beef insulin.
5. Possibly for those diabetics whose need for insulin therapy is temporary and therefore may result in intermittent insulin therapy, e.g., during stress or pregnancy. Since interruption of insulin therapy augments the immune response, patients with an allergic diathesis, as suggested, for instance, by a history of allergy to penicillin or other substances, should be considered for treatment with the purified pork insulins.

*There are no conclusive data demonstrating unique efficacy of chromatographically purified pork insulin in labile diabetes or the prevention of the complications of diabetes.

prolonged period of hyperglycemia and ketonuria. Sodium restriction and diuretic therapy may be needed, although most cases clear spontaneously after a few days.

References

1. Galloway JA and Bressler R: Insulin treatment in diabetes. Med Clin North Am 52:663–80, 1978
2. Koivisto VA and Felig P: Effects of leg exercise on insulin absorption in diabetic patients. N Engl J Med 298:79–83, 1978
3. Galloway JA, Nelson RL, and Spradlin CT: The bioavailability of regular insulin. To be submitted to Diabetes Care
4. Guerra SMO and Kitabchi AE: Comparison of the effectiveness of various routes of insulin injection: Insulin levels and glucose response in normal subjects. J Clin Endocrinol Metab 42:869–74, 1976
5. Nelson RL, Galloway JA, Wentworth SM, et al: The bioavailability, pharmacokinetics, and time action of regular and modified insulins in normal subjects. Diabetes 25:325 (Suppl 1), 1976
6. Molnar GD, Taylor WF, and Langworthy A: On measuring the adequacy of diabetes regulation: Comparison of continuously monitored blood glucose patterns with values at selected time points. Diabetologia 10:139–43, 1974
7. Bolinger RE, Morris JH, McKnight FG, et al: Disappearance of ^{131}I labeled insulin from plasma as a guide to management of diabetes. N Engl J Med 270:767–70, 1964
8. Bolinger RE, Stephens R, Lukert B, et al: Galvanic skin reflex and plasma free fatty acids during insulin reactions. Diabetes 13:600–05, 1964

9. Davidson JK and DeBra DW: Immunologic insulin resistance. Diabetes 27:307–18, 1978
10. Davidson JK: Diabetic ketoacidosis and hyperglycemic hyperosmolar states, in Principles and Practice of Emergency Medicine, Schwartz, GR, and Wagner D (eds), Chapter 46, pp. 1062–75. Philadelphia: WB Saunders Co, 1978
11. Davidson JK: Diabetes mellitus in adults, *In* Current Therapy, Conn HF (ed), pp. 386–409. Philadelphia: WB Saunders Co, 1974
12. Davidson JK: Diabetes mellitus and its treatment with diet, exercise, insulin and sulfonylureas, *In* Practical Drug Therapy, Wang RIH (ed), pp. 417–44. Philadelphia: JB Lippincott, 1979
13. Tattersall RB: Editorial, Home blood glucose monitoring. Diabetologia 16:71–74, 1979
14. Dixon K, Exon PD, and Malins JM: Insulin antibodies and control of diabetes. Q J Med 44:543–53, 1975
15. Wehner H, Huber H, and Kronenberg KH: The glomerular basement membrane of the rabbit kidney on long-term treatment with heterologous insulin preparations of different purity. Diabetologia 9:255–63, 1973
16. Strauss FG, Argy WP, Jr, and Schreiner GE: Diabetic glomerulosclerosis in the absence of glucose intolerance. Ann Intern Med 75:239–42, 1971
17. Ludvigsson J and Heding LG: C-peptide in children with juvenile diabetes. Diabetologia 12:627–30, 1976
18. Karam JH, Grodsky GM, and Forsham PH: Insulin-resistant diabetes with autoantibodies induced by exogenous insulin. Diabetes 18:445–54, 1969
19. Field JB: Chronic insulin resistance. Acta Diabetologica Latina 7:220–41, 1970
20. Feinglos MN and Jegosothy BV: "Insulin" allergy due to zinc. The Lancet, pp. 122–24, 1979
21. Wright AD, Walsh CH, Fitzgerald MG, et al: Very pure porcine insulin in clinical practice. Brit Med J 1:25–27, 1979
22. Wentworth SM, Galloway JA, Davidson JA, et al: The use of the purified insulins in the treatment of patients with insulin lipoatrophy. Presented at the International Diabetes Federation Meeting. Vienna, Austria, September 13, 1979
23. Kumar D, Miller LV, and Mehtalia SD: Use of dexamethasone in treatment of insulin lipoatrophy. Diabetes 26:296–99, 1977
24. Saudek CD, Boulter PR, Knopp RH, et al: Sodium retention accompanying insulin treatment of diabetes mellitus. Diabetes 23:240–46, 1974

15

Oral Hypoglycemic Agents

Fred W. Whitehouse, M.D.
Dorothy M. Kahkonen, M.D.

Though many insulin-using diabetic patients desire an oral drug instead of daily injections of insulin, no pharmaceutical drug exists now that mimics insulin in chemical structure or in precise action. In 1977, because of the alleged heightened incidence of lactic acidosis, the biguanide phenformin became available only in special situations under an Investigational New Drug (IND) process. Thus, only the sulfonylureas are freely available to physicians and patients in the United States.

PHARMACOLOGY AND MECHANISM OF ACTION

Four sulfonylurea drugs are now available for use in the United States. These include:

1. *Tolbutamide:* a short-acting drug detoxified by the liver into a metabolite without hypoglycemic effect. It is best given twice daily to a maximum dosage of 3.0 grams. Trade name: *Orinase.*
2. *Chlorpropamide:* a long-acting drug unchanged by the liver but excreted completely by the kidney. It should be given once a day to a maximum dosage of 500 mg. Trade name: *Diabinese.*
3. *Acetohexamide* and *Tolazamide:* Two intermediate-acting drugs with hepatic detoxification to metabolites

with some hypoglycemic effect. Respective maximum daily dosage is 1.5 grams and 1.0 gram given in divided doses. Trade names: *Dymelor* and *Tolinase*.

After 25 years of study on the mechanism of action of the sulfonylureas, no certainty exists on how these drugs lower the blood glucose level. Following acute administration of a sulfonylurea, one can demonstrate a rapid-component insulin release with hyperinsulinemia and a fall in blood glucose. On the contrary, chronic administration of a sulfonylurea fails to demonstrate hyperinsulinemia, although evidence exists suggesting that the beta cell release of insulin after physiologic stimuli is more sensitive. Olefsky and Reaven[1] have shown that sulfonylurea therapy produces an increase in peripheral insulin receptors. Thus, for a salutary pharmacologic effect, it appears that endogenous insulin must be present; then its peripheral effect will be accentuated by the increased insulin receptors which follow administration of the sulfonylurea. No convincing evidence supports other mechanisms of drug action as: (1) a decrease in secretion of glucagon or other contrainsulin hormones; (2) lessened hepatic gluconeogenesis or glycogenolysis; or (3) an impaired absorption of glucose from the gut. "Second generation" sulfonylureas, such as glyburide and glipizide, have no discernable pharmacologic actions different from those suggested for these "first generation" agents.

INDICATIONS FOR USE

Controversy continues on whether the sulfonylureas should be used in patients with diabetes mellitus. Boyden and Bressler[2] see little reason to use sulfonylureas, while Krall and Chabot[3] believe that they have a place in the management of the older diabetic person. Positive effects of this controversy include a greater emphasis on dietary management of the maturity-onset diabetic patient and a more appropriate selection of patients for sulfonylurea therapy. Inadequate control of hyperglycemia with diet alone suggests the need for a blood glucose-lowering medication. If the patient has noninsulin-dependent diabetes (NIDDM) without evidence of ketosis, and if the patient is not too lean and is over 50 years of age, the sulfonylureas may be effective. Since primary drug failures can occur even in carefully selected patients, monitoring of glucose levels remains important. It has been argued that the steady loss of metabolic control after initial control (secondary drug failure) vitiates the value of the sulfonylureas.

CONTRAINDICATIONS

Sulfonylureas should not be used in the patient with insulin-dependent diabetes (IDDM), since endogenous insulin is needed for a salutary drug effect. In general, the drugs are ineffective in individuals who are below ideal body weight. The presence of parenchymal disease of the liver or kidney precludes their use. Sulfonylureas should not be used during pregnancy or lactation, not only because of possible side-effects on the fetus but also because of their frequent inability to continue to meet the increasing stresses of gestation. It is also prudent to avoid these drugs in patients with severe myocardial disease who are taking multiple medications. Of course, these agents should be avoided when a drug allergy exists.

PRIMARY AND SECONDARY FAILURES

By definition, a primary failure of a sulfonylurea occurs when the blood glucose level remains high after 30 days of drug use. During this period, deterioration of metabolic control and worsening hyperglycemia may occur. These patients lack endogenous insulin and usually have IDDM; they never should have been given a sulfonylurea.

Secondary failure to the drug occurs when initial metabolic control is established, then lost. Reasons for this loss of drug action are complex and may include laxity in dietary control, weight gain, intercurrent stress, infection, or worsening insulin deficiency. While loss of endogenous insulin may occur, often hyperglycemia develops because the patient forgets the demands of the diet. However, it is of interest that the serum of patients with NIDDM who demonstrate successful control with an oral agent at one time and then show a secondary failure may contain islet cell antibodies similar to those found in the serum of patients with IDDM.[4] This observation suggests a possible means by which patients may be selected for successful long-term treatment with an oral agent. Thus, only patients with NIDDM whose serum lacks islet cell antibodies would be advised to use an oral sulfonylurea.

COMPLICATIONS OF DRUG USE

Surprisingly, side-effects secondary to the sulfonylureas occur infrequently. Idiosyncratic reactions may cause gastrointestinal symptoms which vary from vague distress and anorexia to malaise and vomiting. While diffuse skin eruptions may follow use of the sulfonylureas in less than one percent of patients, a more serious, yet rare, side-effect is cholestatic jaundice, which we have identified more often with chlorpropamide. Cholestasis without jaundice may also occur. We have not encountered the reported hematologic reactions of severe leukopenia, thrombocytopenia, and mild anemia, nor have we identified patients with drug-induced aplastic anemia or agranulocytosis. Asymptomatic hyponatremia with water retention has been reported with chlorpropamide. It appears that the antidiuretic hormonal effect on the distal renal tubular cells is potentiated. This drug effect, like its acute action on the pancreatic islet cells, seems related to potentiation of cyclic AMP through inhibition of phosphodiesterase activity.

Hypoglycemia, which may be prolonged and profound, is not an idiosyncratic side-effect but rather a complication related to the therapeutic action of the drug. Individuals with severe hypoglycemia secondary to sulfonylureas generally need to be hospitalized for several days of treatment with supplemental glucose. This complication occurs even with the short-acting preparations. It is avoided by using the drug carefully in the older patient whose eating habits and compliance are erratic. An Antabuse-like intolerance to alcohol with flushing has been reported by patients who use sulfonylureas.* Possible drug in-

---

*This reaction to alcohol in patients taking chlorpropamide (CPAF) has lately been identified as a possible genetic trait in patients with NIDDM.

teractions in patients taking several medications should be remembered.

"SECOND GENERATION" SULFONYLUREAS

In addition to the four sulfonylureas currently available, there are two "second generation" sulfonylurea drugs available in Europe, but now used only in investigational studies in the United States. These agents include glyburide (glibenclamide) and glipizide, which are 100 to 200 times more potent by weight than the "first generation" agents. However, experience suggests that the mechanism of action is similar in both groups of drugs so that no broader application of an oral agent seems possible.[5] It has been suggested that these agents may be effective in patients who experience a secondary failure with a "first generation" drug. Marketing of these "second generation" agents is expected.

UGDP

Since the first reports of the University Group Diabetes Program (UGDP) in 1970, no agreement on the interpretation of the data has developed. These disagreements relate to honest differences in interpretation of presented data, to clinical concerns about unpublished data, and to proffered recommendations of actions emanating from the Food and Drug Administration which were based on the UGDP data. Several summaries of the UGDP are available for the interested reader, including reports from the UGDP,[6] critiques of the study,[7] newer view on the UGDP data,[8] and a recent policy statement by the American Diabetes Association.[9]

The UGDP study has had a positive effect on the practice of clinical diabetes despite publicized differences of opinion. It has reemphasized the importance of diet in the therapy of the patient with NIDDM. Without calorie and weight control in this group of patients, we now recognize the futility of attempting blood glucose control with either insulin or an oral agent. We now understand that the first therapeutic principle for NIDDM must be dietary modification, usually with calorie restriction. Only when this fails to control the hyperglycemia should one consider the use of insulin or a substitute for insulin, one of the sulfonylurea drugs. The physician should decide with the patient when to use the oral sulfonylureas after discussion of their indications and potential side effects. Again, the prevailing opinion on their use suggests that:

1. Only NIDDM patients should be considered as candidates for an oral drug.
2. Oral hypoglycemic agents should be used only after dietary control alone has failed to lower the blood glucose to normal.
3. Oral therapy should be avoided in those patients with parenchymal disease involving the heart, liver, or kidney.
4. If good blood glucose control cannot be achieved and maintained by a sulfonylurea, then insulin should be used. Minimal biochemical goals are fasting plasma glucose levels under 160 mg/dl and postprandial levels below 200 mg/dl, although optimal goals would include a fasting plasma glucose level below 120 mg/dl with a postprandial level below 160 mg/dl, and normal levels of glycosylated hemoglobin.

PERSONAL VIEWPOINTS

Oral sulfonylurea drugs are best reserved for the diabetic person over age 50 who is otherwise healthy. Their action is unreliable in the slender patient with symptomatic diabetes. Insulin is indicated in any patient when the drug fails to control the blood glucose level.

In 1978, one of us (FWW) studied 82 consecutive personal patients who were taking an oral agent. The following summarizes the findings: only three patients were under age 50; almost 50 percent took chlorpropamide; just 17 patients were at normal weight; 19 patients should have taken insulin; 18 patients were blind (a good reason for use of an oral agent). The average fasting plasma glucose at the time of the office visit during the study was 153 mg/dl (range 70–220 mg/dl) with the average postprandial level being 159 mg/dl (range 80–330 mg/dl). Glycosylated hemoglobin levels in these 82 patients were not measured. No patient reported diabetic symptoms. These 82 patients had used a sulfonylurea from less than one year to over 19 years.

CONCLUSIONS

The oral sulfonylurea drugs should be considered only in patients with NIDDM who have tried dietary modification without successful blood glucose control. When more than diet is needed and no specific contraindications exist (parenchymal disease, infection, IDDM, drug allergy), then one of the sulfonylurea drugs may be used as a substitute for insulin. When blood glucose levels are satisfactorily controlled (under 140 mg/dl fasting and under 200 mg/dl postprandially), the drug can be continued. If hyperglycemia recurs despite reemphasis on calorie restriction and a maximal dosage of the drug, then insulin should be advised. When the diabetic state is properly regulated, accentuated cardiovascular morbidity and mortality because of sulfonylurea use does not appear to be significant.[10]

References

1. Olefsky JM and Reaven GM: Effects of sulfonylurea therapy on insulin-binding to mononuclear leukocytes of diabetic patients. Am J Med 60:89–95, 1976.
2. Boyden T and Bressler R: Oral Hypoglycemic agents. Adv Int Med 24:53–70, 1979
3. Krall LP and Chabot VA: Oral hypoglycemic agent update. Med Clin No Amer 62:681–694, 1978
4. Irvine WJ, Gray RS, McCallum CJ, et al: Clinical and pathogenic significance of pancreatic islet-cell antibodies in diabetes treated with oral hypoglycemic agents. Lancet 1:1025–1027, 1977
5. Beck-Nielsen H, Pedersen O, and Lindskov HO: Increased insulin sensitivity and cellular insulin binding in obese diabetics following treatment with glibenclamide. Acta Endocrinol 90:451–462, 1979
6. Klimt CR, Knatterud GL, Meinert CL, et al: The University Group Diabetes Program (UGDP): A study of the effects of hypoglycemic agents on vascular complications in patients with adult-onset diabetes. II. Mortality results. Diabetes 19 (Suppl): 789–830, 1970
7. Seltzer HS: A summary of criticisms of the findings and conclusions of the UGDP. Diabetes 21:976–979, 1972
8. Feinstein AR: How good is the statistical evidence against oral hypoglycemic agents? Adv Int Med 24:71–95, 1979

9. Whitehouse FW, Arky RA, Bell DI, et al: Policy statement, the UGDP controversy. Diabetes 28:168–170, 1979
10. Kilo C, Miller JP, and Williamson JR: The Achilles heel of the University Group Diabetes Program. JAMA 243:450–457, 1980

16

Exercise in Diabetes: Clinical Implications

Veikko A. Koivisto, M.D.
Philip Felig, M.D.

EFFECTS OF EXERCISE ON GLUCOSE HOMEOSTASIS

Normal Man

In normal subjects, uptake of glucose by the exercising leg is increased 7– to 20–fold above the basal level in proportion to the intensity of exercise. The rise in glucose utilization is accompanied by an increase in hepatic glucose production. Consequently, blood glucose remains unchanged or falls only slightly during short-term exercise. Contributing to the maintenance of glucose homeostasis is a decrease in endogenous insulin secretion and an increase in counterregulatory hormones, glucagon, catecholamines, growth hormone, and cortisol. The altered hormonal milieu facilitates the increase in hepatic glucose production. On the other hand, exercise-induced increases in glucose utilization occur in the absence of a rise in serum insulin.

Exercise-Induced Hypoglycemia in Diabetes

In insulin-treated diabetics, exercise-induced hypoglycemia is a well recognized complication. Studies on pancreatectomized dogs and in diabetic patients injected with subcutaneous insulin have demonstrated a rise in plasma insulin levels during exercise. However, when insulin is administered intravenously, no rise is observed in plasma insulin and the tendency to hypoglycemia is decreased.[1,2] These findings suggest that exercise may increase the mobilization of insulin from a subcutaneous injection site. The absorption rate of insulin was consequently determined by measuring the disappearance rate of ^{125}I-insulin from the subcutaneous injection site in the leg, arm, and abdomen during and after leg exercise.[3] Leg exercise caused a 50 to 135 percent rise in insulin absorption rate from the leg. However, leg exercise had no effect on the insulin absorption rate from an injection site in the arm, and it actually decreased the absorption rate from the abdomen during the postexercise recovery period.[3] Furthermore, the exercise-induced fall in plasma glucose is proportional to the insulin absorption rate.[1,3] As compared to leg injection, arm or abdominal injection can markedly reduce the hypoglycemic effect of leg exercise (Figure 16-1).[1,3]

Zinman, et al.[1] have demonstrated that the hypoglycemic effect of enhanced insulin delivery during exercise in insulin-treated diabetics in not due to augmented glucose uptake by exercising muscle but is a consequence of inhibition of the rise in hepatic glucose production which normally occurs in exercise. As a result, the rate of glucose utilization exceeds the rate of production, and hypoglycemia ensues.[1,2]

The clinical implications of these observations are as follows. The tendency to exercise-induced hypoglycemia can be minimized by: (a) taking extra carbohydrate before exercise; (b) using a nonexercised area as the injection site; and (c) if hypoglycemia still recurs, the dose of insulin should be lowered. Unfortunately, the amount of extra carbohydrate needed or the amount by which the insulin dose requires reduction can only be determined by trial and error.

INFLUENCE OF EXERCISE ON INSULIN BINDING AND INSULIN SENSITIVITY

Acute Exercise

The enhanced glucose uptake which occurs in the face of lowered plasma insulin levels in normal man during exercise

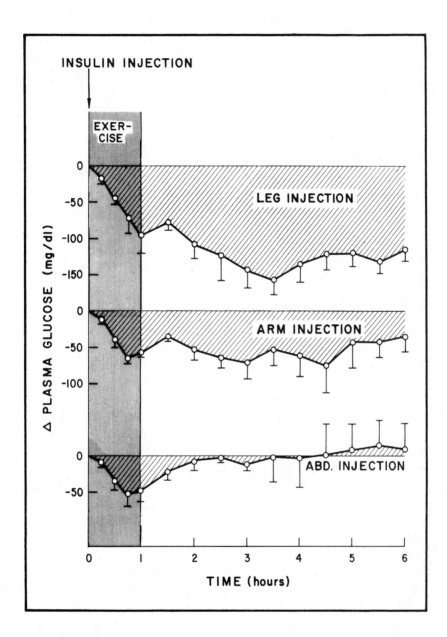

Figure 16-1. Influence of injection site in the plasma glucose response to leg exercise. The shaded areas represent the change in plasma glucose induced by leg exercise as compared to the resting, control day. The area above the curve for abdominal and arm injection was 89% and 57% smaller respectively, than that for leg injection. (From ref 3, with permission).

suggests that exercise may augment body sensitivity to insulin. To examine the mechanism of the enhanced insulin sensitivity during exercise, Soman et al.[4] determined the effect of acute exercise on insulin binding. In normal man, a 3 h submaximal exercise led to a 36 percent increase in specific binding of ^{125}I-insulin to monocytes.[4] The changes in insulin binding caused by acute exercise were mainly due to an increase in receptor affinity rather than a change in binding capacity. Interestingly, the increase in insulin binding was proportional to the fall in plasma glucose during exercise. This raises the possibility that enhanced insulin binding contributes to augmented insulin sensitivity during exercise. In addition to changes in insulin binding, other factors, such as increased blood flow or changes in cellular calcium content, have been suggested as contributing to the stimulation of glucose uptake during exercise.[2]

Physical Training

After physical training, the insulin response to a glucose load is diminished in the face of unchanged glucose tolerance, thus indicating enhanced body sensitivity to insulin.[5] In contrast, physical inactivity, such as bed rest for 1–2 weeks, significantly impairs glucose tolerance in normal man.[6] Recent studies have indicated that in well-trained athletes, insulin binding to monocytes in the basal state is 70 percent higher than in untrained controls.[7] The rise in insulin binding in athletes is due to an increase in the number of receptors rather than any change in binding capacity. Furthermore, elevated insulin binding is proportional to the degree of physical fitness in athletes. In addition, in previously untrained subjects, physical training can increase insulin binding in concert with the increased in vivo insulin sensitivity as measured directly by the insulin clamp technique.[8] These changes in insulin sensitivity occur in the absence of changes in body weight. These findings in normal man suggest that enhanced insulin sensitivity after training may be mediated, at least in part, by augmented insulin binding to receptors.

In maturity-onset diabetics, Saltin et al.[9] have recently reported an improvement in oral glucose tolerance after 3 months of physical training. In a similar study, involving a 6-week training program, Ruderman et al.[10] failed to show any improvement in oral glucose tolerance. The disappearance rate of glucose after intravenous administration was, however, improved.[10]

Anecdotal observations in diabetic children while at summer camp suggest that regular exercise may reduce insulin requirements.[2] In keeping with this, after 6 weeks of intensive training, juvenile-onset diabetics were able to reduce the dose of insulin by 10 to 18 units/day. Simultaneously, their glucosuria and fasting blood glucose levels were decreased.[11] These findings suggest that regular exercise may increase body sensitivity to insulin in diabetic patients and decrease insulin requirements in juvenile-onset diabetics. Whether the training-induced increase in body sensitivity to insulin in diabetic patients is related to the changes in insulin binding to receptors remains to be established.

INSULIN AVAILABILITY AND THE HORMONAL RESPONSE TO EXERCISE

In hyperglycemic, insulin-deficient diabetics, acute exercise causes an exaggerated rise in plasma glucagon, catecholamines, and growth hormone. When patients are treated with multiple daily injections so as to achieve normoglycemia, the growth hormone response is suppressed.[12] Recently, the hormonal response to exercise was evaluated during treatment with an "open loop" type of "artificial pancreas." By employing a portable insulin infusion pump which delivers insulin at a preprogrammed basal rate with pulse dose increments before meals, blood glucose levels were normalized in juvenile diabetics.[13] In these patients, the hormonal response to exercise was determined during conventional treatment and after 2 weeks of treatment with the insulin pump. As shown in Figure 16-2, during conventional treatment the growth hormone response to exercise was 7-fold greater and the catecholamine response 11-fold greater than in normal man. However, after 2 weeks of treatment with the insulin pump, the hormonal response to exercise was virtually normal.[13] These findings thus indicate the importance of adequate insulin availability and metabolic control on the hormonal response to exercise in diabetes.

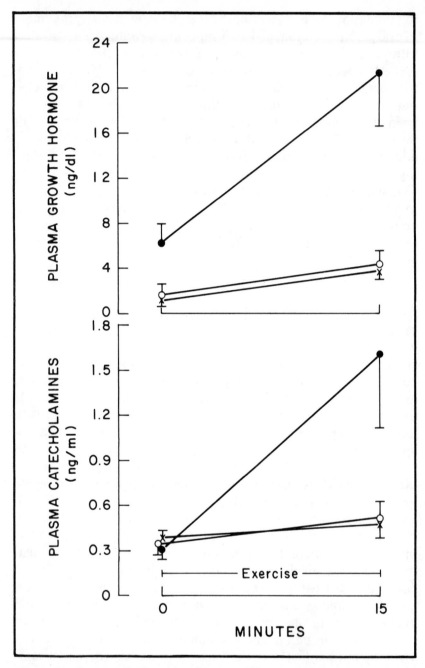

Figure 16-2. Plasma growth hormone and catecholamine (epinephrine plus norepinephrine) response to 15 minute exercise in healthy controls (x) and in insulin-dependent diabetics during conventional treatment (α) and in the same patients after 2 weeks of treatment (O) with a portable, subcutaneous insulin infusion system. Based on the data of Tamborlane, et al.[13]

EXERCISE IN POORLY REGULATED DIABETES

In addition to the exaggerated hormonal response, when blood glucose control is poor in the resting state, exercise may intensify rather than improve hyperglycemia as well as ketogenesis. It has been recognized for over 50 years that, in the absence of insulin administration, if blood glucose levels exceed 300 mg/dl in the resting state, acute exercise will cause a further rise in blood sugar.[14] Furthermore, the rate of ketogenesis is increased during exercise in such poorly regulated diabetics.[14] Blood ketones may, however, remain unchanged because ketone utilization keeps pace with ketone production. Nevertheless, the important clinical implication is that exercise should be viewed as an *adjunct rather than an alternative* to careful management of the juvenile-onset diabetic with proper doses of insulin.

SUMMARY

Based on its blood glucose lowering effect, exercise is traditionally recommended to diabetic patients. However, hypoglycemia is a well-recognized complication of exercise in insulin-dependent diabetics. Exercise-induced hypoglycemia is due to insulin-mediated suppression of glucose production. This complication can be avoided by: (a) increasing carbohydrate intake; (b) using non-exercised insulin injection sites to avoid enhanced insulin mobilization; and (c) where necessary, lowering the insulin dose.

Exercise-induced elevations of counterregulatory hormones are exaggerated in diabetes if insulin treatment is less than optimal. Furthermore, if moderate to severe hyperglycemia (>300 mg/dl) is present in the resting state, exercise will increase rather than ameliorate hyperglycemia and ketogenesis. In contrast, treatment with a portable subcutaneous insulin infusion system, which normalizes blood glucose levels, normalizes the growth hormone and catecholamine response to exercise in juvenile-onset diabetics. These findings underscore the importance of insulin availability in the glycemic and hormonal response to acute exercise in diabetes and indicate that exercise is an adjunct rather than substitute for proper management of diabetes with insulin.

In normal man, physical training results in augmented insulin sensitivity and increased insulin binding to receptors. In adult-onset diabetics, training may improve glucose tolerance. Furthermore, in juvenile-onset diabetes, regular exercise may reduce insulin requirements. Whether augmented insulin sensitivity observed in diabetic patients after training is mediated by augmented insulin binding remains to be established.

References

1. Zinman B, Vranic M, Albisser AM, et al: The role of insulin in the metabolic response to exercise in diabetic man. Diabetes 28 (suppl 1):76–81, 1979
2. Vranic M and Berger M: Exercise and diabetes mellitus. Diabetes 28:147–163, 1979
3. Koivisto VA and Felig P: Effects of leg exercise on insulin absorption in diabetic patients. New Engl J Med 298:79–83, 1978
4. Soman V, Koivisto VA, Grantham P, et al: Increased insulin binding to monocytes after acute exercise in normal man. J Clin Endocrinol Metab 47:216–219, 1978
5. Lohman D, Liebold F, Heilman W, et al: Diminished insulin response in highly trained athletes. Metabolism 27:521–524, 1978
6. Lipman RL, Raskin P, Love T, et al: Glucose intolerance during decreased physical activity in man. Diabetes 21:101–107, 1972
7. Koivisto VA, Soman V, Conrad P, et al: Insulin binding to monocytes in trained athletes: changes in the resting state and after exercise. J Clin Invest 64:1011–1014, 1979
8. Soman V, Koivisto V, Diebert D, et al: Increased sensitivity to insulin and increased insulin binding after physical training. N Eng J Med 301: 1200–1204, 1979
9. Saltin B, Lindgarde F, Houston M, et al: Physical training and glucose tolerance in middle-aged men with chemical diabetes. Diabetes: 28 (suppl 2):30–32, 1979
10. Ruderman NB, Ganda Om P, Johansen K: The effect of physical training on glucose tolerance and plasma lipids in maturity-onset diabetes. Diabetes 28 (suppl 1):89–92, 1979
11. Engerbretson DL: The effects of exercise upon diabetic control. J Assoc Phys Ment Rehab 19:77–78, 1965
12. Tchobroutsky G, Lenormand M-E, Michel G, et al: Lack of post-prandial exercise-induced growth hormone secretion in normoglycemic insulin-treated diabetic man. Horm Metab Res 6:184–187, 1974
13. Tamborlane WV, Sherwin RS, Koivisto V, et al: Normalization of growth hormone and catecholamine response to exercise in juvenile-onset diabetics treated with a portable insulin infusion pump. Diabetes 28:785–788, 1979
14. Felig P and Wahren J: Fuel homeostasis in exercise. N Engl J Med 293:1078–1084, 1975

17

The Team Approach to Patient Education and Management

A. Denise Stevens, BSN, MAT
Robert F. Bradley, M.D.

The Team Approach to treating and educating diabetic patients has gained increasing acceptance in recent years. The burgeoning of diabetes education programs in the United States[1] has already broadened considerably the opportunities for diabetes education in many areas. Recognition of the importance of programs, such as the one described briefly herein, is exemplified by the creation of a key component within the Diabetes Research and Training Centers (Albert Einstein College of Medicine, Indiana University, University of Michigan, Washington University, University of Chicago, Joslin Diabetes Foundation, Inc., Vanderbilt University, University of Virginia) of "Model Demonstration Units." These are intended to emulate some of the existing education and treatment centers in providing a Team Approach to diabetes care and education of the patient and his or her family, as well as a focus for training allied health professionals and physicians. The anticipated ultimate result will be to "spread the word" to the outer reaches of every community in the United States.

The objectives of a treatment and education center are to reduce the overall impact of *acute* and *chronic* complications of diabetes. The ability to reduce the impact of *acute* complications has been demonstrated through the use of allied health professionals trained in the details of daily diabetes management and available through a 24-hour "hot line" at Los Angeles County University of Southern California Hospital.[2] Demonstration of benefit, in terms of preventing or reducing chronic complications, will be no easier than proving to universal scientific satisfaction that careful "control" of blood glucose level will result in a major reduction in these chronic underlying complications. Thus, the issue of "cost effectiveness" as a measure of the worth of the Team Approach in mitigating the adverse effects of "chronic" complications, whether in an in-patient or out-patient setting or both, is irrelevant. On the other hand, impact on *acute* complications, avoidable foot lesions leading to gangrene and change in performance of the individual as a productive member of society, probably can be assessed with some accuracy.

The "Diabetes Treatment Unit" described herein might also be labeled a "Model Demonstration Unit," which, in its current form, has been in existence since 1957. The concept evolved from the utilization many years ago of a "wandering diabetic nurse," whose value to patients and their families in their homes through direct guidance in the use of diet, insulin, and urine testing was recognized by Dr. Elliott P. Joslin. Later, "Teaching Nurses" under the supervision of physicians of the Joslin Clinic and New England Deaconess Hospital and their participation both in the in- and out-patient setting from the early 1930s until 1956 led to the creation by the Joslin Diabetes Foundation of a specific area administered by the New England Deaconess Hospital starting in January 1957. Initially called "Diabetes Teaching Unit," the concept that "education" is "treatment" led to redesignation a few years ago to "Diabetes Treatment Unit."

DIABETES TREATMENT UNIT

This in-patient unit has a capacity of 70 ambulatory diabetic patients. Those patients too ill to be up and about, attending classes or going to a communal dining hall, or with more serious complicating illnesses, are treated in a separate main portion of the New England Deaconess Hospital in Boston. The DTU has some private rooms, but mostly groups of 2 and 4 bedrooms, which are often helpful in assisting a newly diagnosed person to realize he or she is not alone in this situation. Sharing a room with others has also been a stimulus for points of discussion in class, e.g., when a management technique or tool is used by one patient and is suggested to others by one of his/her roommates. The informal atmosphere, with patients dressed in street clothes and an area designated for relaxation and group conversation, provides the camaraderie needed by many for lowering anxiety levels and, therefore, allowing greater concentration on the reason(s) for admission.

The objective is to provide a realistic atmosphere by giving the patients as much responsibility for their own care as possible. This also increases the opportunities for learning by repetition. All individuals and/or their family members are responsible for testing and recording their daily urine tests, injecting their own insulin (if they are insulin-dependent), and selecting their own food from a menu according to their given meal plan. However, the food service will soon be changed to a cafeteria system, which will provide even greater experience in selecting actual foods in correct amounts and learning to identify portion sizes and appropriate substitutions. All patients are first observed by the health professionals to insure their use of correct procedures before placing them in the "independent" category. Anyone requiring additional assistance receives it for as long as necessary.

Units established to treat and educate persons with diabetes involve a variety of health professionals. Each plays an essential and distinct role.

The physician role is shared by the attending physician and one or more physicians in training, usually a Fellow. They will usually make daily rounds together, sharing information and progress about and *with* the patients. The patients are fully involved in discussions and are encouraged to identify their concerns and ask questions. The Fellow remains available to the patients during the day and can, therefore, keep the attending physician informed about any changes in status. He, in turn, provides his/her expertise to the Fellow regarding the possible changes in management as a result of variations in status and is ultimately responsible for the results. The senior physician is also responsible for communication with the referring physician or suitable resource within the community to which the patient is returning.

Attending physicians serve the additional function of being formal educators by conducting daily patient lectures. This task serves several useful purposes. It provides basic information to patients and stresses to them the importance of the education process, identifying that even a busy doctor takes time out to participate in the program. It benefits the physician by allowing him to hear what concerns patients express and what concepts they find difficult to grasp.

Recently a pediatrician who manages many of the juvenile admissions has been added to the Joslin Clinic staff. These young patients frequently are grouped in one area of the unit and are admitted at designated intervals. This grouping allows the juveniles to identify with others of the same age and has proved of great value. The pediatrician is sensitive to the young peoples' needs and is perhaps more "tuned in" to the potential problems of growth and development to which juvenile diabetics are prone.

A recreational director is employed by the hospital to assist and guide the young people in appropriate activities, both within and outside the institution. This provides them not only with supervised activity, but also with on-the-spot teaching in specific situations, e.g., how to eat at a fast food restaurant and remain within the meal plan. A calendar of activities is scheduled for the youth weeks, and preadmission information is sent to the children and parents regarding any specific items to bring related to the activities of that week.

Admitting the juvenile patients at one time has the added advantage that parents may relate to other parents in the same situation, which is often not possible for those who live in small communities. These people are often extremely anxious and require much time, support, and thorough education. The team endeavors to answer these needs with individual and group sessions with the pediatrician, teaching nurses, and social worker.

One other professional who is an integral part of the DTU and many other programs is the podiatrist. He is available for consultation and treatment of any patient requiring his services. In addition, he conducts weekly patient classes on the importance of, and procedures for, proper foot care.

For any major diabetes treatment program, other physicians will also be needed for selected patients. Ophthalmologists of the

William P. Beetham Eye Unit see many of the DTU patients in consultation to allay fears and/or recommend treatment for eye disease. Nephrologists may also be asked to see those with evidence of renal disease. There is a host of other specialists from the New England Deaconess Hospital, or other staffs as needed, who are frequently consulted, such as the gastroenterologist, vascular surgeon, neurologist, cardiologist, urologist, gynecologist, psychiatrist, and dentist.

The role of the nurse in the Joslin unit is shared by two different groups: The primary nurses who staff the unit and the teaching nurses. All are involved in the education process. The primary nurses work with the patients on an individual basis, identifying educational needs related to the mechanics of urine testing and insulin administration. They also provide assessment of the patients' psychosocial adjustment, behavior patterns, and other pertinent data.

The teaching nurses are responsible for assessing the patients' diabetes-related educational needs and implementing a plan to meet them. They see their patients on a daily basis, often rounding with the doctors and primary nurses. During the individual teaching sessions, counseling is given on specific aspects of management not included in the formal classes. Those who need extra help to understand specific concepts receive it at this time.

The teaching nurses are also responsible for conducting afternoon classes. Because people of varying ages and duration of diabetes often have different interests, needs, and goals for management, patients are grouped into small, age-related sessions for the afternoon classes. These small groups are beneficial in promoting discussion and insuring that each individual has his/her questions answered.

Though most programs utilize dietitians for instructing patients in the concepts of a diabetic diet, the bulk of this responsibility is also that of the teaching nurses in our unit. There are obvious advantages and disadvantages to this system. Advantageously, it certainly allows for less fragmentation of personnel, as well as fewer personnel needed to conduct the program. It is also simpler for patients to be able to ask diet-related questions of the person who is instructing them in all other aspects of diabetes management.

On the other hand, dietitians have far greater knowledge of nutrition in general, can more fully assess patient needs, and are an important resource for patients requiring multi-restricted diets.

The dietitians in the DTU are sharing an increasing responsibility for diet instruction. They work with individual patients who require the added time. They also conduct special classes on meal planning and behavioral techniques for weight loss for the noninsulin-dependent patients. Recently, they initiated a class on weekends to discuss the general concepts of good nutrition.

As with any chronic disease, the diagnosis of diabetes affects individuals in a variety of ways and many of them have difficulty adjusting to the diagnosis. A social worker is a team member essential to a diabetes treatment program and should be available to any patient requiring his/her expertise. A specific individual is assigned to the DTU and outpatient program to work with patients on a consultation basis. In addition, she meets weekly with the staff to identify any problem patients to whom she might be of service. She also offers assistance to staff members who might be struggling with the management of a difficult patient.

In some programs, pharmacists play a key role, instructing patients regarding the use of insulin or other hypoglycemic agents. He/she might be the most appropriate health professional to discuss with patients how medications affect diabetes and/or test results.

A physician therapist and/or exercise physiologist might be employed to help with the instruction of exercise and its relation to diabetes. Patients could be assisted in determining the best type of exercise program for them and ways to implement it.

GENERAL CONCEPTS

Certain precepts form a fundamental base for the ongoing success of a Diabetes Treatment and Teaching Program. In a prior essay,[3] *The Importance and Techniques of Patient Education* were outlined in considerable detail, and almost without exception they remain unchanged. At that time it was stated that "the central role of the physician should be maintained." Today, although still ultimately responsible for the performance of the "Team," for the treatment of complicating illness, and for the training of physicians and allied health professionals, the details of day-to-day management, of general health care, and of care of the feet, etc. have rightly been delegated to the allied health professional. In turn, they and some of the support personnel listed above are providing a far more sensitive "ear" to the needs of diabetic patients and their families and the emotional, as well as technical, support so greatly needed.

The Joslin Diabetes Foundation and New England Deaconess Hospital DTU described above represent only the more formally structured portion of the treatment and training program. Patients in the main portion of the New England Deaconess Hospital are in some instances able to travel by wheelchair to formal classes and, when appropriate, receive the same one-on-one exposure to training by teaching nurse, dietitian, etc. The hospitalized diabetic population exposed regularly to the "Team Approach" represents approximately 10 percent of the Joslin Clinic population. Teaching nurses rotate through the outpatient setting where they are available to initiate and review diabetes treatment programs as outlined by the patient's physician.

Through the creation of a Diabetes Treatment Unit where inpatients are ambulatory and at times can be asked to help with specific functions, such as making their own beds, it has been possible to keep the daily cost of the DTU beds at approximately 60 percent of the current costs in the main hospital ($126 versus $200 for a private, $111 versus $170 for a semiprivate).

Whatever portions or all of a DTU or Model Demonstration Unit can be made available to communities throughout the country, the needs of diabetic patients and their families should be the "core" emphasis by physician leadership and all allied health professionals involved. If such programs are to attract well-qualified professionals and provide continuity of effort through a stable "team," third party reimbursement mechanisms recognizing the importance of educational and supportive personnel must supply *dollars*.

References

1. Director of Diabetes Education Programs. American Association of Diabetes Educators. 1978
2. Miller LV and Goldstein J: More efficient care of diabetic patients in a county hospital setting. N Engl J Med 286:1388–91, 1972
3. Bradley RF: Importance and techniques of patient education. *In* Diabetes Mellitus: Diagnosis and Treatment, American Diabetes Association, Inc, 1967, Vol 2, Chapter 16, p. 83

MANAGEMENT PROBLEMS IN DIABETES

18

The Child with Diabetes Mellitus

Allan L. Drash, M.D.

Diabetes mellitus is seen in its purest form in the child. The disease is almost invariably one of primary insulin deficiency, and metabolic derangements are a consequence of this insulin lack. Major disturbances in carbohydrate, lipid, and protein metabolism result, which lead to predictable clinical features. Far less commonly, maturity-onset diabetes with normal or excessive insulin levels, often associated with obesity, is also seen in childhood.

EPIDEMIOLOGY

The true prevalence of diabetes in the United States is not known since most, if not all, estimates are derived from incomplete surveys without medical verification. The few prevalence studies which have been carried out in childhood provide estimates varying from 1 diabetic child per 770 normal children to 1 per 2500 normal children under 16 years of age. The disorder occurs equally in boys and girls over the entire period of childhood and adolescence, but there is variation in sex incidence depending upon age of onset. Although the disease may be diagnosed any time from neonatal period through completion of puberty, there are two age periods where peak of incidence of new cases can be expected. The first is in the 5–6 year age group, coinciding with the beginning of school experience and its associated increase in stress and exposure to infectious disease. The second period is in the immediate preadolescent age group of 11–13 years.

ETIOLOGY

The etiology of insulin-dependent diabetes remains a question of intense research interest. A brief status report indicates that in many cases there appears to be a genetic defect in immunological competence leading to an increased likelihood of viral infections and/or autoimmune damage to the islet cells of the pancreas, either of which, acting alone or in concert, may lead to permanent islet cell destruction and insulin-dependent diabetes mellitus. The finding of an unexpectedly large number of insulin-dependent diabetic individuals with specific HLA types, particularly HLA B8, Bw15, Dw2 and Dw3, provides a technique for studying the genetic features of this disorder in a more sophisticated method than we have ever had available previously.

PRESENTATION AND CLINICAL COURSE

The clinical features of diabetes of the child are a direct result of insulin deficiency. The classical features include polyuria, polydipsia, polyphagia, weight loss, and fatigue. In our experience, 80 percent of our patients have had a recognizable clinical course of less than four weeks in duration, most of these associated with an intercurrent viral illness. At the time of diagnosis, 15–20 percent of the patients are in a marked state of metabolic disturbance characterized by diabetic ketoacidosis. The remainder of the patients have lesser and varying degrees of biochemical disturbance and clinical symptoms. The initial therapy involves insulin administration, development of a diet specific for the needs of the child, and educational and emotional support for the child and family. We try to accomplish these initial phases of therapy during a hospitalization of approximately six days.

Following hospital discharge, the family maintains daily contact with the physician for instruction regarding alteration in the daily insulin dose and any other aspects of management that need discussion. These daily contacts continue for three to six weeks, depending upon the needs of the individual family. The child is returned to school and full activity promptly following hospital discharge. Daily vigorous physical activity is strongly encouraged.

In approximately 90 percent of the patients, a significant decline in insulin requirement occurs two to four months following diagnosis. This period, referred to as the "remission" or "honeymoon" phase, results from a partial recovery of islet cell function. In a small number of patients, possibly 5 percent of the total, insulin administration may be completely discontinued for relatively short periods of time. In these patients, islet cell function has returned essentially to normal. However, invariably islet cell function declines and insulin requirements increase so that by 12–18 months following diagnosis the great majority of children have reached a stage referred to as "total diabetes," at which time their daily insulin requirements are approximately 1 unit/kg/day.

THERAPEUTIC OBJECTIVES

The primary objective of the practice of medicine is prevention and cure of disease. In our current state of knowledge, we are incapable of either preventing or curing insulin-dependent diabetes mellitus. Consequently, the physician, in concert with the patient and family, must establish secondary therapeutic objectives. The control of blood glucose has long been considered the appropriate therapeutic goal in the management of the patient with diabetes. By this is meant that the concentration of blood glucose is continuously maintained within normal limits. However, it is rarely possible to achieve continuous normality of glucose concentration under the varying situations of exercise, emotional stress, food ingestion, food deprivation, etc. in the patient with complete insulin deficiency. Consequently, the physician and patient must compromise from what is ideal to what is possible or what is practically achievable. The concern about the control of blood glucose variation and, more appropriately, the control of the total biochemical alterations associated with insulin deficiency is that there may be a definite relationship between the cardiovascular complications of diabetes and those metabolic derangements.

The physician who cares for the child with diabetes mellitus should attempt to assess realistically what he hopes to achieve in terms of both immediate and long-term goals. He must then constantly redefine his optimal goal for each individual patient based on what he empirically learns is practical and consistently obtainable. Concern about the psychological well-being of the child and his family must be placed into proper context within the overall treatment regimen. A therapeutic program which prevents or minimizes cardiovascular complications but produces an individual who is psychologically incapable of functioning in an adult environment can hardly be judged a successful therapeutic modality.

The therapeutic objectives of our clinic include the following:

1. Complete elimination of the overt acute symptoms of diabetes mellitus including polyuria, polydipsia, and polyphagia.
2. Prevention of ketonuria, ketonemia, and ketoacidosis. (Although ketonuria can be expected to occur transiently in association with intercurrent infections, the development of ketoacidosis in the child with previously diagnosed diabetes mellitus should not occur. It is a treatment failure, the responsibility of which should be borne by the physician as well as the patient and his family.)
3. Prevention of hypoglycemia.
4. Control of hyperglycemia and glucosuria to the extent that caloric losses are minimized; a 24-hour urinary glucose loss of less than 7 percent of the ingested carbohydrate (20–25gm glucose per day) is a reasonable goal which can be achieved in a high percentage of patients who have received dietary advice.
5. Maintenance of blood lipid concentrations within the normal limits for age.

6. Achievement of normal growth development, including the normal timing of secondary sexual development.
7. Maintenance of a high level of physical fitness.
8. Avoidance of obesity.
9. Full participation in all activities appropriate to age and interest.
10. Acceptance of the diet that helps to minimize postprandial hyperglycemia and to prevent hyperlipidemia.
11. Education of the patient and family regarding diabetes and its treatment so that they can effectively participate in all management decisions.
12. Assumption by the patient of progressively more responsibility for insulin administration, urine testing, and dietary and other daily management activities.
13. Development by the patient of sound psychological acceptance of diabetes, including a positive outlook for the future.
14. Eventual achievement of full intellectual, physical, and emotional potential as a contributing member of society.
15. Prevention of cardiovascular complications of diabetes, including atherosclerosis and microvascular disease.

THERAPY

Insulin

The therapy of insulin-dependent diabetes has changed minimally over the past thirty years. The basic treatment program involves the daily administration of insulin by injection. This may be given as a single injection once daily, usually as a mixture of intermediate and rapid-acting insulin or as multiple injections before meals. There is considerable controversy over the relative effectiveness of single versus split-dose insulin therapy in terms of both day-to-day glucose control and long-term complications. In the majority of our children, NPH insulin and regular insulin is given once daily before breakfast. In 20–30 percent of our patients, most of whom are adolescents, we find that two insulin injections daily, NPH and regular insulin, before breakfast and supper, provide better symptomatic and biochemical control. There is currently great excitement that the open-loop subcutaneous insulin infusion pump may provide a clinically applicable technique for achieving near normality of energy metabolism. We share this enthusiasm, but suggest cautious and careful investigation of the total response to this method before its widespread clinical application. Certainly, the psychological response to dependency upon a mechanical device must be evaluated.

Diet

Diet is critically important in the management of insulin-dependent diabetes. We recommend the use of the exchange technique with adequate total calories and nutrients to meet the changing energy demands of the growing child. The child's appetite is a more reliable indicator of need than any of the techniques for estimating calorie requirements. We recommend a diet with 50–55 percent of calories from carbohydrate, 30–35 percent from fat, and 15–20 percent from protein. The carbohydrate component is approximately 70 percent complex starches and 30 percent from a mixture of lactose, sucrose, and fructose. The fat component has a P/S of greater than 1.0 and cholesterol content of less than 250 mg/day. The calories should be distributed over the entire waking hours in order to minimize hyperglycemia and hyperlipidemia and prevent hypoglycemia. The younger child usually requires 3 meals and 3 snacks, while the older child responds well to a 3-meal, 2-snack schedule, more characteristic of the eating habits of American children.

Exercise and Physical Fitness

The place of physical fitness in diabetic therapy is attracting increasing attention in both the clinical and research areas. The highly fit organism is a more efficient metabolic machine. In general, insulin requirements are lower and metabolic variations are closer to normal in the physically fit diabetic. Whether this prevents or minimizes cardiovascular complications remains to be determined. We strongly urge our children and adolescent patients to exercise daily, and we endorse their participation in competitive athletics.

EMOTIONAL ADJUSTMENT

Serious psychological disturbances are common in the child with diabetes, particularly during adolescence. Why does this occur? Chronic illness of any sort increases family stress and the likelihood of psychological maladjustment. Many examples from the pediatric experience can be cited: leukemia, nephrosis, congenital heart disease, asthma, rheumatoid arthritis, and others have been associated with emotional disability. It is my opinion that insulin-dependent diabetes carries with it very special psychological hazards for both the patient and family. We expect that our patients by age 10 years, if not earlier, will carry out chemical analysis multiple times daily on urine specimens, on which life-sustaining medical judgments will be made. Indeed, we not only expect these children to make these judgments, but to actually administer the necessary medication by injection. Food, a source of pleasure for all of us, takes on special meaning with restrictions and limitations. A reward and punishment system, utilizing food, invariably becomes entangled in daily management decisions. Not the least of our problems is the fact that we do not have an effective, reliable technique for ascertaining the success of therapy. The children are very aware of this. Most of them are also aware that there is considerable confusion and controversy among the "diabetic experts" as to the best mode of therapy. The child with diabetes learns early that he has a power tool which he can use as either a crutch or weapon to manipulate his environment. Is it any wonder that problems follow?

CONCLUSIONS

The child with diabetes presents a special challenge. Optimal therapy requires a team approach to the entire family. The variables of growth and maturation, changing nutritional requirements, the metabolic alterations of emotional stress and intercurrent infections, and the ever-present concerns of impending vascular complications require a skillful, patient, and attentive physician. The rewards of assisting a child with diabetes through the vicissitudes of adolescence and placing him on the road to a meaningful adult life in a state of good health are well worth the effort.

References

1. Drash AL and Becker D: Diabetes mellitus in the child: course, special problems and related disorders. *In* Diabetes, Obesity, and Vascular Disease, Chapter 18, Katzen, HM and Hahlen RJ, (eds), New York. Hemisphere Publishing Corporation, 1978
2. Drash AL: The etiology of insulin deficiency diabetes mellitus. N Engl J of Med 300:1211–13, 1979
3. Craig O: Childhood diabetes and its management. Postgraduate Pediatrics Series. Apley J (ed), Butterworths, 1977
4. Traisman HS: Management of juvenile diabetes mellitus. St. Louis, CV Mosby Co, 1971
5. Sandler R and Sandler M: Daily Management of Youth-Onset Diabetes Mellitus: An Integrated Guide for Patients and Physicians. Pub by Charles C Thomas, Springfield, 1977

19

Management of Diabetes and Pregnancy

Jay S. Skyler, M.D.
Daniel H. Mintz, M.D.
Mary Jo O'Sullivan, M.D.

INTRODUCTION

The management of pregnancy complicated by diabetes mellitus provides the physician and patient an unparalleled opportunity in terms of both immediate impact and overall therapeutic dimension. The immediate survival of the mother can be assured and that of the unborn child brought close to that of the child of the nondiabetic gravida. Further, such relatively remote events as intellectual and psychological performance in offspring from these pregnancies may be jeopardized by inadequate attention to details of medical management during pregnancy. Finally, an opportunity is presented to both physician and patient to influence beneficially future diabetes therapy. The intense motivation of the mother, together with her positive experiences, can be channeled to promote an enduring attitudinal and behavioral approach to future diabetes care.

A number of factors can be cited as having importance in lessening the impact of diabetes during pregnancy in terms of fetal and neonatal morbidity and mortality. Three critical variables are: (1) control of maternal glycemia; (2) perinatal obstetrical care; (3) neonatal intensive care. The first two, which relate to management of the diabetic pregnant woman, will be addressed in this chapter. Our current management scheme will be reviewed both for diabetes mellitus antedating pregnancy (pregestational diabetes) and gestational-onset diabetes mellitus. Selected references are provided for the interested reader, to serve as an entry into the extensive literature on this subject, for both a broader basis of understanding current notions about therapy and to help gain further insights into the controversies that still remain.

RATIONALE FOR CONTROL OF MATERNAL GLYCEMIA

Control of maternal gylcemia is the most important factor influencing fetal outcome. Fetal glucose levels are a direct function of maternal glucose levels, since glucose is transported across the placenta to the conceptus by facilitated diffusion. When maternal diabetes mellitus is not well regulated and hyperglycemia is present, the fetus will be exposed to either sustained or meal-related intermittent waves of hyperglycemia. As a consequence, albeit by mechanisms that remain unresolved, the fetal pancreatic beta cell adapts to this setting by developing a linkage between its glucose sensors and the insulin-secretory mechanism. The result is prematurely induced and inappropriately sustained or intermittent fetal hyperinsulinemia that parallels the prevailing blood glucose in the mother and fetus. Many of the physical and morbid complications experienced by infants of mothers with diabetes mellitus can be attributed to fetal hyperglycemia and hyperinsulinemia. Thus, fetal hyperinsulinemia can result in increased fetal body fat (macrosomia), accounting for the cherubic appearance of those infants at birth and possibly complicating vaginal delivery due to dystocia. Fetal hyperinsulinemia may also inhibit the pulmonary maturation processes required for surfactant production, and contribute, by this mechanism, to the increased incidence of respiratory distress syndrome experienced by these neonates. Additionally, a persistence of enhanced responsivity of the fetal beta cell into neonatal life also contributes to the propensity for the development of neonatal hypoglycemia once the fetus is removed from a constantly delivered maternal source of glucose.

Unstable maternal glucose levels may be associated with the sudden and unexpected intrauterine deaths characteristic of diabetes in pregnancy. Ketoacidosis, in particular, has been associated with intrauterine demise. In addition, it has been suggested that preconceptional and early pregnancy maternal hyperglycemia, during early embryogenesis, may contribute to the increased rate of congenital malformations encountered in the offspring of diabetic women. Finally, maternal ketonuria has been associated with significant lowering of intelligence quotient (IQ) and the occurrence of neuropsychiatric deficits in offspring, particularly if the ketonuria is manifested during the third trimester.

The standards of assessment of diabetic control during pregnancy should be the plasma glucose values found in nondiabetic pregnant women. Pregnancy is normally associated with a significant progressive lowering of fasting plasma glucose from a mean of 73 ± 9 mg/dl, in early pregnancy, to a mean of 65 ± 9 mg/dl near term. Diurnal plasma glucose values in nondiabetic women rarely exceed 100 mg/dl, except in the first hour postprandially. Mean diurnal plasma glucose normally is 82 ± 5 mg/dl in early pregnancy and 85 ± 5 mg/dl in late pregnancy. Maximum diurnal plasma glucose in nondiabetic early pregnancy is 107 ± 10 mg/dl and in late pregnancy is 114 ± 8 mg/dl. The range of plasma glucose excursions normally is 37 ± 8 mg/dl in early pregnancy and 46 ± 7 mg/dl in late pregnancy. Thus, our goals for gylcemic control in diabetic women during pregnancy are: fasting plasma glucose, 60–90 mg/dl; preprandial plasma glucose less than 105 mg/dl; and postprandial plasma glucose less than 120 mg/dl.

CLASSIFICATION AND DIAGNOSIS

White's clinical classification of diabetes in pregnancy (Table 19-1) is based primarily in the patient's condition prior to pregnancy, particularly the duration of diabetes and the presence of vascular disease. It is useful for risk assessment and for comparison of data between groups. Also useful for risk assessment in terms of fetal jeopardy are Pedersen's prognostic bad signs of pregnancy (PBSP, Table 19-2). In Pedersen's series, higher mortality was encountered if PBSP were present in each of White's classes except F.

Table 19-1. White's Classification of Diabetes in Pregnancy.

Class A:	Glucose Tolerance Test abnormal. No symptoms. Euglycemia maintained with treatment by appropriate diet, but without insulin; any duration or onset of age.
Class B:	Adult onset (age 20 or older) *and* short duration (less than 10 years).
Class C:	Relatively young onset (age 10–19) *or* relatively long duration (10–19 years).
Class D:	Very young onset (age less than 10) *or* very long duration (20 years or more), *or* evidence of minimal vascular disease (e.g., background retinopathy), *or* hypertension (not preeclampsia).
Class E:	Pelvic vascular disease (by x-ray).
Flass F:	Renal disease (with over 500 mg/day proteinuria).
Class R:	Proliferative retinopathy.
Class RF:	Both renal disease and proliferative retinopathy.
Glass G:	Women with multiple failures in pregnancy. (This class is used in conjunction with one of the other classes, e.g., CG, RG, etc.).
Class H:	Arteriosclerotic heart disease.
Class T:	Pregnancy after renal transplantation.

Table 19-2. Prognostically Bad Signs During Pregnancy (PBSP).

1. *Clinical Pyelonephritis*
   Urinary tract infection (culture positive) with acute temperature elevation exceeding 39°C.

2. *Precoma or Severe Acidosis*
   Precoma: diabetic acidosis with venous bicarbonate below 10 mEq/1.

   Severe acidosis: venous bicarbonate 10–17 mEq/1.

3. *Pregnancy-induced Hypertension* (Toxemia)

4 *Neglectors*
   Pregnant diabetic women who are in labor when first admitted or who are psychopathic or of low intelligence; or women in poor social circumstances who present themselves less than 60 days before term.

   With the exception of class H patients, where pregnancy
threatens maternal survival and thus indicates that pregnancy
should be avoided, the White classification is obsolete in terms
of management of maternal glycemia and the pregnancy itself. In
the other White classes, maternal mortality has been virtually
excluded with current treatment programs, and vigilant fetal
monitoring is necessary in all classes. From the standpoint of
glycemic management, we have found the scheme outlined in
Table 19-3 to be useful. The categorization is based primarily on
the lability of glycemia, which influences both the insulin regimen used and the mode of monitoring of therapy. Patients with
labile, pregestational insulin-dependent diabetes mellitus form
one category. A second category includes patients with stable,
pregestational noninsulin-dependent diabetes mellitus *and* patients with gestational-onset diabetes mellitus.

   Gestational-onset diabetes is diagnosed by oral glucose tolerance test according to the criteria of O'Sullivan and Mahan,
which were recently endorsed by the National Diabetes Data
Group. These are summarized in Table 19-4. Because even mild
decompensation of carbohydrate tolerance is associated with in-

Table 19-3. Classification of Diabetes in Pregnancy Based on Glycemic Management.

	Pregestational Diabetes Mellitus		Gestational-Onset Diabetes Mellitus		
	Insulin-Dependent	Noninsulin-Dependent	Fasting PG <105	Fasting PG 105–120	Fasting PG >120
Usual pattern of glycemia	Labile	Stable	Stable	Stable	Stable or labile
Insulin therapy	Multiple component	Single or multiple component	Some may be con-trolled with diet alone	Single or multiple component	Multiple component
Blood glucose monitoring	Daily	Weekly	Weekly	Weekly	Weekly or Daily

Table 19-4. Criteria for Diagnosis of Gestational-Onset Diabetes Mellitus.

	Two or more of the following values after a 100 gm oral glucose challenge must be met or exceeded:	
	Plasma	Whole blood
Fasting	105 mg/dl	90 mg/dl
One-Hour	190 mg/dl	170 mg/dl
Two-Hour	165 mg/dl	145 mg/dl
Three-Hour	145 mg/dl	125 mg/dl

creased perinatal mortality, it is desirable to detect such abnormalities whenever present. A still unresolved question is whether to survey all pregnant women or only those thought to be at increased risk of developing gestational-onset diabetes. The latter group is defined by having the presence of any of the following screening criteria: a family history of diabetes; the presence of obesity, hypertension, or hydramnios; multiparity; maternal age over 35; glycosuria; and a past obstetric history including unexplained perinatal mortality, recurrent prematurity or abortion, macrosomia, or congenital anomalies.

DIETARY MANAGEMENT

Weight Gain: Current recommendations are for weight gain during pregnancy of 10 to 12 kg (22 to 26 1/2 pounds), distributed in an appropriate pattern, i.e., 1 to 2 kg during the first trimester, and a progressive, linear rate of weight gain of approximately 350 to 400 grams per week throughout the second and third trimesters. This degree of weight gain will insure the adequacy of nutrition to both mother and fetus. The presence of diabetes should not influence the projection of weight gain in any way. Likewise, the presence of obesity should not influence the degree of weight gain during pregnancy, although excessive gain is firmly discouraged.

Nutrient Needs: Caloric requirement is dependent on maternal age, activity, height, prepregnancy weight, and stage of pregnancy. An increment of about 300 kcal per day above basal requirements, or a total of 36 to 50 kcal per kg ideal body weight, should provide calories sufficient to meet the nutritional needs of pregnancy. At least 45 percent of calories should be in the form of carbohydrate, including no less than 200 grams, and approximately 50 gm per day above nonpregnancy needs. Adequate protein intake is essential because of the special requirements in pregnancy to synthesize new tissue in great abundance. Thus, 30 gm of protein per day are prescribed to supplement the usual nonpregnant allowance. In a mature woman, 1.3 gm per kg of body weight will meet this requirement. Higher intakes (1.5–1.7 gm/kg body weight) are recommended for adolescent pregnancies. The remainder of the calories are provided as fat. Other nutrient requirements include: iron, 18 mg per day; folic acid, 800 μg per day; calcium, 1200 mg per day. Sodium restriction generally should be avoided.

Meal Planning: The goal of meal planning is to limit the extent of hyperglycemia and to minimize hypoglycemia, while providing nutrients in a pattern throughout the day in an attempt to coincide with the time course of action of exogenously administered insulin. The importance of regular meals and snacks must be emphasized. A bedtime snack is essential and should include both 25 gm carbohydrate and some protein. This will help avert both overnight hypoglycemia and starvation ketosis. Some women will need two evening snacks, if there is a long interval between supper and bedtime. In addition, if morning ketosis develops despite the bedtime snack described, an additional 3:00 a.m. snack may sometimes be required. Rapidly absorbed, concentrated simple carbohydrate should be avoided from regular meal planning in order to minimize hyperglycemic excursions. The Exchange Lists for Meal Planning facilitate the development of a meal plan with consistency and regularity of nutrient consumption.

INSULIN THERAPY

Labile, Pregestational Insulin-Dependent Diabetes Mellitus: In order to achieve adequate glycemic control in labile, pregestational insulin-dependent diabetic patients, insulin must be provided in a regimen with multiple components of insulin action, each having a peak at a different time of the day. A number of multiple component regimens have been used (Table 19-5). The regimen most commonly used in the past has been the split-and-mixed regimen (number 1 in Table 19-5), so designated because it both splits the insulin into two doses (one in the morning before breakfast and the other in the evening before supper) and mixes short-acting insulin (e.g., regular) and intermediate-acting insulin (e.g., NPH or Lente) in each injection. As a guideline, initial daily dosage during pregnancy approximates 0.7 units per kg ideal body weight, distributed as two-thirds of the total daily dose in the morning (divided as one part short-acting insulin to two parts intermediate-acting insulin) and one-third of the total daily dose in the evening (divided in equal parts between short-acting and intermediate-acting insulin). Each component of the insulin regimen is then titrated to achieve glycemic control as close as possible to the goals stated earlier. In most women, better results may be obtained if the evening intermediate-acting insulin is delayed until 10:00 p.m., as per regimen number 2 in Table 19-5.

Through daily home blood glucose monitoring, it is possible to attain our glycemic goals in the majority of women. Such monitoring entails daily determinations of four blood glucose levels—fasting, prelunch, presupper, and bedtime. In addition, at least twice weekly, patients obtain at least three additional samples two hours postprandial breakfast, lunch, and supper. Blood glucose determinations are made with the Ames Dextrostix/Eyetone method or the Biodynamics Stat-Tek method. Both methods utilize reagent strips impregnated with glucose oxidase to determine true blood glucose in a drop of

Table 19-5. Multiple Component Insulin Regimens.

	AC Breakfast	AC Lunch	AC Supper	Bedtime
1.	REG/NPH		REG/NPH	
2.	REG/NPH		REG	NPH
3.	REG/NPH	REG	REG/NPH	
4.	REG	REG	REG/NPH	
5.	REG	REG	REG	REG
6.	REG	REG	REG	NPH

capillary blood obtained by fingerstick. The colorimetric change on the reagent strip is quantitated with an electronic device. Accuracy can be maintained within 10 to 15 percent if careful attention is paid to proper technique. Initially, patients maintain daily telephone contact with the professional staff (physicians and diabetes nurse specialists) of the Diabetes Unit, who, together with the patient, make appropriate adjustments in insulin dosage to achieve euglycemia. As the patient becomes more familiar with the adjustment program, an algorithm for insulin dose alterations is developed and telephone contacts with the professional staff can be less frequent. Weekly, the patient is seen in the Diabetes Unit for full evaluation of diabetes regulation, review of progress, and discussion of any questions that have risen. An example of the glycemic regulation that can be achieved with this approach is shown in Figure 19-1.

Stable, Noninsulin-Dependent Diabetes Mellitus: Glycemic control in pregnant women with noninsulin-dependent diabetes mellitus and in most patients with gestational-onset diabetes generally shows much less day-to-day variability than that seen in the labile, pregestational diabetic woman. Thus, insulin regimens may be different, and there is not a need for daily blood glucose monitoring.

When commencing insulin therapy during pregnancy, we have attempted to use the least immunogenic insulin available, which is highly purified pork (single-component) and the Lente insulins in lieu of NPH. This is in the theoretical attempt to obviate excessive antibody production, since there is transfer of immunoglobulins across the placenta. If fasting plasma glucose is less than 120 mg/dl and postprandial excursions are not high, we have generally commenced insulin therapy with an evening injection of pork Lente insulin of approximately 0.3–0.4 units per kg ideal body weight in nonobese patients or 0.5–0.7 units per kg ideal body weight in obese patients. Often, if we attain control of fasting glycemia with such evening insulin, additional daytime insulin is unnecessary. Once fasting plasma glucose is less than 90 mg/dl, diurnal glycemic excursions are examined to determine if additional morning insulin (regular and/or Lente) or evening regular insulin is required, and these are added as necessary. If initial fasting plasma glucose is greater than 120 mg/dl or postprandial excursions are high (i.e., greater than 200 mg/dl),

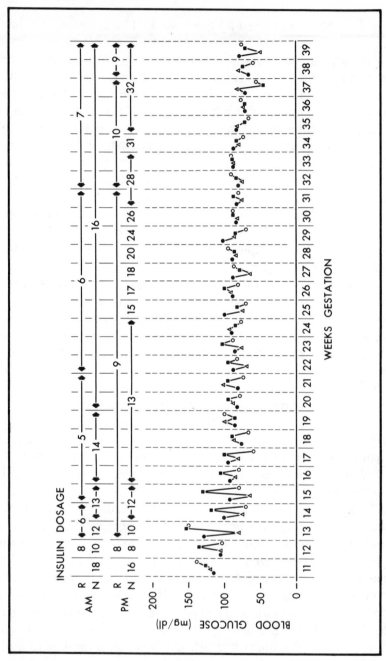

Figure 19-1. Summary of mean weekly preprandial and bedtime home blood glucose determinations for a 21-year-old pregnant woman with Class C diabetes. She monitored her home blood glucose from the eleventh week of gestation until term. Average morning and evening insulin dosage is listed at the top of the figure. Closed circles represent mean fasting blood glucose for each week. Triangles represent mean prelunch blood glucose for each week. Squares depict mean presupper blood glucose for each week. Open circles depict mean bedtime blood glucose for each week. Each symbol represents 4–7 determinations. There was no significant hypoglycemia throughout the course.

the patient is initiated on a multiple component insulin regimen, as done for women with pregestational insulin-dependent diabetes.

Unless glycemic control is labile, once it is attained weekly blood glucose determinations (at home or at a laboratory) are generally adequate for monitoring, although daily fasting determinations (at home) may be considered desirable. Patients with stable glycemia are seen every two weeks during the first half of pregnancy and weekly thereafter. Target glucoses remain fasting 60–90 mg/dl, preprandial less than 105 mg/dl, postprandial less than 120 mg/dl.

All women continue to monitor their urine for glucose and ketones. Glucose is determined by a specific glucose oxidase method (e.g., Diastix), and glycosuria is generally not seen. Its presence indicates that diurnal glycemic patterns should be further assessed. Urine ketones, particularly fasting, are determined to indicate potential starvation ketosis and to help detect potential unrecognized nocturnal hypoglycemia.

ANTEPARTUM FETAL MONITORING

Ultrasonography provides valuable and reliable information concerning fetal maturity, growth, and size. Between six and twelve weeks' gestation, crown-rump length is exponential, and variation from week to week is within narrow limits. Between thirteen and twenty weeks' gestation, ultrasonic measurement of fetal biparietal diameter may be used as a reasonably accurate measure of gestational age. An objective early determination of gestational age is vital in the event that a decision is necessary about early elective delivery prior to term. Serial ultrasonography subsequently provides valuable information concerning the rate of fetal growth, since growth pattern deviations—both macrosomia and intrauterine growth retardation—may complicate diabetic pregnancies. The development of macrosomia is indicative of inadequate control of maternal hyperglycemia. The detection of a reduced rate of fetal growth is indicative of placental insufficiency and forecasts the need for specialized techniques and procedures required for the management of fetuses at high risk. Differential serial ultrasonography is useful for the demonstration of disparity in growth of tissues, with an increase in abdominal circumference being an early feature of macrosomia. Monthly serial ultrasonography, therefore, provides a powerful noninvasive tool for antepartum fetal monitoring and can be accomplished on an outpatient basis. Adequate interpretation is dependent on an experienced ultrasonographer.

Urinary Estriol: The most widely used and frequently abused test of fetoplacental function is the 24-hour urinary excretion of estriol. The clinical value of estriol determinations remains controversial. Variations in urinary excretion should be corrected by calculating an estriol/creatinine ratio. A rising estriol/creatinine ratio is indicative of fetal well-being. Fetal compromise must be suspected if there is a significant fall in estriol excretion (greater than 35 percent drop) or if estriol levels consistently fall two standard deviations below the mean for diabetic pregnant women. Since day-to-day variability in estriol excretion may be substantial, a fall in estriol excretion requires comparison with the antecedent stable excretion in the individual patient. To establish a baseline, twice-weekly or thrice-weekly estriol determinations may be commenced between 30 and 32 weeks' gestation, with daily estriols begun around 35 weeks' gestation. Daily determinations are necessary if the test is to have maximum value. They should be performed in a reliable laboratory with rapid turn-around time. In women with renal disease (class F or RF), unconjugated plasma estriol levels might be more reliable, since they are not influenced by alterations in maternal renal function.

Cardiography: Antepartum fetal heart rate monitoring enjoys wide acceptance as a noninvasive procedure to rapidly assess the respiratory functional reserve of the placenta. Uterine contractions can transiently interfere with uteroplacental blood flow and represent a transient ischemic challenge to the fetus. If there is associated compromise of uteroplacental blood flow or placental dysfunction, transient fetal hypoxia may result in an alteration of fetal heart rate. Two approaches are used. One is the contraction stress test (CST) or oxytocin challenge test (OCT) in which uterine contractions are induced by intravenous oxytocin infusion. The other approach is that of nonstress testing (NST) which is more easily performed, involving monitoring during spontaneous fetal movements and spontaneous uterine contractions.

A negative CST is a reassuring prognostic signal that the fetus is not in imminent jeopardy. A positive CST consists of delayed deceleration of the fetal heart rate following uterine contractions. Other indices of fetal hypoxia are absence of beat-to-beat variability, absence of acceleration with fetal movement, or persistent tachycardia. A reactive NST is indicative of fetal well-being and allows pregnancy to continue, and is indicated by acceleration of 15 beats per minute for 10–15 seconds, induced by fetal movement. A nonreactive NST is one in which there is no increase of fetal heart rate with activity or an absence of fetal activity. There may be associated late decelerations with spontaneous uterine activity. An undulating heart rate or sinusoidal pattern is a questionably ominous sign. It has been associated with high fetal morbidity and mortality in severely Rh-sensitized pregnancies.

A negative CST should be followed by repeated assessment on a weekly basis. A reactive NST appears to be predictive of good fetal condition for one week. These tests may be accomplished as an outpatient. Long-term experience with NST in diabetes is not as extensive as with CST, however. Therefore, a nonreactive NST should be confirmed by a CST. A negative CST is reassuring of good fetal condition. A positive CST serves as a catalyst for hospitalization and further action, including review of the estriol excretion pattern and assessment of fetal lung maturation (vide infra) with a view towards potential early delivery. If urinary estriol levels are low in the presence of a positive CST, pregnancy probably should be terminated. If urinary estriols are good, in the presence of a positive CST, delivery should only be considered if there is fetal lung maturation. Consideration might be given to inducing lung maturation with steroids. However, careful evaluation of diabetic status will be essential, as disturbance of carbohydrate metabolism could be even more detrimental to the fetus. In the absence of fetal lung maturation, careful monitoring should be continued.

Fetal Lung Maturation: The measurement of amniotic fluid phospholipids is a valuable tool in the assessment of fetal lung maturation. The lecithin/sphingomyelin (L/S) ratio has been the most widely used test, since the maturation process is associated with increase in amniotic fluid lecithin, phosphatidylinositol, and phosphatidylglycerol. The importance of assessing fetal lung maturation is related to the fact that respiratory distress syndrome (RDS) and hyaline membrane disease, prominent causes of neonatal morbidity and mortality, are related to inadequate surfactant production, an ultimate product of maturation of the fetal lung. A mature L/S ratio is indicative of minimal risk of RDS. In infants of a nondiabetic population, an L/S ratio of 2.0 is indicative of maturity. This probably holds true for diabetic pregnancies as well, although some authors have suggested that a ratio of 2.5 be used. The presence of phosphotidylglycerol appears to be the most reassuring indicator of fetal lung maturation. The shake test has also been used as an index of fetal lung maturation. It appears to be associated with few false-positive results.

LABOR AND DELIVERY

Our goal is for spontaneous labor at term and vaginal delivery. With careful control of maternal hyperglycemia and the documentation of euglycemia, coupled with careful continued weekly antepartum fetal monitoring, the need for early induction is virtually obviated. Nevertheless, hospital admission may be desirable for mothers in classes B, C, D, F, and R, and in class A, at term. If euglycemia cannot be documented, and/or fetal monitoring either cannot be accomplished or is aberrant, early admission and consideration of preterm delivery is necessary.

Fetal Monitoring in Labor: Intrapartum fetal cardiotachometry and fetal blood sampling (by scalp vein) provide useful indices of surveillance of the fetus during this vulnerable period. There are good correlations among innocuous cardiotachometric patterns, minimal alteration in pH, and good fetal outcome. Interruption of placental function causes asphyxia revealed by a rising $_pCO_2$, and a falling pH, $_pO_2$ and base excess.

Glycemic Management During Labor and Delivery: Our approach to glycemic control during labor and delivery is to provide simultaneous continuous infusions of glucose and insulin (Figure 19-2). Glucose infusion rate is 300 mg/kg/hour as 5 or 10 percent dextrose in water. This rate provides adequate substrate

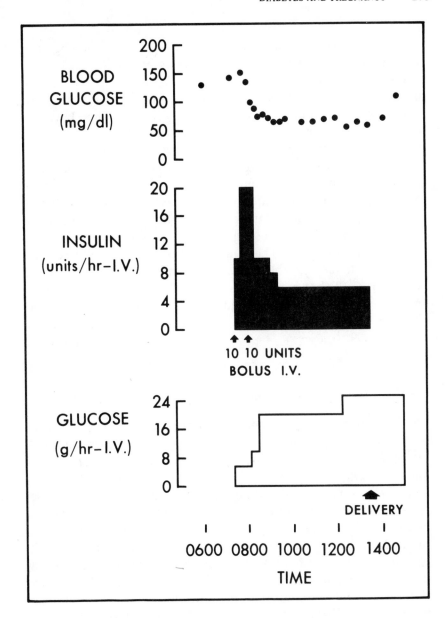

Figure 19-2. Record of insulin and glucose infusion rates and blood glucose responses during labor and delivery, for the patient described in Figure 19-1. Patient was admitted to the hospital after commencement of spontaneous labor. Vaginal delivery was accomplished.

for the energy requirements of labor. Insulin infusion rate is initiated at 0.06–0.07 units per kg per hour, after a loading dose of 0.1 units per kg is given by intravenous bolus. Rate of insulin delivery is carefully regulated by an infusion pump. This is adjusted on the basis of blood glucose determinations carried out half-hourly on samples obtained through an indwelling butterfly needle with heparin lock and bedside glucose analyzer. This often is the very machine the patient has used for home blood glucose monitoring during gestation. Our goal is maintenance of blood glucose between 60 and 100 mg/dl. With the delivery of the placenta, insulin infusion is discontinued in order to obviate maternal hypoglycemia during the postpartum period of exquisite sensitivity to insulin, a consequence of removal of placental counterinsulin factors. The glucose infusion is maintained until there is evidence of stable or rising blood glucose (usually one to two hours). At that point, glucose infusion is also discontinued. Insulin therapy is then withheld until significant hyperglycemia (greater than 200–250 mg/dl) reappears or three days have elapsed.

CONCLUSIONS

The management of pregnancy in patients with diabetes requires a specialized team of an obstetrician specializing in high-risk pregnancy, a diabetologist, and a neonatologist. This team should be experienced in the frequent management of pregnancy in diabetic women, and should be supported by modern laboratory and inpatient facilities and a well-equipped and well-staffed intensive care nursery. With meticulous monitoring and control of maternal hyperglycemia and careful antepartum and intrapartum surveillance of fetal well-being, fetal mortality and morbidity can approach that seen in nondiabetic women. The prevention of congenital malformations and other long-term complications in the offspring will require both better understanding of the nature of their development and carefully planned pregnancies with meticulous control achieved prior to conception so that euglycemia can be accomplished during early embryogenesis.

Finally, although the prospects for successful pregnancy in diabetic women have never been brighter, the management of

such women poses a continuing challenge and requires persistent vigilance by both the patient and the management team.

References

1. Ciba Foundation Symposium 63. Pregnancy Metabolism, Diabetes and the
   Fetus. Amsterdam, Excerpta Medica, 1979
2. Gabbe SG, Mertman JH, Freeman RK, et al: Management and outcome of
   pregnancy in diabetes mellitus, Classes B to R. American Journal of
   Obstetrics and Gynecology 129:723–732, 1977
3. Gugliucci CL, O'Sullivan MJ, Opperman W, et al: Intensive care of the
   pregnant diabetic. American Journal of Obstetrics and Gynecology
   125:435–441, 1976
4. Jovanovic L, Peterson CM, Saxena BB, et al: Feasibility of maintaining
   euglycemia in insulin dependent pregnant women. American Journal of
   Medicine, 68:105–112, 1980
5. Karlsson K, Kjellmer I: The outcome of diabetic pregnancies in relation to
   the mother's blood sugar level. American Journal of Obstetrics and
   Gynecology 112:213–220, 1972
6. Merkatz IR, Adam PAJ (eds): Diabetes in pregnancy. Seminars in
   Perinatology 2:287–339, 1978
7. Mintz DH, Skyler JS, Chez RA: Diabetes and pregnancy. Diabetes Care
   1:49–63, 1978
8. Pedersen J: The Pregnant Diabetic and Her Newborn. Second Edition.
   Baltimore, Williams and Wilkins, 1977
9. Skyler JS, O'Sullivan MJ, Robertson EG, et al: Blood glucose control
   during pregnancy. Diabetes Care 3:69–76, 1980
10. Sutherland HW, Stowers JM (eds): Carbohydrate Metabolism in Preg-
    nancy and the Newborn. Berlin, Springer, 1979
11. Tyson JE, Hock RA: Gestational and pregestational diabetes: an approach
    to therapy. American Journal of Obstetrics and Gynecology 125:1009–
    1027, 1976

20

The Infant of the Diabetic Mother

Richard K. Raker, M.D.
Lawrence M. Gartner, M.D.

INTRODUCTION

Perinatal morbidity is significantly increased in pregnancies complicated by diabetes mellitus. The frequency of intrauterine death, fetal congenital malformations, and neonatal morbidity and mortality is related to the duration, severity, and mode of management of maternal diabetes. Despite intensive recent advances, we are perhaps only slightly beyond the situation prevailing twenty years ago when Farquhar remarked that the "changes which characterized the infant of the diabetic mother (IDM) resulted from intrauterine indiscretions of which we know nothing."[1] The profound influence that maternal diabetes has on the growing fetus has been only partially explained by hormonal and metabolic changes occurring during gestation.

METABOLIC STATE

Pregnancy has been described as a metabolic state analogous to semistarvation. Maternal energy substrates: free fatty acids, triglycerides, and ketone bodies are elevated several fold, mediated by human somatomammotrophin (HCG).[2] Fetal glucose supply is maintained in part by the anti-insulin effect of HCG. Progesterone and adrenal, ovarian, and placental steroids further support fetal glucose needs. Thus, insulin "resistance" and carbohydrate "intolerance" stress overt diabetes and ultimately reveal latent or chemical diabetes (gestational).

IDENTIFICATION OF THE DIABETIC

Attempts have been made to correlate the severity of diabetes with fetal outcome. White emphasized that early age of onset, prolonged duration, and severity of angiopathy worsened perinatal outcome.[3] Pedersen showed perinatal morbidity increased when the diabetic pregnancy was complicated by pyelonephritis, acidosis, toxemia, and/or medical neglect.[4] Fetal wastage, macrosomia, and respiratory distress syndrome are reduced by early identification of diabetes, antenatal fetal surveillance, and rigid control of maternal blood sugar.[5]

The gestational diabetic is identified by screening for a family history of diabetes mellitus, obesity, previous neonate with birth weight over 4,000 grams, unexplained stillbirths, neonatal deaths, and congenital malformations.[6] Since glycosuria in pregnancy is not a reliable sign of hyperglycemia, O'Sullivan recommends a one-hour oral glucose tolerance test as an initial screen. If the plasma glucose level exceeds 130 mg percent, a three-hour tolerance test is then performed.[6] These tests may be repeated during the second and third trimesters, if originally negative when a high suspicion of diabetes persists. Recently, HbA_{1c}-glycohemoglobin has been recognized as marker of chronic hyperglycemia.

FETAL HEALTH

Fetal well-being is assessed by fetal ultrasonography at midtrimester for documentation of age and by estriol determination after the 30th week for fetal-placental function. Antepartum electronic fetal monitoring by either nonstress or oxytocin stimulation techniques is employed during the third trimester.

The timing and mode of delivery are individualized with particular attention placed on documentation of fetal lung maturity and avoidance of fetal stress. The well-controlled *gestational* diabetic is allowed to await onset of labor. Patients requiring predelivery hospitalization for control of unstable diabetes should have weekly amniocentesis for evaluation of fetal lung maturity (lecithin/sphingomyelin; L/S ratio) starting at 36 weeks or earlier if there is hypertension, poor obstetric history, or fetal instability. An L/S ratio 2 or > in a *non*diabetic pregnancy indicates fetal lung maturity, in which case neonatal respiratory distress syndrome (RDS; hyaline membrane disease) is very unlikely to develop. In the diabetic, however, a "mature" L/S ratio may still indicate a risk for RDS. Judgments must balance risk for fetal demise against risk for neonatal morbidity and mortality, along with maternal risks in determining time of delivery.

Perinatal mortality, fetal macrosomia, and neonatal hypoglycemia are significantly reduced when maternal mean blood sugar concentration is maintained below 100mg/dl throughout pregnancy.[7] Rigid dietary control, insulin utilization, early and liberal hospitalization, and maternal education have all demonstrated beneficial effects on blood sugar stability.[5] Pedersen hypothesized that the pathophysiological changes seen in the IDM, such as macrosomia and hypoglycoma, were explained by maternal hyperglycemia, producing fetal hyperglycemia, which, in turn, induces fetal hyperinsulinemia.[8] Glucose crosses the placenta by the process of facilitated diffusion.[9] There is pathologic evidence of this mechanism seen as hypertrophy and hyperplasia of the islets of Langerhans and β-cells of the fetal pancreas. Insulin content of pancreas is elevated.[10] Insulin has profound fetal growth-promoting effects,[11] with length, body, and visceral weight at least 20 percent greater in the IDM than in gestational-age controls.[8] Naeye demonstrated that both cellular hyperplasia and hypertrophy were responsible for organ enlargement.[12] Infants born to mothers with vascular disease (White's classification DRF) are growth retarded, however, as a result of fetal malnutrition. Normosomia is ideal and should be strived for through use of "tight control" of blood glucose concentrations.[5]

NEONATAL HEALTH

A common problem in the IDM is early postnatal hypoglycemia. Although there has not been a strong association between cord blood insulin levels and neonatal hypoglycemia, neonatal plasma insulin levels are higher and glucose removal increased in IDMs. Neonatal hypoglycemia (blood glucose levels less than 30mg/dl in any infant regardless of birth weight or gestational age) occurs in 20–30 percent of IDMs. Most hypoglycemic IDMs are asymptomatic, but may display a wide range of symptoms, such as tremors, irritability, convulsions, hypothermia, poor feeding, tachypnea, congestive heart failure, apnea, cyanosis, and limpness. Hypoglycemia should be anticipated during the first 12 hours of life and blood glucose determined at birth and every 4 hours thereafter for the first 48 hours of life.

Oral feedings of 5 percent or 10 percent glucose solution should be started within 4 to 6 hours of birth in healthy infants, and gavage or intravenous 10 percent dextrose in sick or low-birth-weight infants. Human milk or prepared formula feedings should be started by 8 hours of age in otherwise healthy infants.

RDS is a major cause of neonatal mortality and morbidity in the IDM. Although the incidence of RDS in IDM has been reported as high as 37 percent,[13] more recent incidences may be much lower because of the current practice of extending pregnancy until the fetal lung is mature. The unreliability of the L/S ratio of 2 as an indication of fetal lung maturity in the IDM has been noted. Recently, Gluck[14] has demonstrated that fetuses of gestational diabetics differ from those of other classes of diabetes and of normals. The appearance of phosphatidyl glycerol (PG) is delayed while phosphatidyl inositol (PI) persists. In those pregnancies where PG was found in amniotic fluid, RDS did not occur, presumably because PG is the *effective pulmonary surfactant*. While the L/S ratio is adequate for most uncomplicated pregnancies, the more detailed lung profile,[14] including L/S ratio, percentage of disaturated acetone precipitated lecithin, percentage of PG and percentage of PI should be performed for absolute determination of fetal lung maturity in the diabetic pregnancy. Neonatal pulmonary complications are related to diabetic class, length of gestation, the route of delivery, and duration of rupture of membranes. Criteria for diagnosis of RDS and its differentiation from transient tachypnea of the newborn, also common in the IDM, should be familiar to the staff caring for the infant. If sophisticated neonatal care is not available, transfer of the mother to a level III perinatal center is indicated.

Congenital anomalies, including neural-vertebral, cardiac, and caudal regression, are found in as many as 9 percent of IDM.[17] Although the etiology is unknown, metabolic derangements due to hypoglycemia, hyperglycemia, acidosis, hypoxia, and insulin treatment may affect embryogenesis.

Other manifestations of neonatal morbidity are common in IDM, although much less so in those born to gestational diabetics. Excessive hyperbilirubinemia (total bilirubin > 15mg/dl) and hypocalcemia (total calcium < 7.0mg/dl) may be noted as early as at 24 hours. Hyperbilirubinemia also tends to be prolonged, persisting is some cases for 3 to 4 weeks. Polycythemia (venous hematocrit 65 or greater during the first 4 hours of life) and associated hyperviscosity, poor feeding, cardiomegaly, renal vein thrombosis, and meconium plug syndrome often prolong the IDM's hospitalization.

Many factors are critical in the successful outcome of the diabetic pregnancy. Early diagnosis, prompt and careful maternal treatment, reliable estimation of fetal well-being, and evaluation of lung maturity improve perinatal mortality and morbidity. Individualization of delivery timing and route, early recognition of neonatal complications, and recent advances in neonatal care have dramatically reduced neonatal mortality for the IDM and improved the outlook for good health in childhood.

References

1. Farquhar JW: The child of the diabetic woman. Ar Dis Child 34:76–96, 1959
2. Bleicher SJ, O'Sullivan JB, and Freinkel N: Carbohydrate metabolism in pregnancy. V. The interrelations of glucose, insulin and free fatty acids in late pregnancy and postpartum. N Engl J Med 271:866–872, 1964
3. White P: Pregnancy complicating diabetes. Am J Med 7:609–616, 1949
4. Pedersen J and Pedersen LM: Prognosis of the outcome of pregnancies in diabetics. A new classification. Acta Endocrinol (Kdh) 50:70–78, 1965
5. Gyves MT, Rodman HM, Little AB, et al: A modern approach to management of pregnant diabetics: A two year analysis of perinatal outcomes. Am J Obstet Gynecol 128:606–616, 1977
6. O'Sullivan JB, Mahan CM, Charles D, et al: Screening criteria for high risk gestational diabetic patients. Am J Obstet Gynecol 116:895–900, 1973
7. Karlsson K and Kjellmer I: The outcome of diabetic pregnancies in relation to the mother's blood sugar level. Am J Obstet Gynecol 112:213–220, 1972

8. Osler M and Pedersen J: The body composition of newborn infants of diabetic mothers. Ped 26:985–992, 1960

9. Crawford JS: Maternal and cord blood at delivery. IV. Glucose, sodium, potassium, calcium and chloride. Biol Neonat 8:222–237, 1965

10. Steinke J and Driscoll SG: The extractable insulin content of pancreas from fetuses and infants of diabetic and control mothers. Diabetes 14:573–578, 1965

11. Susa JB, McCormick KL, Wildness JA, et al: Primary hyperinsulinemia in the rhesus monkey fetus. Effects on fetal growth and hepatic composition. Ped Res 13:482, 1979

12. Naeye RL: Infants of diabetic mothers: A quantitative morphologic study. Ped 35:980–988, 1963

13. Gellis S and Hsia O: The infant of the diabetic mother. Am J Dis Child 97:1–41, 1959

14. Kulovich MV and Gluck L: The lung profile. II. Complicated pregnancy. Am J Obstet Gynecol 135:64–70, 1979

15. Gabbe SG: Congenital malformations in infants of diabetic mothers. Obstet Gynecol Surv 32:125–132, 1977

21

Diabetic Ketoacidosis

J. Denis McGarry, Ph.D.
Daniel W. Foster, M.D.

DIABETES AND COMAS

The diabetic patient is vulnerable to three types of metabolic comas (the term "coma" is used loosely to mean a diabetic crisis with unconsciousness or an altered state of mental function):

1. Hypoglycemia
2. Diabetic ketoacidosis
3. Hyperosmolar, nonketotic coma

This discussion will concentrate on diabetic ketoacidosis, the complication expected when insulin-dependent (Type I) diabetes goes out of control. It should be recognized that patients with the insulin-dependent form of the disease ordinarily do not progress to the extreme hyperglycemia and dehydration that characterizes hyperosmolar coma because the nausea, vomiting, and acidosis of severe ketosis ordinarily exert their effects before there is time to develop major volume depletion. However, it is known that hyperosmolar, nonketotic coma can develop in a patient with Type I diabetes when enough insulin is available to block ketogenesis but not to prevent hyperglycemia.

PATHOPHYSIOLOGY OF DIABETIC KETOACIDOSIS

While the effects of uncontrolled diabetes are many, for practical purposes two should be emphasized:

1. Hyperglycemia—which leads to osmotic diuresis, volume depletion, and dehydration
2. Accelerated ketogenesis—which causes metabolic acidosis

Hyperglycemia and Its Effects

Hyperglycemia is due to accelerated glucose production by the liver (increased gluconeogenesis) coupled with diminished peripheral utilization, the consequence of insulin deficiency. In the absence of insulin, glucose acts osmotically across the plasma membrane, resulting in water shifts from the intracellular space into the ECF. As glycosuria worsens, an osmotic diuresis supervenes with shrinkage of the ECF volume; the loss of water is greater than the loss of electrolytes during diuresis, resulting in dehydration as well as volume depletion.

Ketogenesis

Considerable new information is now available regarding the mechanisms by which the liver overproduces acetoacetate and β-hydroxybutyrate during diabetic ketoacidosis. In order to fully activate the system, changes must occur in two hormones and two organ systems (Figure 21-1). The substrate for the ketone bodies is long-chain fatty acids delivered from adipose tissue stores. Accelerated lipolysis is initiated by a fall in circulating insulin levels. Mobilization of free fatty acids is not sufficient to cause ketosis, however. There must be a change in the biochemical makeup of the liver as well, such that fatty acids taken up are preferentially oxidized to ketones rather than entering the normal pathway of re-esterification and very low density lipoprotein formation. This biochemical change is induced by a rise in glucagon concentration (an increased glucagon:insulin ratio). Thus full-blown ketosis requires *both* an activation of the liver and

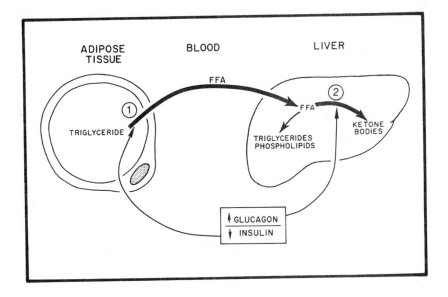

Figure 21-1. Bihormonal model for the regulation of ketogenesis. Site 1 represents the primary site of insulin action in the adipocyte, while site 2 indicates the locus of glucagon acyltransferase. (Reprinted from McGarry JD, Diabetes 28:517–523, 1979. By permission of the American Diabetes Association.)

increased delivery of free fatty acids to hepatic tissue. Once the liver is activated, the rate of ketone body production is determined solely by the rate at which fatty acids reach the oxidation site. (It is important to note that fasting also activates the liver for ketone formation because lack of food produces a fall in insulin and a rise in glucagon in the plasma. Fasting ketosis is mild because free fatty acids in plasma are low. If free fatty acids increase above the normal fasting level, as occurs in alcoholic ketoacidosis, simple starvation ketosis is converted into a severe metabolic acidosis equivalent to that of uncontrolled diabetes.)

The site of activation in the liver has now been identified. It is the enzyme called carnitine acyltransferase I (CAT I), which is located in the outer aspect of the inner mitochondrial membrane (Figure 21-2). Long chain fatty acids are immediately esterified to coenzyme A on arrival in the liver, but the CoA derivative cannot cross the mitochondrial membrane. For this to be accomplished, a transesterification with carnitine has to be carried out by CAT I. The carnitine ester then passes into the mitochon-

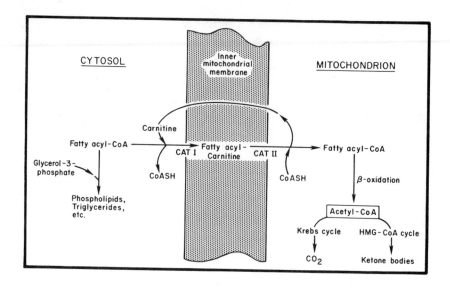

Figure 21-2. The mitochondrial fatty and transport system. CAT stands for carnitine acyltransferase. (Reprinted from McGarry JD, Diabetes 28:517–523, 1979.)

drion where the esterification reaction is reversed by CAT II. Once inside the mitochondrion, the fatty acid is oxidized almost exclusively to ketone bodies (only a small portion enters the Krebs cycle for CO_2 production).

Glucagon excess activates this system in two ways. *First,* it causes a marked increase in liver carnitine content, favoring the formation of fatty acylcarnitine esters. *Second,* it removes the inhibition of carnitine acyltransferase I that is present in the normal fed state when insulin levels are high and glucagon concentrations are low. It turns out that the physiological inhibitor of carnitine acyltransferase I is the compound malonyl-CoA, which is the first committed intermediate in the synthesis of fat from glucose (i.e., all other intermediates have alternative pathways of metabolism available, but malonyl-CoA can only be used to synthesize long-chain fatty acids). An overview of the system is shown in Figure 21-3. Briefly, in the fed state, insulin values are high, glucagon values are low, and glucose is oxidized through the Krebs cycle with the production of citrate. Citrate leaves the mitochondrion, is split to acetyl-CoA and oxaloacetate, and the acetyl-CoA is utilized for malonyl-CoA formation.

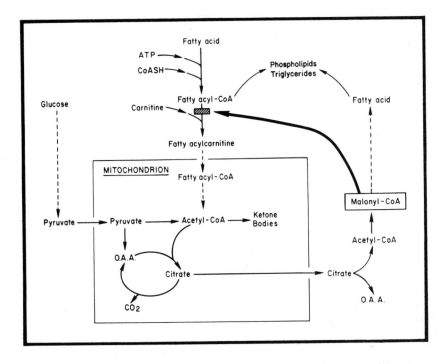

Figure 21-3. The interrelationship between glucose metabolism, fatty acid synthetase, and fatty acid oxidation. O.A.A. stands for oxaloacetate. (Reprinted from McGarry, et al, J Clin Invest 60:265–270, 1977. By permission).

The high concentrations of malonyl-CoA inhibit carnitine acyltransferase I and stimulate fatty acid synthesis. Thus, fatty acid synthesis is brisk, fatty acid oxidation does not occur, and a wasteful futile cycle of simultaneous fat synthesis and fat breakdown is avoided. During fasting or uncontrolled diabetes, glucagon rises, with the immediate result that malonyl-CoA formation is blocked. As a consequence, fatty acid synthesis stops, fatty acid oxidation is disinhibited, and ketosis supervenes. The overall model is shown in Figure 21-4.

OTHER METABOLIC ABNORMALITIES

Other metabolic abnormalities result from the osmotic diuresis and ketoacidosis just described.

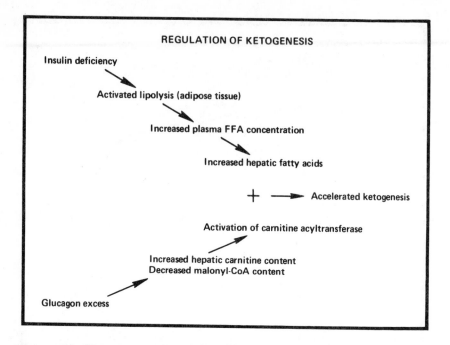

Figure 21-4. The regulation of ketogenesis. (Modified from McGarry and Foster, Amer J Med 61:9–13, 1976).

Total body potassium deficiency: Total body potassium deficiency is always present although the plasma potassium may be initially elevated due to shifts from the intracellular space under the influence of metabolic acidosis.

Total body phosphate depletion: As with potassium, phosphate stores are markedly depleted although the plasma phosphate on arrival may be low, normal, or high. One major consequence is that red cell 2,3-diphosphoglycerate concentration is decreased, shifting the oxygen dissociation curve to the left. Oxygen delivery in peripheral tissues would be impaired were it not for the compensating effect of severe acidosis which shifts the curve to the right, neutralizing the effect of 2,3-DPG deficiency.

Increased serum lactate: While not well recognized, lactate elevation is the usual accompaniment of ketoacidosis, with levels of up to 6 mM being found in the absence of shock or other cause for lactic acidosis.

Hypertriglyceridemia: Elevated triglyceride levels (usually VLDL) are due both to hepatic overproduction and diminished peripheral utilization (the latter a consequence of decreased lipoprotein lipase activity, an insulin-dependent enzyme). Occasionally chylomicrons are present if the patient has eaten in proximity to the onset of acidosis. High triglyceride levels may account for an artefactual lowering of the serum sodium.

CLINICAL PICTURE

Patients with diabetic ketoacidosis usually present with anorexia, nausea, and vomiting coupled with polyuria, rapid respiration, and, in severe cases, altered consciousness. Children may develop a syndrome of relatively pure acidosis (with little volume depletion) but the usual picture is that of acidosis and dehydration. The biochemical findings in three large series are shown in Table 21-1.

TREATMENT

The treatment of ketoacidosis has to be individualized.

Table 21-1. Clinical Characteristics of Ketoacidosis.

	Dallas[1]	Los Angeles[2]	Washington[3]
Age	38	36	43
Glucose (mg/100 ml)	476	675	733
Sodium (mM)	132	131	132
Potassium (mM)	4.8	5.3	6.0
Bicarbonate (mM)	<10	6	10
BUN (mg/100 ml)	25	32	42
Acetoacetate (mM)	4.8	—[4]	—
β-hydroxybutyrate (mM)	13.7	—	—
Free fatty acids (mM)	2.1	—	2.3
Lactate (mM)	4.6	—	—
Osmolarity (milliosmol/L)	310	323	331

[1]McGarry and Foster, unpublished series of 88 consecutive patients.
[2]Beigelman, Diabetes 20:490, 1971.
[3]Gerich, et al., Diabetes 20:228, 1971.
[4]No data.

Insulin: Always use regular insulin. At the present time in this country almost all patients are treated with "low dose" insulin schedules (5 to 10 units per hour intravenously). While most patients respond well to this procedure, a few patients are resistant (largely because of insulin antibodies and hormonal factors). Since such patients cannot be identified ahead of time, we prefer standard treatment with 50 units of regular insulin per hour until ketosis has broken. If the low dose schedule is used and the patient has not begun to respond with a fall in ketones (and a rise in pH) within 3 to 4 hours, *large doses of insulin should be given.* (Note: A fall in glucose is unimportant since it always precedes reversal of ketosis. Insulin resistance manifests itself in the acidosis component.)

Fluids: The average deficit is 3 to 5 liters. Fluid therapy should be started with a balanced salt solution (Ringer's lactate) or 0.9 percent sodium chloride. Glucose solutions should be initiated when the plasma glucose is about 250–300 mg percent to provide free water, to avoid hypoglycemia, and to minimize the chance of cerebral edema.

Potassium: Potassium shifts intracellularly as glucose is metabolized. Ordinarily, replacement therapy becomes necessary about 4 hours into treatment as plasma levels begin to fall. If the initial potassium concentration is normal or low, replacement should be started immediately. In general, 100–200 mEq will be required over the first 24 to 36 hours.

Phosphate: In view of the invariable phosphate depletion present in ketoacidosis, the initial potassium should be given as the phosphate salt (commercially available).

Bicarbonate: Sodium bicarbonate should be restricted to those patients with a pH of 7.0 or below. If used, the infusion of bicarbonate should be stopped when the pH reaches 7.2 in order to avoid a metabolic alkalosis as ketosis is reversed. Alkalosis is detrimental because it shifts the oxygen dissociation curve of hemoglobin to the left, rendering tissue oxygenation more difficult and predisposing to development of superimposed lactic acidosis.

Supportive measures: If infection is present, antibiotics will be required. Leukocytosis is not a sign of infection since very high white blood cell counts may normally be present in ketoacidosis. The presence of fever, on the other hand, strongly suggests infection, since uninfected patients tend to be slightly hypothermic in the ketoacidotic state. Blood and urine cultures should be obtained in any patient with fever who does not have an obvious site for infection. Hypertriglyceridemia need not be specifically addressed during the acute episode, since this will usually respond to insulin therapy.

References

1. Clements RS and Vourganti B: Fatal diabetic ketoacidosis: major causes and approaches to their prevention. Diabetes Care 1:314–325, 1978
2. Kreisberg RA: Diabetic ketoacidosis: new concepts and trends in pathogenesis and treatment. Ann Int Med 88:681–695, 1978
3. McGarry JD and Foster DW: Regulation of ketogenesis and clinical aspects of the ketotic state. Metabolism 21:471–489, 1972
4. McGarry JD and Foster DW: Hormonal control of ketogenesis. Biochemical considerations. Arch Int Med 137:495–501, 1977
5. McGarry JD, Leatherman GF, and Foster DW: Carnitine palmitoyltransferase I. The site of inhibition of hepatic fatty acid oxidation by malonyl-CoA. J Biol Chem 253:4128–4136, 1978
6. Padilla AJ and Loeb JN: "Low-dose" versus "high-dose" insulin regimens in the management of uncontrolled diabetes. A survey. Am J Med 63:843–848, 1977

22

Hyperosmolar Nonketotic Coma

Stephen Podolsky, M.D.

Hyperosmolar nonketotic coma is a life-threatening emergency with an extremely high mortality rate. It is a clinical syndrome with four major features: (1) severe hyperglycemia (blood glucose greater than 600 mg/dl); (2) absence of ketoacidosis (plasma Acetest® less than 2+ at 1:1 dilution); (3) profound dehydration; and (4) variable neurologic signs, such as depressed sensorium or frank coma. Plasma or serum osmolality is elevated to greater than 350 milliosmol/kg of water.

This syndrome is most common in the elderly diabetic, and often develops insidiously in patients without previously diagnosed diabetes. It probably accounts for 10 to 20 percent of cases of severe hyperglycemia with or without ketoacidosis.[1] Slightly more women are affected than men, reflecting both their increased longevity and the fact that diabetes mellitus is more prevalent in women.

There were a number of clear reports of the syndrome of hyperosmolar nonketotic coma in the preinsulin era and even in the 19th century medical literature.[2] Such reports disappeared from the literature after the first decade following the discovery of insulin, perhaps as a result of the introduction of insulin therapy. The reason(s) for the apparent disappearance of hyperosmolar nonketotic coma for 25 years, and especially for its reappearance when it was rediscovered in 1957,[3] are not clear.

PATHOPHYSIOLOGY

A variety of underlying medical conditions have been found in patients with hyperosmolar nonketotic coma, including pancreatitis, severe infections, myocardial infarction, renal failure, surgical stress, burns, peritoneal dialysis, hemodialysis, and hyperalimentation.

The typical patient is brought to the hospital in a sleepy or confused state, or actually comatose, with a history of days or even weeks of polyuria and increasing thirst. As the syndrome progresses, thirst is impaired, possibly due to alteration of the hypothalamic thirst center secondary to hyperosmolality or severe hyperglycemia. Physical examination reveals a striking and profound dehydration, shallow respiration, and there is no odor of acetone on the breath.

These patients often present with a variety of neurologic signs, including grand mal seizures, hemiparesis, Babinski reflexes, aphasia, muscle fasciculations, hyperthermia, hemianopsia, nystagmus, visual hallucinations, and so forth, suggesting diffuse cortical and subcortical damage. Not infrequently, a cerebrovascular accident is suspected and the patient is admitted to a neurology ward, particularly when diabetes has not been previously diagnosed.[4] Treatment with phenytoin may be hazardous. Not only is it ineffective in relieving seizures associated with hyperosmolar states, but it may worsen the hyperglycemia by impairing release of endogenous insulin. Many of the localizing neurologic signs are completely reversed with successful treatment. Occasionally, prolonged and persistent mental confusion has followed treatment, but correction of the dehydration and hyperglycemia often results in disappearance of even the most alarming neurologic signs.

The profound osmotic diuresis results in loss of water in excess of electrolytes. Plasma concentrations of sodium and potassium are of no value in estimating the magnitude of net ion losses, except for the fact that initial hypokalemia indicates very severe potassium loss. In the absence of severe hyperglycemia, serum sodium levels would be considerably higher at the same serum osmolality levels. Hyponatremia develops when hyperglycemia causes water to be withdrawn from the cells into the plasma in an attempt to maintain a normal serum osmolality.

Serum sodium concentration is also affected by urinary loss of sodium. When fluid loss and dehydration become severe, hypernatremia gradually ensues.

The hyperglycemia-induced osmotic diuresis causes a shift in intracellular potassium into the plasma followed by urinary loss, which results in considerable depletion of body potassium, from 400 to 1000 mEq.[5] Even if initial hyperkalemia is present, iatrogenic hypokalemia may be precipitated later when insulin therapy drives potassium as well as glucose into the cells. Elderly patients frequently receive long-term therapy with potassium-wasting diuretic drugs and so are particularly susceptible to hypokalemia in diabetic coma. Potassium depletion itself results in impaired insulin secretion, which may worsen hyperglycemia and cause a vicious cycle of further osmotic diuresis and potassium loss in hyperosmolar nonketotic coma.

One reason for this syndrome's prevalence in the geriatric population may be the widespread use of hyperglycemia-inducing and other pharmacologic agents in this age group. Table 22-1 lists drugs or medical procedures which have caused the syndrome.

There is no single answer to the question, "Why is there no ketosis with such severe hyperglycemia?" Patients with hyperosmolar nonketotic diabetes invariably have some circulat-

Table 22-1. *Therapeutic Agents or Procedures Which Have Caused Hyperosmolar Nonketotic Diabetic Coma.*

Hydrochlorothiazide and thiazide diuretics
Glucocorticoids
Propranolol
Chlorthalidone
Phenytoin
Furosemide
Diazoxide
Ethacrynic acid
Cimetidine
Chlorpromazine
1-asparaginase
Immunosuppressive agents
Peritoneal dialysis
Hemodialysis
Intravenous hyperosmolar alimentation

---

ing endogenous insulin present, usually 5 to 20 μU/ml. While these insulin levels are insufficient to transport blood glucose across cell membranes and into the cells or to prevent endogenous glucose production, they may be high enough to block lipolysis in adipose tissue and thus prevent subsequent ketosis. The mechanism of blockage of free fatty acid release from fat stores and masking of severely uncontrolled diabetes by prevention of ketosis probably accounts for the attacks of hyperosmolar nonketotic coma provoked by administration of high doses of propranolol.[6]

Plasma levels of growth hormone and cortisol are generally lower than in patients with diabetic ketoacidosis.[7] Cortisol and growth hormone are lipolytic hormones. Plasma glucagon levels are markedly elevated in hyperosmolar nonketotic coma.[8] Some patients with the syndrome have plasma-free fatty acid levels as high as in diabetic ketoacidosis, indicating impaired hepatic synthesis of ketones from the free fatty acids, without any inhibition of lipolysis. Furthermore, dehydration itself may also impair free fatty acid release from adipose tissue, thus contributing to the absence of ketogenesis.

Depressed sensorium closely parallels hyperosmolality in hyperglycemic nonketotic diabetes.[9] Intracellular dehydration of the brain leads to neurological abnormalities. Hemoconcentration may be followed by arterial and venous thromboses, which often complicate hyperosmolar nonketotic coma.[1,2,4]

Virtually all of these patients have some degree of prerenal azotemia. Many patients with hyperosmolar nonketotic coma have an increased "anion gap," with varying degrees of acidosis.[10] In some, lactic acidosis occurs, complicating the syndrome. Often the cause of the acidosis is not known. Occasionally the patient actually has unsuspected ketoacidosis due entirely to accumulation of beta-hydroxybutyrate, a ketone body which is not detected by the Acetest® tablet.

THERAPY

Treatment of hyperosmolar nonketotic coma is directed toward: (1) correction of the extreme degree of volume depletion; (2) correction of the hyperosmolar state; and (3) detection and correction of any underlying precipitating cause, such as associated illness or drug administration.

Fluids

There has been some controversy about the appropriate type of intravenous fluid to be administered, with a bewildering array of fluids being recommended at various times. Balance studies suggest that the fluid lost in hyperosmolar nonketotic coma contains about 60 mEq/L of sodium plus potassium, which closely approximates half-normal saline (77 mM NaCl). I believe this is the fluid of choice.

After confirmation of the diagnosis, two liters of hypotonic (half-normal) saline should be infused very rapidly, i.e., to run in within two hours. Thereafter, one liter of hypotonic saline should be administered every two hours, titrating according to the central venous pressure (CVP). The infusion solution should be changed to 5 percent dextrose in water when the blood glucose has fallen to 250 mg/dl. Half the estimated water deficit, including urinary losses, should be replaced in the first 12 hours and the remainder in the next 24 hours. At least six, and as many as 18, liters of fluid may be required, with nine liters being the average amount retained.

If hypotension or tachycardia is present, isotonic saline should be infused until the CVP begins to rise. Blood or plasma should be given if the systolic blood pressure remains below 80 mm Hg. Intravenous furosemide (50 to 100 mg) has resulted in a marked increase in urine volume in patients in whom acute renal failure has developed.

Insulin

Widely varying regimens for insulin therapy are recommended in the literature. I advise 25–50 U regular insulin administered intravenously as an initial dose.[1,2,4] Insulin may be administered every two hours in the same quantity as the initial dose, if the blood glucose has not fallen by at least 100 mg/dl. Often no additional insulin will be required after the initial dose. No additional regular insulin should be given after the blood glucose reaches 300 mg/dl. Insulin should not be added to the intravenous infusion bottles because a large amount may be lost by adsorption to bottles and tubing, unless precautions are taken such as the addition of sterile albumin or some of the patient's own blood, which are absorbed in place of the insulin.

It seems likely that the recent low-dose insulin regimens for treating diabetic ketoacidosis are appropriate for hyperosmolar nonketotic coma also. Twenty units of regular insulin may be administered intramuscularly as an initial dose, followed by 5 units intramuscularly every hour until the blood glucose level reaches 300 mg/dl.

After recovery from the acute episode, the patient should be given a daily subcutaneous injection of Lente or NPH intermediate-acting insulin. Many of these patients can be gradually changed from diet plus insulin therapy to diet alone or diet plus sulfonylurea therapy after discharge from the hospital.

Potassium

Potassium therapy should be started earlier in the therapy of nonketotic diabetic coma than it would be in diabetic ketoacidosis, because of the greater prodromal potassium loss as well as the sometimes precipitous and fatal fall in serum potassium level which follows insulin therapy in these patients. Addition of at least 20 to 40 mEq of potassium chloride to each liter of parenteral fluid should be accomplished early, once adequate urinary output has been established, unless the patient presents with hyperkalemia. Infusion of potassium can be stopped if serum potassium levels rise above 5.0 mEq/L, or doubled if levels fall below 4.0 mEq/L.[1] As much as 200 to 300 mEq of potassium may be required during the first 36 hours of treatment, and even more may be needed in some cases.

Potassium replacement can be started from the beginning of treatment if the patient presents with hypokalemia, provided the heart is monitored with electrocardiograms and the urinary output is adequate. These patients also have phosphate deficits, and potassium phosphate, 5 mM/L, can be infused instead of potassium chloride. Red blood cell 2,3-diphosphoglycerate is depleted in phosphate deficiency states, affecting the affinity of hemoglobin to bind oxygen.

While it is neither possible nor necessary to replace the total body potassium deficit acutely, therapy with oral potassium chloride or potassium phosphate may be advisable for short periods of up to one week after apparent recovery.

It cannot be overemphasized that adjusting the therapeutic regimen to the needs of the individual patient, with meticulous clinical care, the vigorous replacement of fluid and potassium, and correction of precipitating factors or associated illnesses are just as important as the details of insulin therapy. Finally, because of the propensity of these patients to develop arterial and venous thromboses, consideration should be given to early use of heparin therapy.[2,4,11]

References

1. Podolsky S: Hyperosmolar nonketotic coma in the elderly diabetic. Med Clin North Am 62:815–828, 1978
2. Podolsky S: Hyperosmolar nonketotic coma: Underdiagnosed and undertreated. *In* Podolsky S (ed): Clinical Diabetes: Modern Management. Appleton-Century-Crofts, New York, pp. 209–236, 1980
3. Sament S and Schwartz MD: Severe diabetic stupor without ketosis. S Afr Med J 31:893–894, 1957
4. Podolsky S: Hyperosmolar nonketotic coma: Death can be prevented. Geriatrics 34 (3):29–42, 1979
5. Podolsky S and Emerson K, Jr: Potassium depletion in diabetic ketoacidosis and in hyperosmolar nonketotic coma. Diabetes 22:299, 1973
6. Podolsky S and Pattavina CG: Hyperosmolar nonketotic diabetic coma: A complication of propranolol therapy. Metabolism 22:685–693, 1973
7. Gerich JE, Martin MM and Recant L: Clinical and metabolic characteristics of hyperosmolar nonketotic coma. Diabetes 20:228–238, 1971
8. Lindsey CA, Faloona CR and Unger R: Plasma glucagon in nonketotic hyperosmolar coma. JAMA 229:1771–1773, 1974
9. Fulop M, Rosenblatt A, Kreitzer SM, et al: Hyperosmolar nature of diabetic coma. Diabetes 24:594–599, 1975
10. Arieff AE and Carroll HJ: Nonketotic hyperosmolar coma with hyperglycemia: Clinical features, pathophysiology, renal function, acid-base balance, plasma-cerebrospinal fluid equilibria and the effects of therapy in 37 cases. Medicine (Balt) 51:73–94, 1972
11. Mather HM: Management of hyperosmolar coma. J Roy Soc Med 73:134–138, 1980

23

Lactate Homeostasis and Lactic Acidosis

Robert A. Kreisberg, M.D.

INTRODUCTION

Lactic acidosis is now the most common cause of metabolic acidosis in clinical medicine. While it usually develops in situations where tissue perfusion is inadequate, it may also be encountered when oxygenation is not obviously impaired (Table 23-1).

Lactic acid is a strong metabolic acid (pKa, 3.8) that is completely dissociated at body pH. For each mEq of lactic acid produced there will be one mEq each of hydrogen ion and lactate liberated. The hydrogen ion reduces the bicarbonate concentration and the body pool of buffer. Lactate is the anionic residue of previously buffered lactic acid and, when present in increased concentration, indicates that the production and/or utilization of lactic acid/lactate has been altered.

METABOLISM

Lactate is a metabolic by-product of glycolysis and is in equilibrium with pyruvate by virtue of the reaction catalyzed by lactic dehydrogenase:

Equation 1: Pyruvate + NADH + H$^+$ $\underset{\longleftarrow}{\overset{LDH}{\rightleftharpoons}}$ Lactate + NAD$^+$

Table 23-1. Classification of Lactic Acidosis.

Impaired tissue perfusion and oxygenation

1. Carbon monoxide
2. Hemorrhage
3. Hypovolemia
4. Myocardial infarction/failure
5. Pancreatitis
6. Pulmonary embolism
7. Sepsis
8. Trauma

Tissue perfusion and oxygenation not obviously impaired

1. Associated disorders
   a. Anemia
   b. Diabetes mellitus
   c. Hepatic disease
   d. Neoplasia
   e. Renal failure
   f. Fasting

2. Drugs
   a. Biguanides
   b. Catecholamines
   c. Cyanide
   d. Dithiazinine
   e. Ethanol
   f. Ethylene glycol
   g. Fructose/sorbitol/xylitol
   h. Isoniazid
   i. Methanol
   j. Salicylates
   k. Streptozotocin

3. Hereditary forms
   a. Glucose 6—phosphate dehydrogenase deficiency
   b. Fructose 1,6—diphosphatase deficiency
   c. Pyruvate carboxylase deficiency
   d. Pyruvate dehydrogenase deficiency
   e. Defective oxidative phosphorylation

Modified from References 2 and 6.

The concentration of lactate is determined by the concentrations of pyruvate, NADH, NAD^+ and hydrogen ion:

$$\text{\textit{Equation 2:} Lactate} = K\ \frac{(\text{Pyruvate})\ (\text{NADH})\ (H^+)}{(NAD^+)}$$

in which K is the equilibrium constant for the reaction, and NADH and NAD$^+$ are the concentrations of the free (unbound) reduced and oxidized nucleotides. The NADH/NAD ratio reflects the cellular cytosol redox state, and it and the pyruvate concentration are the major determinants of the lactate concentration.

The NADH/NAD ratio is primarily dependent upon mitochondrial activity. While the availability of oxygen is critical, it is not the only determinant of cellular redox, and a variety of factors altering mitochondrial function are also very important. Consequently, alterations in NADH and NAD do not solely reflect tissue oxygenation. NADH is generated during glycolysis and reoxidized to NAD by the mitochondria. When mitochondrial function is impaired, NADH accumulates, cellular ATP concentrations decrease, and the generation of pyruvate and its conversion to lactate are accelerated (Figure 23-1). As ATP concentrations decrease, phosphofructokinase, the rate limiting enzyme of glycolysis, is activated and there is increased flux of substrate down the pathway to pyruvate. The shift in cellular redox and the accumulation of NADH accelerate the conversion of pyruvate to lactate. The conversion of pyruvate to lactate permits reoxidation of NADH to occur in the cytosol instead of in the mitochondrial compartment. The NAD regenerated by this mechanism is utilized at the glyceraldehyde phosphate dehydrogenase step of the glycolytic pathway and is necessary if increased flux is to occur.

Pyruvate plays a central role in lactate homeostasis, and factors that regulate its concentration have a profound effect on lactate homeostasis. The balance between pyruvate production and pyruvate utilization is critically important. Pyruvate is primarily produced by glycolysis and the transamination of alanine. Pyruvate utilization is dependent upon intramitochondrial processes, cellular redox, and the availability of ATP. In adipose tissue, brain, muscle, and other tissues, pyruvate is converted to acetyl CoA by the enzyme pyruvate dehydrogenase (PDH). NAD is an important co-factor in this reaction. If insufficient quantities of NAD are available, the conversion of pyruvate to acetyl CoA will be inhibited and its conversion to lactate will be augmented. PDH is inhibited by starvation and diabetes mellitus, in addition to conditions that impair NADH reoxida-

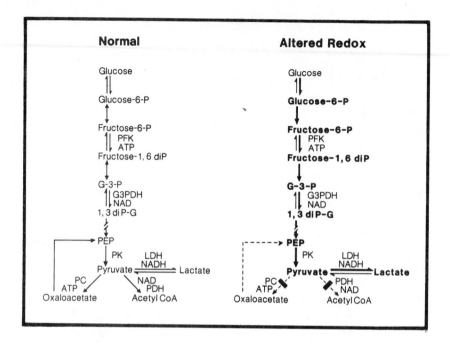

Figure 23-1. Heavy lettering and arrow (———→) indicate increased concentration, flux or activity. Normal lettering and arrow (———→) indicate normal concentration or activity. Interrupted arrow (— — — —→) indicates decreased flux or activity. Abbreviations: PFK=phosphofructokinase; G3PDH=glyceraldehyde 3-phosphate dehydrogenase; PK=pyruvate kinase; LDH=lactic dehydrogenase; PC=pyruvate carboxylase; PDH=pyruvate dehydrogenase; G-3-P=glyceraldehyde 3-phosphate; 1, 3 diP-G=1,3-diphosphoglycerate; NAD and NADH=oxidized and reduced forms of the nicotinamide adenine dinucleotide; ATP=adenosine triphosphate.

tion. In the liver and in the kidney, pyruvate is utilized predominantly for gluconeogenesis. The first and rate-limiting step in this sequence, the conversion of pyruvate to oxaloacetate, catalyzed by pyruvate carboxylase (PC), requires an adequate supply of ATP. Impairment of mitochondrial function influences the activity of both PDH and PC and the subsequent disposition of pyruvate. Thus, factors that increase lactate production generally decrease lactate utilization.

LACTATE HOMEOSTASIS AND QUANTITATIVE ASPECTS OF LACTATE METABOLISM

Lactate is produced by virtually all tissues, but brain, erythrocytes, skeletal muscle, and, perhaps, skin account for most of the lactate synthesized; minor contributions are made by leukocytes, platelets, and renal medulla. Lactate is utilized predominantly by the liver and the kidneys, although other tissues have the capacity to metabolize lactate. When lactate is oxidized or used for glucose synthesis (the Cori cycle), bicarbonate is regenerated and/or hydrogen ions are consumed. Thus, acid-base homeostasis and lactate utilization are intimately related. Lactate serves as substrate for replacement of the bicarbonate which was lost when lactic acid was synthesized. The acid-base considerations of the Cori cycle are every bit as important as those dealing with glucose homeostasis.

Lactic acidosis may be viewed as an imbalance between lactic acid production and lactate utilization. Controversy currently exists over the relative importance of these factors in clinical conditions associated with lactic acidosis. It has been traditional to attribute lactic acidosis to the overproduction of lactic acid by hypoxic tissues, even in the absence of obvious poor tissue perfusion. Since splanchnic, as well as peripheral, blood flow is reduced in such situations, the delivery of lactate to the liver and kidneys and its extraction would also be expected to be reduced. Thus, overproduction as well as underutilization appear to contribute to the development and/or maintenance of lactic acidosis in low flow states. The relative importance of these processes in idiopathic lactic acidosis and in lactic acidosis due to metabolic abnormalities and toxic substances has not been defined.

The basal rate of lactic acid production is not precisely known. Resting lactate production, determined by isotopic dilution, is 0.9–1.0 mMoles/kg/hr or approximately 20 to 25 mMoles/kg/day, while that calculated from lactate balance across tissue beds is 15 to 20 mMoles/kg/day. Maximum rates of lactate production can be estimated in situations where there is intense muscle contraction of brief duration (strenuous exercise, convulsions, etc.). Plasma lactate concentrations may reach 20 to 30 mM after maximum work of short duration, representing lactate production rates of 10 to 20 mMoles/kg/min for 30 seconds. When this quantity of lactate is distributed in the lactate space (60 percent of total body weight), a lactate concentration of 8 to 10 mM is produced. Thus, under certain circumstances, there can be little doubt that lactic acidosis is due to the overproduction of lactic acid.

It also seems reasonable that inhibition of lactate utilization can produce lactic acidosis in a relatively short period of time. Lactic acid production at a rate of 0.9 mMoles/kg/hr (basal lactate turnover) would generate approximately 60 to 70 mEq each of hydrogen ion and the lactate anion per hour for the 70 kg reference individual. The body bicarbonate pool for such an individual would be reduced by 50 percent within 6 to 7 hours and the concentration of lactate in body water would approach 13 mM.

DEFINITION AND DIAGNOSIS OF LACTIC ACIDOSIS

Although a number of definitions are available, lactic acidosis can be considered to be present when lactate concentrations are $\geq$ 4–5 mM, plasma bicarbonate concentrations are comparably reduced and there is significant lowering of the arterial pH ($\leq$ 7.35). The precipitous development of unexplained severe hyperventilation and the presence of an increased anion-gap metabolic acidosis in a critically ill patient with compromised cardiovascular function, in the absence of ketoacidosis and/or chronic renal failure, will generally permit a firm early diagnosis of lactic acidosis. The anion gap is determined by substracting the sum of the plasma chloride and bicarbonate concentrations from the sodium concentration $[(Na)-(Cl+HCO_3)]$. The difference, normally 12 to 15 mEq/L, represents unmeasured anions, including albumin, present in plasma. Occasionally, exclusion of diabetic ketoacidosis will be difficult because the nitroprusside color reaction, dependent primarily on acetoacetate, will be weakly positive or negative in the presence of severe ketoacidosis when the predominant ketoacid is beta-hydroxybutyrate. Under these circumstances and in the absence of rapid lactate measurements, the increased anion gap will be falsely attributed to lactate. Ketoacidosis and lactic acidosis may occasionally coexist, particularly in patients with alcoholic ketoacidosis or in patients with diabetic ketoacidosis in whom there is coexistent poor tissue perfusion. In the absence of lactate measurements, these combinations may be difficult to detect.

DIABETES MELLITUS

The relationship between diabetes mellitus and lactic acidosis has been an intriguing one that has defied resolution. Approximately 50 percent of the reported cases of idiopathic lactic acidosis have occurred in patients with diabetes mellitus. In my experience, idiopathic lactic acidosis in patients with diabetes mellitus has become virtually nonexistent since the removal of phenformin from the market. Macrovascular disease, microangiopathy, altered affinity of hemoglobin for oxygen (due to increased 2,3-DPG and/or the presence of increased quantities of glycosylated hemoglobin), abnormal platelet function, and altered blood viscosity could individually and collectively predispose to inadequate tissue oxygenation. The possibility that a metabolic lesion may exist in addition to, or instead of, the above possible causes must also be considered. Skeletal muscle PDH and lactate oxidation are reduced and lactate production is increased in experimental diabetes mellitus and in patients with insulin-dependent diabetes mellitus deprived of insulin for 24 hours.

In patients with diabetic ketoacidosis, clinically significant lactic acidosis is uncommon. Those patients with the severest degree of acidosis, hyperglycemia and hypovolemia, have the highest initial lactate concentrations, while those with milder abnormalities have lower lactate concentrations. With therapy, lactate concentrations decline in the former while they increase in the latter, but in no instance does clinical lactic acidosis develop. In experimental ketoacidosis, blood lactate concentrations are normal or minimally decreased but tend to increase with insulin therapy. This increase is attributed to inhibition of gluconeogenesis by insulin and reduced hepatic extraction of lactate rather than increased extrahepatic lactate production.

ETHANOL

Hyperlactatemia is a well recognized consequence of ethanol consumption, but it is seldom severe, and lactate concentrations in excess of 3 mM are rare. The hyperlactatemia that is associated with the use of ethanol is a result of decreased hepatic lactate extraction rather than increased lactate production. Lactic acidosis may occasionally be encountered in alcoholic patients with or without elevated blood ethanol concentrations. Ethanol interferes with lactate clearance, and lactic acidosis may occur when other factors, such as seizures or hyperventilation, strain homeostatic mechanisms by accelerating lactic acid production. Lactic acidosis has also been reported after the parenteral administration of ethanol. While lactic acidosis usually occurs with active ethanol consumption and ketoacidosis with ethanol withdrawal or abstinence, they occasionally occur together and may be associated with hypoglycemia. It is stated that ethanol is more likely to induce lactic acidosis in diabetic than in nondiabetic patients.

TREATMENT

The most important aspect of the therapy of lactic acidosis is to identify and, where possible, correct predisposing factors. Recovery, however, is usually limited by the underlying disorder (i.e., myocardial infarction, sepsis, etc.). The appropriate use of inotropic, vasopressor and/or vasodilator agents, fluids, colloid, blood, and bicarbonate is indicated. Early and accurate assessment does not guarantee success since the remedies for some problems are not currently available. In idiopathic lactic acidosis and with lactic acidosis associated with drugs and/or toxic agents, cardiovascular function is usually preserved initially. With protracted or intractable acidosis, myocardial contractility fails and tissue perfusion becomes inadequate. While the aggressive use of bicarbonate at the outset to maintain hemodynamic stability is warranted, a variety of complications may develop (volume overload, worsening acidosis, and rebound alkalosis). It has been suggested that alkalinization can be associated with enhanced lactic acid production and a worsening of the acidosis. At present, the dilemma concerning the use of bicarbonate cannot be resolved. In the absence of specific therapy, and when there cannot be a reasonable expectation of recovery without the use of bicarbonate, withholding it seems irrational.

Because the subtle metabolic abnormalities that exist in the diabetic may predispose to the development of lactic acidosis, the use of insulin in the treatment of lactic acidosis has been recommended under certain circumstances. Although phenformin-associated lactic acidosis should no longer be a problem, uncontrolled studies in such patients suggested that improved recovery could be expected with the use of insulin, presumably because insulin served to correct or ameliorate the predisposing metabolic abnormalities. While this evidence is circumstantial at best, aggressive management of diabetes in the diabetic patient with lactic acidosis would seem to be indicated, even in the absence of phenformin. The continuous infusion of insulin, used for treatment of diabetic ketoacidosis, can easily be modified for use in the patient with uncontrolled or poorly controlled diabetes and lactic acidosis.

References

1. Alberti KGMM, Nattrass M: Lactic acidosis. Lancet 2:25–29, 1977
2. Cohen RD, Woods HF: Clinical and biochemical aspects of lactic acidosis. Blackwell Scientific Publication 1976 London WC 1
3. Cohen RD, Iles RA: Lactic acidosis: some physiological and clinical considerations. Clin Sci Mol Med 53:405–510, 1977
4. Krebs HA, Woods HF, Alberti KGMM: Hyperlactatemia and lactic acidosis. Essays Med Biochem 1:81–103, 1975
5. Oliva PB: Lactic acidosis. Am J Med 48:209–225, Feb 1970
6. Relman AS: Lactic acidosis. *In* Acid-base and Potassium Homeostasis, Brenner BM and Stein JH (eds), Chapter 3, pp. 65–100. New York: Churchilll-Livingstone, 1978
7. Waters WC, Hall JD, Schwartz WB: Spontaneous lactic acidosis. Am J Med 35:781–793, Dec 1963

24

Infection in the Diabetic Patient

Stanley G. Rabinowitz, M.D.

GENERAL

Because infection in the diabetic can precipitate marked pertur-
bations in insulin-dependent metabolic functions, it is of
paramount importance that attention be directed to rapidly diagnosing and treating infections in the diabetic patient. In this
chapter, emphasis will be placed on the more common infections
seen in diabetic patients.

HOST DEFENSE MECHANISMS IN THE DIABETIC

Much effort has been expended experimentally in evaluating
host defense mechanisms in the diabetic. In particular, some
studies have suggested that in the diabetic whose glucose
metabolism is poorly controlled, there are abnormalities in neutrophil chemotaxis and phagocytosis, as well as lymphocyte
mitogenic responses. Antibody synthesis, complement, and op-
sonin levels appear normal. What role these immunologic alterations play in explaining the increased incidence of infection in
the well-controlled diabetic is not at all clear.

Since cellulitis and vascular ulcers of the lower extremities
are the commonest infections experienced by diabetics, it is
probable that local vascular and/or neurological impairments ex-

plain the enhanced susceptibility to infection. By compromising local blood flow and oxygenation of tissues, vascular lesions are critical to the pathogenesis of such infections. Finally neurological deficits contribute to the enhanced susceptibility to infection by permitting repeated episodes of trauma.

Cutaneous: Patients with diabetes mellitus are prone to the recurrent development of furunculosis and carbuncles. The reasons for this susceptibility are not entirely clear, but presumably are associated with white blood cell defects induced by hyperosmolarity and excessive ketone body production. Since staphylococci are responsible for the production of furunculosis, therapy must incorporate a penicillinase-resistant penicillin along with surgical drainage whenever appropriate. Local care with warm compresses can be used as long as it is emphasized that hot compresses applied to areas where preexisting vascular insufficiency is present may markedly exacerbate infection and further compromise the blood flow to that extremity.

Cellulitis alone, or in association with vascular ulcers of the lower extremities, represents another common infection in the patient with diabetes mellitus. Frequently the leg ulcers are colonized by mixed gram-positive and gram-negative bacterial organisms, including *S. aureus,* streptococci, Proteus species, and *Pseudomonas aeruginosa.* Increasingly, anaerobes are incriminated as important pathogens in cellulitis and ulcers in the diabetic patient. When anaerobes are present, gas formation is often detected by routine x-rays and by finding crepitus during the examination of the affected area. Infected ulcers with surrounding cellulitis present particular problems for the patient with diabetes mellitus. Aggressive therapy with antibiotics appropriate to the bacteria recovered from the infected site, as well as surgical débridement and drainage, are essential. It cannot be overemphasized how important early therapy is in such cutaneous infections if loss of a portion of an extremity is to be prevented. Since vascular impairment in such infected areas is common, a combination of high-dose penicillinase-resistant penicillin with an aminoglycoside or clindamycin is administered intravenously until the infection appears well-controlled and resolving.

If infection spreads to underlying bone, osteomyelitis will develop. These infections are difficult to treat successfully and often eventuate in amputation.

Urinary Tract Infections: Colonization of the urinary tract with gram-negative bacteria is common in diabetic patients. In fact, asymptomatic bacteria (greater than 10^6 organism/ml) are found in 10 to 20 percent of diabetic patients. If autonomic dysfunction exists secondary to the diabetes, then neurogenic bladder with retention of urine may be present. Such a urologic condition makes the patient particularly susceptible to urinary tract infection and sepsis. It is probably worthwhile to attempt to eradicate bacteriuria in diabetic patients. Although there are no definitive studies to support the hypothesis that bacteriuria in patients with diabetes mellitus requires therapy, it is probably prudent to do so.

Clearly, if pyelonephritis supervenes, therapy with antimicrobial agents is mandatory. Pyelonephritis in diabetics can be a particularly devastating condition marked by high fever, shaking chills, flank pain, and hematuria. In fact, diabetics are particularly prone to developing renal papillary necrosis, a severe complication associated with significant morbidity and mortality. Urinary tract infection in the diabetic requires prompt hospitalization and initiation of antimicrobial therapy. Because diabetic patients often have received antimicrobial therapy for previous urinary tract infections, treatment should include use of an aminoglycoside until a definitive etiologic agent is recovered and its antimicrobial susceptibilities determined. During the course of hospitalization, studies directed at excluding obstructive uropathy should be performed. If the diabetic patient is responding poorly or not at all to appropriate antimicrobial therapy, then renal or perinephric abscess should be suspected and evaluated. In these conditions, surgical drainage is of paramount importance.

Finally, genitourinary tract manipulation or instrumentation should be scrupulously avoided in diabetics. As already outlined, urinary tract infections may follow a virulent course in the diabetic and, hence, such instrumentation should only be done where indications are compelling. Such patients, furthermore, should probably be given antimicrobial therapy prophylactically just before, during, and immediately after the procedure. Ampicillin or an aminoglycoside antibiotic administered for a total course of 48 hours may be considered if genitourinary tract instrumentation must be done.

Pulmonary Infections: The most frequent infection seen in the diabetic patient is pneumonia. The commonest bacterial organism recovered from diabetic patients with pneumonia is *Streptococcus pneumoniae.* Nevertheless, a substantial number of cases of pneumonia in diabetics is caused by gram-negative bacterial organisms. Thus, initial clinical evaluation of all diabetics with infection should include a chest roentgenogram, sputum smear (gram and acid-fast stains), and culture. If no sputum is being produced, prompt translaryngeal aspiration should be performed to obtain adequate material for sputum smear and culture. Presumptive therapy can begin, based on the initial gram stain of sputum or the translaryngeal aspirate. If gram-positive organisms are seen, penicillin is the therapy of choice unless staphylococci are suspected on the basis of smear morphology. The detection of predominantly gram-negative bacteria in the sputum smear suggests an aminoglycoside antibiotic as the treatment of choice. If mixed gram-positive and gram-negative bacteria are encountered, as occurs in aspiration pneumonia, therapy with clindamycin and an aminoglycoside is prudent.

Malignant External Otitis: This is a disease seen in elderly diabetics who present with severe and sudden pain from a chronically draining ear. The etiologic agent is usually *Pseudomonas aeruginosa.* This infection has been associated with a number of complications, including osteomyelitis of the base of the skull, cranial nerve paralysis, brain abscess, and meningitis. The mortality is generally about 50%, and, thus, prompt recognition and treatment is essential. Treatment consists of administration of an aminoglycoside and carbenicillin along with appropriate surgical débridement wherever appropriate.

Unusual Infections: Although a lot of attention in the literature has been directed at rhinocerebral mucormycosis complicating diabetic ketoacidosis, this disease is very rare. Clinical findings in such patients include black necrotic nasal turbinates, bloody nasal discharge, and periorbital edema with or without ptosis or proptosis. Systemic findings include headache, stupor, and mental obtundation. One must be suspicious of this condition in any diabetic with ketoacidosis who develops a nasal discharge or unilateral eye findings or mental obtundation. Fever is an inconstant finding in these patients. The diagnosis requires a biopsy of the nasal turbinate to demonstrate the typical branched, irregular, nonseptate hyphae of mucor. Therapy includes surgical débridement combined with administration of amphotericin B.

References

1. Beigelman PM: Severe diabetic ketoacidosis: 482 episodes in 251 patients. Experience of three years. Diabetes 20:490, 1971
2. Abramson E, Wilson D, and Arky RA: Rhinocerebral phycomycosis in association with diabetic ketoacidosis. Ann Int Med 66:735, 1967
3. Vejlsgaard R: Studies of urinary infections in diabetics III. Significant bacteriuria in pregnant diabetics and in matched controls. Acta Med Scand 193:337, 1973
4. Maibach HI, Hildick-Smith G (ed): Skin bacteria and their role in infection. New York, McGraw-Hill, 1965
5. Kleeman CR, Hewitt WL, and Guze LB: Pyelonephritis. Medicine 39:3, 1960
6. Zaky DA, Bentley DW, Lowy K, et al: Malignant external otitis: A severe form of otitis in diabetic patients. Am J Med 61:298, 1976
7. Molenaar DM, Palumbo PJ, Wilson WR, et al: Leukocyte chemotaxis in diabetic patients and their non-diabetic first-degree relatives. Diabetes 25:880, 1976
8. Bagdade JD: Infection in diabetics: Predisposing factors. Postgrad Med 59:160, 1976

25

Host Defense Abnormalities in Diabetic Patients

Joan I. Casey, M.D., F.R.C.P. (C)

INTRODUCTION

From current literature, one could defend the position that diabetic persons have an increased incidence of infections compared to a nondiabetic population. One could defend as easily the opposite argument. Despite this confusion, there is agreement that, once infected, the diabetic has a poorer prognosis with most infections when compared to the nondiabetic person. This chapter will present a brief review of host defenses, in general, and possible reasons for the occurrence of certain infections will be presented.

HOST DEFENSES

Grossly, from the mechanical coverage by the skin to the intracellular components of our white cells, the body is geared to protecting itself from invasion by microbial parasites. The neuropathy seen in the diabetic is the first abnormality which may allow a breakdown in host defenses. Since avoidance of trauma is essential in keeping the skin intact, the diabetic with neuropathy is at a major disadvantage. This is especially important in the sole of the foot, as the decreased sense of pain occurs in an area which is seldom visualized.

Because of the small vessel disease which occurs in diabetic patients, blood flow to the periphery is compromised. This results in a diminished oxygen supply as well as a diminished supply of those host defense factors carried in the bloodstream. The cellular and humoral factors of the blood constitute the major bulwark of the host defense system. White blood cells have to leave the blood and collect at the area of inflammation. The thickened capillary basement membrane of the diabetic blood vessels may slow down leukocyte movement and decrease diffusion of nutrients to cells already outside the vessels. The problem may be compounded by decreased sticking of the leukocytes to the endothelial wall of the vessel.[1]

In addition to the normal flow of blood past an area of inflammation, there are more specific host factors activated. Neutrophils and macrophages are attracted to an area by chemotaxis, that is, the directed migration of cells to an area of inflammation. Chemotaxis of cells has been shown to be diminished not only in the diabetic patients,[1] but in first-degree kindred of diabetic patients.[2] Once at the area of infection, phagocytosis and intracellular killing of microorganisms must take place. Both of these host defense factors are diminished in diabetic patients. Nolan et al. have recently reported further studies to clarify some of the data relevant to the problems of neutrophil phagocytosis and killing.[3] They showed that engulfment and intracellular killing of bacteria were less than in normal controls. Their data suggested that control of hyperglycemia improved leukocyte function. To date, macrophage function has not been fully studied.

Cell-mediated immunity has been studied and it appears that the diabetic patient has a diminished response to staphylococcal antigen as measured in the lymphocyte transformation assay,[4] as well as to Candida antigen as measured by skin testing.[5] Data relating to humoral immunity is mainly from early literature, suggesting that antibody responses to certain antigens may be less in children with severe diabetes, but relatively normal in well-controlled subjects. There is very little literature in recent years relevant to this interesting topic, and newer methods of studying humoral immune responses might shed some light on some of the disease associations in which humoral immunity may be as important as cellular immunity.

INFECTIONS

Consideration of some of the above related defects may explain the severe and relentless progression of certain of the more unusual infections which afflict diabetic persons.

A decreased oxygen supply to an area, particularly to a traumatized area, may allow multiplication of anaerobic organisms. A high incidence of infections with these organisms has been found in diabetic skin ulcers.[6] A much more lethal infection seen frequently in diabetic persons is that of synergistic gangrene or necrotizing fasciitis. In this condition, one usually sees a combination of anaerobic (Bacteroides or anaerobic streptococcus) and aerobic (gram-negative rods or staphylococcus) organisms. These infections may progress to such severity that the affected limb must be sacrificed to save the patient. When these infections occur in the perineal area or the abdominal wall, they are extremely difficult to eradicate and wide surgical excision is a must to prevent the excessive mortality now reported. It has been suggested by Roberts and Hester that Bartholin cyst abscesses in diabetic patients should be considered for surgery as soon as the diabetes is under control.[7] In their series, mortality in such infections was 50 percent. Gas is not infrequently encountered in these synergistic infections, and they may be mistaken for clostridial infections. The importance of recognizing the different entities is in the need for different antibiotics.

Another infectious problem simulating gas gangrene and seen in diabetic patients is emphysematous pyelonephritis, a very severe, suppurative infection of the kidneys. This may be localized to the renal pelvis, or it may involve the cortical and perirenal areas. A less serious form of the disease may involve only the ureters or the urinary bladder. The gallbladder may also be the site of serious, suppurative emphysematous infection. The organisms involved in these infections are gas-producing aerobic gram-negative rods, usually *E. coli*. A high index of suspicion is needed to diagnose this infection and x-rays of the involved organs confirm the diagnosis. Appropriate surgical intervention is the main therapy, with antibiotics playing a complementary role. Nonclostridial gas-producing infections are much more common than clostridial, as seen in Bessman and

Wagner's series. Of 49 gas-producing infections, only one yielded clostridial organisms.[8]

In the adult population, the number of diabetic persons among patients with Group B streptococcal infections is much higher than in any other group.[9] The reason for this unusual predilection in diabetes remains unexplained.

Malignant otitis externa is a rare but severe infection, seen in diabetic persons in whom the mortality approaches 100 percent.[10] The organism, *Pseudomonas aeruginosa*, is able to invade blood vessels. Since the vessels in the area of the ear are similar to those of the extremities, it is possible that the combination of a diseased vessel and a vessel-invading organism is responsible for the very high mortality seen in this disease in diabetic persons. A similar reason could exist for the predilection for mucormycosis seen in the diabetic patient. That organism also invades the capillary vessels, with the resulting thrombosis of vessels and ischemia and infarction of the affected area.

Mucormycosis may be related to the deficient cell-mediated immune responses as well, since resistance to fungal infections is cell mediated. Other fungal infections, such as candidiasis and cryptococcosis, also occur with increased frequency in diabetic persons and one can assume that deficient cell-mediated immunity is at least partly responsible.

In summary, one could explain both an increased incidence and an increased severity of infections among diabetic patients on the basis of deficiencies which have been described in their host defenses. Although there may not be one single overwhelming problem, the numerous small deficiences noted could account for some major problems.

References

1. Robertson HD and Polk HC: The mechanism of infection in patients with diabetes mellitus: A review of leukocyte malfunction. Surgery 75:123–128, 1974
2. Molenaar DM, Palumbo PJ, Wilson WR, et al: Leukocyte chemotaxis in diabetic patients and their nondiabetic first degree relations. Diabetes 25:880–883, 1976

3. Nolan, CM, Beaty HN, Bagdade JD: Further characterization of the impaired bactericidal function of granulocytes in patients with poorly controlled diabetes. Diabetes 27:889–894, 1978

4. Casey JI, Heeter B, Klyshevich K: Impaired response of lymphocytes of diabetic subjects to antigen of *Staphylococcus aureus*. Journ Infect Dis 136:495–501, 1977

5. Plouffe JT, Silva J Jr, Fekety R, et al: Cell mediated immunity in diabetes mellitus. Infection and Immunity. 21:425–429, 1978

6. Louie T, Bartlett J, Tally FP, et al: Aerobic and anaerobic bacteria in diabetic foot ulcers. Ann Int Med 85:461–465, 1976

7. Roberts DB, Hester LL, Jr: Progressive synergistic bacterial gangrene arising from abscesses of the vulva and Bartholin's gland duct. Amer Journ Obs Gyn 114:285–291, 1972

8. Bessman AN and Wagner W: Nonclostridial gas gangrene. JAMA 233:958–963, 1975

9. Bayer AS, Chow AW, Guze LB: Serious infections in adults due to Group B streptococci. Am J Med 61:498–503, 1976

10. Zaky D, Bently D, Lowy K, et al: Malignant external otitis: A severe form of otitis in diabetic patients. Am J Med 61:298–302, 1976

26

Surgery in the Patient with Diabetes

Karl E. Sussman, M.D.
Orville G. Kolterman, M.D.

Diabetes mellitus is not a protective factor in terms of surgical illnesses. It is thus fortunate that, with the advent of modern anesthetic techniques and the appropriate use of antibiotic therapy, the well-controlled diabetic can tolerate surgery almost as well as the nondiabetic patient, including such difficult surgical procedures as open-heart, thoracic, and brain surgery. Nevertheless, the health care team can ill afford to be complacent regarding management of a diabetic patient through a potentially stressful operative procedure.

PREPARATION OF THE PATIENT FOR SURGERY

In scheduling a patient for admission to the hospital and setting the day of surgery, a reasonable period of time should be planned to allow for additional studies, if indicated, and also the institution of appropriate medical treatment. The diabetic patient undergoing surgery should be in the best general condition obtainable and the nutritional-metabolic state of the patient should be as close to normal as possible. In addition, an effort should be made to assess the presence and severity of diabetic complications, particularly those involving the heart and kidneys, as these may affect the outcome of the surgical procedure.[1]

Because of the emergent nature of certain surgical problems, it is not feasible to take the time required to assess the total nature of the patient's diabetes, the presence of complications, or to institute a reasonable degree of diabetic control. It must be realized that this may exert an unfavorable influence on the outcome of the surgery,[2] but is counterbalanced, at least in part, by the fact that the indicated surgical treatment often helps to restore the metabolic balance by alleviating some factor(s) aggravating or contributing to the unstable metabolic state.

ANESTHESIA

The choice of anesthesia should be governed in large part by the type of surgery being undertaken as well as the experience of the anesthologist and the surgeon with the methods currently available.

In operations involving the lower extremities and lower abdomen, anesthesiologists may prefer utilizing spinal or epidural anesthesia.[3] Theoretically, this will produce less adrenergic stimulation and will result in more stable diabetic control.

When a general anesthetic is required, the anesthesiologist may employ a nitrous oxide-oxygen mixture supplemented by neurolept-analgesia.[3] Neurolepsis (i.e., suppression of subcortical and central autonomic activity) is induced with droperidol or diazepam and analgesia with fentanyl. Neurolept-analgesia does not provide muscle relaxation. Therefore, muscle relaxants may be required. Again, the rationale for using this combination of agents is that it will produce the least disruption in the state of metabolic control.

MANAGEMENT ON THE DAY OF SURGERY

All members of the health care team should share common therapeutic goals which apply, not only during surgery, but also in the postoperative period, regarding the maintenance of both diabetic control and normal fluid and electrolyte balance. The general goals to be sought in managing the diabetic patient through a surgical illness are: (1) prevention of hypoglycemia; (2)

prevention of diabetic ketoacidosis; (3) control of hyperglycemia and glycosuria (random blood glucose levels obtained during surgery and in the postoperative period should be approximately 200 mg/100 ml); (4) maintenance of normal electrolyte and fluid balance; and (5) resumption of oral alimentation as soon as tolerated. Given these therapeutic goals, it is almost always possible to devise an appropriate therapeutic regimen which can be employed in the diabetic patient who must undergo an operative procedure. The proposed management regimen should be discussed by the various members of the health care team prior to the initiation of the planned surgery to assure a unified approach, as this maximizes the chances for successful management of the diabetic patient during this period of stress.

We have found the following guidelines to be most helpful in designing successful therapeutic regimens for diabetic patients undergoing surgical procedures.

1. In general, operations on diabetic patients are best scheduled in the morning as this will cause only modest alteration in the patient's state of metabolic balance and will allow the clinician an opportunity to restore closer diabetic control following completion of the operative procedure. Some hospitals will delay surgery in diabetic patients with infections until other operative procedures have been completed within a given operating room. This is done to avoid bacterial cross-contamination between patients.

2. On the day of surgery, an intravenous infusion of 5 percent dextrose in water should be initiated. If the patient is showing ketonuria in addition to glucosuria, it may be necessary to use a dextrose and saline solution with additional electrolytes, as needed, in order to compensate for urinary losses. Additional insulin may also be required in this situation.

3. At the time that the intravenous glucose infusion is initiated, one-half of the usual daily dose of insulin is given subcutaneously as intermediate acting insulin. For example, if the patient had been receiving 10 units of regular plus 40 units of NPH insulin as part of his daily therapeutic program, one could administer 20 units of

NPH insulin as the initial dose on the day of surgery. It is preferable to give the insulin subcutaneously rather than by adding the insulin to the infusion bottle, as infusion bottles may be changed during the surgical procedure as well as during the postoperative period. This may lead to some uncertainty as to how much insulin has indeed been administered.

4. The intravenous infusion is continued during and following surgery. An attempt is made to give approximately 100 to 150 grams of glucose as well as 2 to 4 liters of fluid during a 24-hour interval unless contraindicated by some clinical circumstance.

5. Following completion of the surgical procedure and the return of the patient to the recovery room, a second dose of intermediate acting insulin may be administered, approximately the same dose as that given initially.

6. Blood glucose and serum electrolyte determinations should be obtained at appropriate intervals in order to evaluate the patient's metabolic control and fluid and electrolyte status. Certain changes may be necessary in the therapeutic program, including the administration of regular insulin, as needed, to achieve reasonable blood glucose levels. The practice of prescribing a sliding scale insulin dosage (i.e., fixed doses of regular insulin for specified urine glucose readings) has no place in the management of the diabetic patient during the postoperative period. (a) This approach tends to relegate a major portion of the patient's metabolic control to the nursing staff without thoughtful clinical assessment of the patient's status. (b) The health care team finds itself treating the patient's metabolic state of the past 6-hour period during the ensuing 6-hour period. This may result in much larger fluctuations in the patient's blood glucose level. (c) Urine glucose readings are not nearly as precise a reflection of the subject's control as are blood glucose determinations.

With careful attention to a well-structured therapeutic program, hypoglycemia is relatively uncommon. It is imperative, however, that the patient with diabetes mellitus be covered with a dextrose infusion and that the infusion be continued during surgery and in the postoperative period until the patient is able to resume oral alimentation. During this period, it is preferable to err on the side of mild hyperglycemia (blood glucose 150–250 mg/100 ml) rather than risk hypoglycemia in an attempt to achieve tight control.

CONSTANT INTRAVENOUS INFUSION

With the use of the constant intravenous insulin infusion for the treatment of ketoacidosis,[4,5] it was only a matter of time before a similar procedure would be employed in patients undergoing surgery. Thus far, there have been few prospective random trials to evaluate the efficacy of the constant intravenous insulin infusion technique in the management of diabetic patients undergoing surgery. In one study, the degree of diabetic control was better in those patients receiving a constant infusion of regular insulin (2 units per hour) in comparison to a group of patients who received two-thirds of their daily maintenance dose of NPH insulin.[6] However, in this therapeutic trial, the threat of hypoglycemia in 2 of the 8 patients who received 2 units per hour resulted in increasing the rate of dextrose infusion and decreasing the rate of insulin administration.[6] Preoperative NPH insulin and then one unit per hour of regular insulin appeared to produce satisfactory diabetic control.[6]

It would seem that the use of constant intravenous infusion of insulin might present a more quantitative means of administering insulin to the diabetic patient in surgery. However, this method of insulin administration necessitates careful monitoring of the blood glucose level, and controlled studies are needed to evaluate this particular therapeutic approach in the management of the diabetic patient through surgery. Use of the artificial endocrine pancreas to manage diabetic patients through surgery should, in theory, allow precise control of the patient's hyperglycemia without the risk of hypoglycemia, since constant monitoring of the blood glucose level is an integral part of this device. Preliminary reports indicate that this is, in fact, the case.[7] If these observations are confirmed and these units become generally available, this approach could well prove to be the ideal method by which to achieve excellent metabolic control in diabetic patients undergoing the stress of major surgery.

PATIENTS TAKING ORAL HYPOGLYCEMIC AGENTS

In patients being maintained on oral hypoglycemic agents, the usual practice is to discontinue these drugs during the period of acute stress. The patients are then given a small dose of insulin in the preoperative and postoperative period, approximately 10 to 20 units of NPH once or twice daily. After postoperative recovery, patients can be replaced on oral hypoglycemic agents, provided satisfactory control had been achieved previously. In some patients with very mild carbohydrate intolerance, specific hypoglycemic therapy during the course of surgery may not be required.

DIABETES ASSOCIATED WITH COMPLICATIONS

If the patient has diabetes complicated by either renal or cardiac disease, problems may arise in the postoperative period. Clearly, in the face of renal insufficiency, the problem of fluid and electrolyte management may indeed pose a major challenge. In the patient with coronary heart disease, the incidence of myocardial infarctions occurring during the postoperative period is significantly increased in the diabetic population. Indeed, in this group of patients, painless myocardial infarction may occur and be difficult to diagnose.[1] Since diabetic patients often have advanced atherosclerotic disease, all possible efforts should be made to avoid a period of hypotension during the operative procedure in order to minimize the effects of decreased perfusion on major organs such as the brain, heart, and kidneys.

SUMMARY

In the days before insulin therapy was available, surgical procedures resulted in significant morbidity and mortality. Because of the availability of insulin administration in conjunction with the use of effective antibiotics, better knowledge concerning fluid-electrolyte therapy, and the wide range of anesthetic agents which are utilized, surgery for the patient with diabetes no longer presents a problem of major magnitude.

References

1. Partamian JO and Bradley RF: Acute myocardial infarction in 258 cases of diabetes: Immediate and 5-year survival. N Engl J Med 273:455, 1965
2. Marble A and Steinke J: Physiology and pharmacology in diabetes mellitus. Anesthesiology 24:442, 1963
3. Collins VJ: Principles of Anesthesiology. Second Edition. Philadelphia, Lea and Febiger, 1976
4. Page MM, Alberti KGMM, Greenwood R, et al: Treatment of diabetic coma with continuous low-dose infusion of insulin. Brit Med J 2:687, 1974
5. Kidson W, Casey J, Drayen E, et al: Treatment of severe diabetes mellitus by insulin infusion. Brit Med J 2:691, 1974
6. Taitelman U, Reece EA, Bessman AN: Insulin in the management of the diabetic surgical patient: continuous intravenous infusion vs. subcutaneous administration. JAMA 237:658, 1977
7. Schwartz SS, Horwitz DL, Zehfns B, et al: Use of glucose controlled insulin infusion system (artificial beta cell) to control diabetes during surgery. Diabetologia 16:157, 1979

LONG-TERM PROBLEMS

27

Control of Diabetes and Long-Term Complications

Harold Rifkin, M.D.
Herbert Ross, M.D.

There are compelling reasons to consider keeping the diabetic patient's blood sugar level as close to normal as possible, but, hopefully, without inducing severe hypoglycemia. A major aim of therapy is to keep the patient symptom-free. Additionally, the prevention of diabetic ketoacidosis and hyperosmolar nonketotic coma, particularly in the patient with persistent hyperglycemia, is a most cogent reason for striving for control of diabetes. Good control also appears to decrease the incidence of refractive changes; to prevent certain types of infection; to promote normal growth and development of the diabetic; and to decrease perinatal morbidity, mortality, and possibly inhibit the development of congenital defects in the newborn of the pregnant diabetic mother.

Whether control of diabetes will prevent or inhibit the rapidity of development or actually reverse the dreaded sequelae of diabetes—namely, neuropathy, microangiopathy, and macroangiopathy—is still uncertain. The possibility exists that not all of these "chronic" complications have the same pathogenetic basis. Genetic factors may play an important role in the pathogenesis of these long-term complications, and hyperglycemia may simply be the critical influence which brings these factors to clinical expression. In the present state of our knowledge, there is really no direct evidence that hyperglycemia per se is responsible for these complications. It may well be that deficiency or inappropriate delivery of insulin is a major factor, and that some other abnormality of metabolism, rather than an elevated blood glucose, is responsible for these complications.

Furthermore, the existing criteria for "good," "fair," or "poor" control of diabetes appear to be arbitrary, since the definition of diabetic "control" varies so widely among diabetologists throughout the world. Indeed, even the definition of diabetes mellitus itself has recently come under close scrutiny.

Proponents of good control believe that the goals of appropriate therapy for the patient with diabetes should include an all-out effort to obtain euglycemic levels, both fasting, as well as pre- and postprandially, throughout the day. This concept may be correct, but, in actual practice, with present-day conventional therapy, it is most difficult to sustain over prolonged periods of time. Such control may occasionally be achieved in patients with noninsulin-dependent diabetes, and has been possible, to some extent, in insulin-dependent and pregnant diabetics, with a program of patient-monitored glucose determinations, diet, and exercise. Various factors, moreover, limit good chemical control in the insulin-dependent diabetic.[7] These include factors such as variations in food intake; altered gastrointestinal motility and absorption; variations in exercise; emotional and physical stresses; factors affecting the availability and effectiveness of administered insulin, such as variable absorption rates from injection sites, variable antibody titers, uncertain rate of release of insulin from antibodies, variability of receptor-binding sites in their affinity for insulin; existing insulin-secretory reserve; hypoglycemia induced by exogenous insulin injection with rebound hyperglycemia caused by a variety of counterregulatory hormones; and, finally, the physiologic fact that exogenous insulin is delivered into the peripheral circulation, in contrast to the secretion of endogenous insulin directly into the portal circulation.

A major problem in attempting to relate hyperglycemia to the development of long-term complications is the demonstration that "monitoring" of the blood or plasma glucose in diabetic patients supposedly in "good" control has frequently indicated wide fluctuations from hour to hour and day to day. Little or no correlation may exist between blood glucose concentrations obtained during a clinic or office visit and values obtained in the school playground, in the classroom, at home, or at business.[7,8,11] In addition, neuropathy, microvascular, as well as macrovascular, complications may be presenting manifestations of diabetes, often in the presence of mild glucose intolerance or even normal glucose tolerance. Heterogeneity, in terms of development of vascular disease, has also recently been described in insulin-dependent juvenile diabetics, related possibly to such phenomena as HLA genotypes, islet cell antibodies, autoimmunity, and insulin-binding titers.[8]

The variability of the relationship of chemical control of diabetes to the development of chronic complications is further demonstrated by the fact that significant microvascular disease and neuropathy have been shown to be absent in 20 to 40 percent of insulin-dependent diabetics who have survived for 40 years.[7]

In spite of these observations, there is a large body of evidence, based on prospective clinical studies, data on spontaneous and experimental diabetes in animals, and biochemical and functional changes in early diabetes, which indicate that persistent hyperglycemia or deficient or inappropriate delivery of insulin may well be responsible for long-term diabetic complications, particularly microangiopathy and neuropathy. Furthermore, these accumulated studies provide fairly strong evidence to suggest that good control may prevent or slow the development of such complications.

Recent epidemiologic studies suggest that the risk of microvascular diabetic complications becomes significant only in patients with a 2-hour venous plasma glucose concentration exceeding 200 mg per 100 ml following a 75 gm oral glucose load or a capillary whole blood glucose level greater than 200 mg per 100 ml after a 50 gm oral glucose load.[7] Recently, this correlation has applied also to fasting plasma glucose concentrations greater than 200 mg per 100 ml.

Retinal and glomerular capillary lesions have been observed in patients with secondary diabetes, namely chronic pancreatitis and hemochromatosis. Serial studies over a mean interval of 5 years of quadriceps muscle basement membrane in patients with chronic pancreatitis and fasting hyperglycemia have revealed a significant increase in capillary basement membrane width.[6] The possibility always exists, of course, that such patients may indeed have coexisting genetic diabetes which was responsible for these changes. A recent study from the University of Minnesota revealed afferent and efferent arteriolar hyalinization in every transplanted kidney that had been in a diabetic host for at least three years, while transplanted kidneys in nondiabetic control patients of the same age and type were relatively unaffected.[4] These findings have been attributed to the presence of the transplanted kidneys in a persistent diabetic environment. No such histologic changes, however, have been noted in the transplanted kidney of a patient with long-standing diabetes who survived for a period of 4 years and 2 months, but with relative normoglycemia following segmental pancreatic transplantation. Such an interpretation of negative findings in a single patient must be treated as conjecture, and more clinical studies are being patiently awaited.

In the past, prospective studies have not been altogether conclusive in terms of relating the prevention of the development of neuropathy or vascular disease to strict chemical control.[7,8,11] However, the recent monumental study in Brussels of 4,400 patients observed by Pirart between 1947 and 1973 would support at least the relationship between higher levels of hyperglycemia and more frequent and/or more severe complications.[5]

Biochemical studies indicate that hyperglycemia or insulin deficiency produce alterations in vascular basement membrane composition, as well as accumulation of glucose-derived substances, such as sorbitol in the lens, the Schwann cell, and the aorta.[1,7,8,9,11] Various glycoproteins have been found to be elevated in diabetes.[1,3] Elevations of glycolysated hemoglobin (HbA_{1c}) have been found in the blood of diabetic mice as well as in human diabetic patients. The glycosylation of hemoglobin is a postsynthetic modification of HbA, which is dependent on the degree of duration of hyperglycemia.[3,7,8] This minor hemoglobin comprises 3 to 6 percent of normal human hemoglobin but is increased in uncontrolled diabetics. The measurement of this minor hemoglobin may be a better marker of diabetic control over a sustained period (at least 4 to 12 weeks) than hyperglycemia per se, and appears to be a most useful approach to the monitoring of the diabetic patient. Serial measurements of HbA_{1c}

concentrations may ultimately allow a real assessment of the control of diabetes to the development of acute or chronic complications. Studies of structural or enzymatic changes of other body proteins resulting from specific glycosylation reactions will probably give increased insight into the pathogenesis of capillary basement membrane thickening. Decreased reactivity of HbA_{1c} with 2,3-diphosphoglycerate may also impair oxygen unloading in poorly controlled diabetics and contribute to tissue hypoxia, which, in turn, may have pathogenetic implications in the development of diabetic angiopathy.[3]

Electron microscopic studies of capillary basement membrane of muscle from diabetic patients have yielded conflicting results. Some investigators suggest that basement membrane thickening is genetically predetermined, while others relate capillary basement membrane thickening to duration of diabetes.[6,8,11] Patient age, site of muscle biopsy, methodology of techniques, unknown actual duration of existing diabetes, as well as definitive criteria for the diagnosis of early or latent or chemical diabetes remain to be clarified before definite conclusions are drawn.

Lesions in the kidney, retina, and muscle have been described in experimentally induced diabetes of rats, dogs, and rhesus monkeys as well as in spontaneous diabetes of Chinese hamsters, KK mice, and Celebes apes. Retinal and glomerular capillary lesions in diabetic dogs appear to have been prevented by good chemical control with insulin therapy over a period of 5 years.[8] Studies of rats with long-standing chemically induced diabetes have been of great current interest.[3] Such rats ultimately develop glomerular mesangial lesions with immunoglobulin and complement deposition. These glomerular changes are reversible when an affected kidney is transplanted from the diabetic rat into a normal host. Transplantation of the pancreatic islets can reverse the diabetic state. In contrast, similar diabetic renal changes develop in normal kidneys transplanted into diabetic rats. These animal experiments suggest that nephropathy in these animals results from the diabetic state itself. Criticisms have been leveled against these animal studies, largely because the lesions produced in both small and large animals are not the counterparts of those found in human diabetics. Also, it has been noted that glomerular basement membrane thickening, which is one of the essential components of human diabetic nephropathy, has not been demonstrated in experimentally induced diabetes in animals.

A variety of functional and physiologic changes have been noted in diabetic patients.[3,11] These include increased red blood aggregation, decreased deformability of red blood cells, more intense platelet aggregation, decreased spontaneous fibrinolytic activity, and alterations in a variety of plasma proteins, all of which may exert an effect on blood viscosity and blood flow that may play a role in accelerating the rate of progression of diabetic angiopathy. Additionally, a number of functional abnormalities are present in the kidneys of patients with early diabetes, especially during poor control.[3] Normalization of these functions, namely glomerular filtration rate and albumin excretion, as well as changes in renal and glomerular size have been observed as a result of control of diabetes.

Elevation in growth hormone has been considered to be of significance in the pathogenesis of diabetic angiopathy, particularly retinopathy.[3,8] Exaggerated growth hormone response to exercise has been noted in poorly-controlled, insulin-dependent diabetics. Recently, normalization of growth hormone, as well as the catecholamine response to exercise, has been seen in juvenile-onset diabetic patients treated with a portable subcutaneous insulin infusion system.[10] Similar changes have been observed in glucagon levels after glucoregulation with an insulin infusion system.[12]

CONCLUSION

Whether reversal of hyperglycemia will affect the development of diabetic microangiopathy is far from settled. Consideration must be given to more intense regulation of dietary factors and exercise; availability and effectiveness of growth hormone-inhibiting agents; the use of substances which can interfere with the postribosomal steps of basement membrane assembly; use of selective glucagon inhibitors; and, finally, to improvements in the delivery of insulin, whether it be by closed- or open-loop insulin infusion systems or by increased knowledge of immunologic and other biologic defenses in the use of pancreatic transplantation.

References

1. Brownlee M and Cahill GF: Diabetic control and vascular complications. Atherosclerosis Reviews 4:30–69, Raven Press
2. Gliedman ML, Tellis VA, Rifkin H, et al: Pancreatic transplantation in human diabetes: long term results. Diabetes Care, 1, No 1: 1–9, Jan/Feb. 1978
3. McMillan DE and Ditzel J: Proceedings of a Conference on Diabetic Microangiopathy. Diabetes, 25, Supp 2: 805–930, 1976
4. Mauer MS, Barbosa J, Vernier RL, et al: Vascular lesions transplanted into diabetes, New Engl J Med 295:916–920
5. Pirart J: Diabetes mellitus and its degenerative complications: a prospective study of 4400 patients observed between 1947 and 1973. Diabetes Care, 1, No 3: 168–188, May–June 1978
6. Raskin P: Diabetes regulation and its relationship to microangiopathy, Metabolism, 27, No 2: 235–250, Feb 1978
7. Rifkin H: Why Control Diabetes? Med Clin N Amer 62: 4, 747–752, July 1978
8. Ross H and Rifkin H: Metabolic control and vascular disease in diabetes mellitus. *In* Clinical Diabetes: Modern Management 36–46, Podolsky S, (ed), Appleton-Century-Crofts, New York, 1980
9. Spiro RG: Search for a biochemical basis of diabetic microangiopathy. Diabetologia 12:1–14, 1976
10. Tamborlane WV, Sherwin RS, Koivisto V, et al: Normalization of the growth hormone and catecholamine response to exercise in juvenile-onset diabetic subjects treated with a portable insulin infusion pump. Diabetes, 28, No 8: 785–788, Aug 1979
11. Tchobroutsky G: Relationship of diabetic control to development of microvascular complications. Diabetologia 15:143, 1978
12. Raskin P, Pietri A, Unger RH: Changes in glucagon levels after four to five weeks of glucoregulation by portable insulin infusion pumps. Diabetes 28:1033–1035, 1979

28

Clinical Significance of Glycosylated Hemoglobin

Kenneth H. Gabbay, M.D.
Rudolf Flückiger, Ph.D.

In the last three decades, considerable controversy has arisen regarding the relationship of blood glucose control to the development of diabetic complications.[1] Our inability to accurately assess the degree of hyperglycemia has contributed to the lack of a consensus on a convincing long-term beneficial relationship. Knowles,[2] in his evaluation of the relationship of diabetic control to complications, concluded: "The most doubtful measurement of all is that of control. Herein, all studies falter, for it is impossible to determine with certainty the chemical state of patients during their day-to-day life and activity."

Recent investigations of the structure and biosynthesis of glycosylated hemoglobins have provided a means to objectively assess long-term blood glucose regulation in the diabetic patient. Although methodological problems and difficulties in interpretation of results still exist, the use of glycosylated hemoglobin levels as an integrated index of long-term blood glucose control represents a significant tool in our research and therapeutic armamentarium.

STRUCTURE AND BIOSYNTHESIS

Cation exchange chromatography of hemolysates of red blood cells resolves four minor hemoglobin components from the main

Hb A fraction. These minor components—Hb A_{1a1}, Hb A_{1a2}, Hb A_{1b}, and Hb A_{1c}—collectively referred to as the Hb A_1 fraction, result from post-translational non-enzymatic modification of Hb A and comprise about 7 percent of the total hemoglobin in normal subjects. Hb A_{1c} is the most abundant of the minor components and is present in increased amounts in patients with diabetes mellitus as a consequence of increased blood glucose levels. In Hb A_{1c}, a glucose molecule is attached to the N-terminal amino group of the β chains, initially as a Schiff base, which subsequently undergoes an Amadori rearrangement to a stable ketoamine linkage.[3] This process represents a post-translational glycosylation of Hb A within the red blood cell, occurring continuously throughout its 120-day life span in the circulation.

Hb A_{1a1} and Hb A_{1a2} are the β chain N-terminal adducts of fructose-1, 6-diphosphate, and glucose-6-phosphate, respectively, while Hb A_{1b} is thought to result from a deamidation in the β chain of Hb A_{1c}. In addition, glycosylation also occurs at the α chain N-terminal amino group as well as the ϵ-amino groups of lysine residues in both α and β chains. The extent of glycosylation at the various sites increases proportionately, indicating that hemoglobin glycosylation is a general and nonspecific process, with its extent determined primarily by the prevailing glucose concentration and the relative reactivities of the various amino groups.

GLYCOSYLATED HEMOGLOBIN AND DIABETIC CONTROL

From the structural and biosynthetic information available, it is clear that glycosylated hemoglobin is formed slowly and irreversibly by the condensation of two abundant reactants within the red blood cell, namely glucose and hemoglobin. With continuous accumulation of glycosylated hemoglobin, it is evident that the amount of this component should be a reflection of the average glucose concentration seen by the red blood cells during their life span. Direct evidence for this relationship derives from at least three lines of evidence, which include: (1) a reduction in glycosylated hemoglobin levels a few weeks after diabetic patients are brought under optimal blood glucose control; (2) a plethora of studies which demonstrate a relationship between glycosylated hemoglobin levels and a variety of diabetic control indices, and (3) excellent correlations between clinical evaluation of the patient's level of control and glycosylated hemoglobin levels (for detailed reviews, see References 3–5).

MEASUREMENT OF GLYCOSYLATED HEMOGLOBIN LEVELS

Hemoglobin glycosylation is currently estimated by two basic methodologies which operate on two different principles and which yield independent results that are, nevertheless, related. The chromatographic methodologies depend on a net change in the charge of the hemoglobin molecule when the N-terminal position of the β chain is glycosylated. Thus, the minor components Hb A_{1a-c} are eluted readily from a cation exchange resin and can be quantitated and expressed as a percentage of total hemoglobin. It should be realized that hemoglobin molecules glycosylated at sites other than the β N-termini do not have sufficiently altered net charge to enhance their mobilities and are hence not estimated by these techniques. These chromatographic separations are exquisitely sensitive to minor changes in pH and temperature, which can significantly affect the values obtained.

Separation based on charge differences is the basis for the standard Biorex-70 column chromatography, iso-electric focusing, high performance liquid chromatography, and the popular commercial minicolumn kits. The latter columns measure the sum of Hb A_{1a-c} (referred to as "fast hemoglobins"), and are particularly sensitive to temperature and pH changes. In general, the methodologies that depend on charge change are not readily amenable to standardization and long-term quality control procedures.

The other general type of methodology involves direct chemical measurement of total glycosylation. In one procedure,[6] furfural compounds are generated from the ketoamine-linked carbohydrate moieties on heating under acidic conditions and are quantitated colorimetrically with 2-thiobarbituric acid (TBA method). This test has many advantages (see below), provides an easily performed and reliable assessment of total glycosylation, and is particularly suited to quality control procedures and laboratory standardization.[7-9]

Finally, a radioimmunoassay has been described[10] for the determination of Hb A_{1c}. No information about its clinical application has been published to date.

LIMITATIONS OF THE ASSAY

Conditions such as uremia, the presence of fetal hemoglobin (Hb F), and certain unusual variants such as Hb H, Hb I and Hb $N_{Baltimore}$, aspirin intake, and alcoholism can all lead to falsely elevated glycosylated hemoglobin levels by the chromatographic techniques. These effects are caused by changes in charge of the hemoglobin molecule brought about by mechanisms other than glycosylation. In contrast, patients with variant hemoglobins such as Hb S, C, or D have erroneously low values because these hemoglobins bind more tightly to the cation exchange resin. In addition, glycosylated hemoglobin levels will be significantly reduced in patients with decreased red cell life span (e.g., anemia, uremia) or patients with active erythropoiesis (e.g., pregnancy).

It is now common practice to chromatograph whole blood hemolysates which may give rise to artifacts in two circumstances. In hyperlipemic blood samples, an increased "fast" hemoglobin fraction may result from interference by lactescence. In addition, when rapid column methods are used to measure Hb A_1, variable amounts of the labile aldimine species of Hb A_{1c} will be measured along with the stable ketoamine Hb A_{1c}. This problem does not arise if the hemolysates are dialyzed prior to chromatography. Specific determination of total hemoglobin glycosylation by chemical means (e.g., TBA method) circumvents all the above complications with the exception of the effect resulting from the decreased red blood cell life span.

INDICATIONS FOR USE OF GLYCOSYLATED HEMOGLOBIN

Clearly, estimation of glycosylated hemoglobin levels provides an important tool for clinical research in diabetes, particularly in the insulin-dependent diabetic patients where blood glucose levels may be subject to wide fluctuation. Such fluctuations in blood glucose seldom occur in noninsulin-dependent diabetic individuals under dietary and/or oral hypoglycemic agent therapy. The overall degree of glucose intolerance in such patients can be readily and more economically estimated by fasting blood glucose measurements. Of course, glycosylated hemoglobin levels can always be performed with the patient in the nonfasting state and, hence, may be more convenient in the management of diabetic patients, in general, and in office practice, in particular.

Glycosylated hemoglobin levels, indeed, have an important role to play in the routine management of insulin-dependent diabetic patients. For the first time, the physician can independently and objectively assess average diabetic control with minimal patient cooperation. Similarly, objective results may have a positive motivating influence on the patient by providing a target number of average blood glucose control. Comparisons of different treatment regimens or patient groups are now facilitated. As a diagnostic tool, estimation of glycosylated hemoglobins are not as discriminating in detecting subclinical borderline diabetes as the standard oral glucose tolerance test or even the fasting blood glucose level. Nevertheless, its convenience and lack of acute dependence on such variables as patient cooperation, time of day, stress, exercise, food intake, and renal threshold makes it an attractive screening test, particularly in population studies.

References

1. Cahill GF Jr, Etzwiler DD, and Freinkel N: "Control" and diabetes. Editorial, New Engl J Med 294:1004, 1976
2. Knowles HC Jr: The problem of the relation of the control of diabetes to the development of vascular disease. Trans Am Clin and Climatological Assoc 76:142–147, 1964
3. Bunn HF, Gabbay KH, and Gallop PM: The glycosylation of hemoglobin: Relevance to diabetes mellitus. Science 200:21–27, 1978
4. Gonen B and Rubenstein AH: Hæmoglobin A_1 and diabetes mellitus. Diabetologia 15:1–8, 1978
5. Bunn HF: Non-enzymatic glycosylation of hemoglobin and other proteins. Contemporary Hematology, Gordon AS, Silber R, LoBue J (eds), Plenum Press, 1980
6. Flückiger R and Winterhalter K: In vitro synthesis of hemoglobin A_{1c}. FEBS Letters 71:356–360, 1978

8. Saibene V, Brembilla L, Bertoletti A, et al: Chromatographic and colorimetric detection of glycosylated hemoglobins: A comparative analysis of two different methods. Clin Chem Acta 93:199–205, 1979

7. Gabbay KH, Sosenko JM, Banuchi GA, et al: Glycosylated hemoglobins: Increased glycosylation of hemoglobin A in diabetic patients. Diabetes 28:337–340, 1979

9. Pecoraro RE, Graf RJ, Halter JB et al: Comparison of a colorimetric assay for glycosylated hemoglobin with ion-exchange chromatography. Diabetes 28:1120–1125, 1979

10. Javid J, Pettis PK, Koenig RJ, et al: Immunologic characterization and quantification of hemoglobin A_{1c}. Brit J Hæmatol 38:329–337, 1978

29

Functional and Early Structural Changes in Diabetic Microangiopathy

Jørn Ditzel, M.D., Ph.D.
Donald E. McMillan, M.D.

INTRODUCTION

In recent years it has become increasingly apparent that functional rather than structural changes are the first alterations to occur in the microvasculature of diabetics (Figure 29-1). The concept that "functional microangiopathy" is an early event in diabetes, which both precedes and accompanies the anatomic small vessel changes of more advanced degenerative microangiopathy, has resulted.[1, 2]

THE DIABETIC RETINA

Normal retinal vessels are essentially impermeable to protein-bound fluorescein. When fluorescein is used to study the eye's vascular pattern, a healthy retina does not have any extravascular fluorescence. Before diabetic retinopathy is ophthalmoscopically detectable, fluorescein angiography may show venous dilatation, a more distinctly outlined capillary network in the macular area, and localized extravascular leakage.[3] These changes may be present prior to evidence of capillary closure and the subsequent appearance of microaneurysms. Using fluorescein angiography, we found evidence of an early breakdown of the blood-retinal barrier in 20 percent of glucose-intolerant subjects;

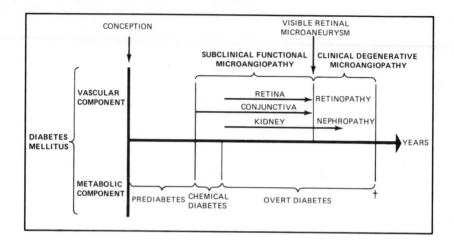

Figure 29-1. The vascular changes of diabetes begin with the readily reversible (subclinical) functional microangiopathy which precedes and accompanies the formation of permanent degenerative microangiopathy.

43 percent had fluorescein dots.[4] The technique of vitreous fluorophotometry has been applied to short-term diabetics without background retinopathy. It has shown that a breakdown of the blood-retinal barrier is the earliest detectable intraocular abnormality of diabetes. This permeability defect may be reversible with long-term regulation of blood glucose.[5] Thus, functional changes in the retinal vessels manifested by increased transvascular macromolecular passage may occur shortly after the onset of abnormalities in carbohydrate tolerance.

THE DIABETIC KIDNEY

Glomerular filtration rate (GFR) has been found increased by 25 to 30 percent in several studies of short-term juvenile diabetic subjects compared to nondiabetic subjects. A significantly increased filtration fraction (GFR/renal plasma flow) has also been noted in the early diabetics. These changes in renal function are compatible with the presence of a variable constrictive state of the efferent system leading to an increase in filtration pressure and with the increased total area of glomerular filtration surface also present.[6] The GFR elevation is nearly reversed by strict

regulation of carbohydrate metabolism. Acute insulin administration decreases both renal plasma flow and glomerular filtration rate.[7] Investigations of the permeability of microvessels to
macromolecules have also been performed in newly diagnosed
and short-term diabetics to test whether changes in permeability
precede or follow the developing basement membrane thickening. Ultrastructural thickening of the basement membrane is not
measurable in the glomerular capillaries at the onset of diabetes
but is detectable after one and a half year's duration. After that,
the basement membrane thickening increases with longer duration of disease.[6] Renal glomerular permeability to macromolecules has been assessed from the urinary excretion rate of
albumin (^{U}alb), and the entire circulation's microvascular permeability to plasma protein has been evaluated, using the transcapillary escape rate of albumin (TER), the fraction of intravas-
cular mass of albumin that passes to the extravascular space per
unit time.[8] Studies under poor metabolic control (TER) and during exercise (^{U}alb)[9] suggest that increased vascular plasma protein loss and water filtration both precede and accompany morphologic changes in the glomerulus. Both ^{U}alb and TER have
been reported as normal in adult short-term diabetics examined
during rest and in good metabolic control. These reversible
dynamic changes occur in kidneys of recent-onset juvenile
diabetics.

THE DIABETIC CONJUNCTIVA

Since study of a peripheral vascular bed could further understanding of the pathogenesis of the microangiopathy, one of us
(JD) has examined the cutaneous vessels of the bulbar conjunctiva. These vessels can be observed directly, and repeated
studies can be performed without interference with normal function. Studies using refined photographic techniques have demonstrated changes in these blood vessels at the earliest detectable disturbance in glucose tolerance. The early functional
changes include a labile microcirculation with variable arteriolar, capillary, and, particularly, venular dilatation, evidence of
increased volume flow, and augmented transcapillary plasma
fluid exchange. Many of these microvascular changes have been
shown to be reversible and improved by prolonged optimal regu-

lation of diabetes. Insulin administration induces acute vaso-constriction of both conjunctival arterioles and venules. The degree of conjunctival functional vascular change appears linked to the incidence and rate of development of diabetic retinopathy, suggesting that the functional changes may be the precursor of more advanced degenerative microangiopathic lesions.

BLOOD CHANGES LINKED TO FUNCTIONAL MICROANGIOPATHY

The reason for readily reversible responses in the small blood vessels is, at present, unknown. The reaction pattern of the microcirculation suggests a fluctuating condition of relative tissue hypoxia. One of us (JD) has described a defect in the oxygen delivery system of erythrocytes in both nonacidotic and acidotic diabetics.[10] An abrupt increase in hemoglobin-oxygen affinity affects the venous part of the microcirculation in a way similar to venous stasis. Other factors tend to act synergistically with the oxygen delivery defect in the microcirculation—increased blood viscosity, increased aggregation of erythrocytes, and decreased erythrocyte deformability. The combined hemorrheologic and oxygen affinity changes in the retina appear to give rise to dilatation of capillaries and venules, altering flow-pressure relations to favor opening of the interendothelial junctions, leading, in turn, to increased plasma protein and water passage through the walls of the small blood vessels. The administration of insulin in inappropriate dosage may induce sudden hypophosphatemia with secondary adverse effects on the microcirculation. Retinal venous dilatation is rapidly reversed by improved control. As duration of diabetes increases, the reversible functional alterations gradually become replaced by irreversible anatomic microvascular stiffening that limits the ability of the microcirculation to respond adaptively. Retinopathy will not develop as long as autoregulatory dilatation of the retinal arterioles can supply the metabolic needs of the tissue. When sclerosis has developed in the arterioles to a degree that will prevent their dilatation and the augmentation of blood flow, the retinal tissue will be permanently exposed to poorly compensated local hypoxia. This tissue hypoxia may act as a triggering mechanism for the development of capillary closure, endothelial proliferation, capillary microaneurysms, and neovascularization—the major components of diabetic retinopathy.

References

1. Ditzel J: Functional microangiopathy in diabetes mellitus. Diabetes 17:388–97, 1968
2. McMillan DE: Deterioration of the microcirculation in diabetes. Diabetes 24:944–57, 1975
3. Dorchy H and Toussaint D: Mise en évidence d'un trouble précoce de la perméabilité des capillaires rétiniens diabétiques par angiographic fluorescéinique. Journées Annuelles de Diabétologic de L'Hotel-Dieu, Flammarion Med Sc Paris: 35–45, 1979
4. Nielsen NV, Sørensen PN, and Ditzel J: Retinal fluorescein angiography and hemoglobin A_{Ic} in borderline diabetes. Diabete et Metabolisme 5:97–102, 1979
5. Cunha-Vaz JG, Fonseca JR, Abreu JF et al: A follow-up study by vitreous fluorophotometry of early retinal involvement in diabetes. Am J Ophthal 86:467–73, 1978
6. Kloustrup JP, Gundersen HJG, and Østerby R: Glomerular size and structure in diabetes mellitus. III Early enlargement of the capillary surface. Diabetologia 13:207–210, 1977
7. Mogensen CE, Christensen NJ, and Gundersen HJG: The acute effect of insulin on renal hæmodynamics and protein excretion in diabetics. Diabetologia 15:153–158, 1978
8. Mogensen CE and Vittinghus E: Urinary albumin excretion during exercise in juvenile diabetics. A provocation test for early abnormalities. Scand J Clin Lab Invest 35:295–300, 1975
9. Parving HH, Noer I, Deckert T, et al: The effect of metabolic regulation on microvascular permeability to small and large molecules in short-term juvenile diabetics. Diabetologia 12:161–66, 1976
10. Ditzel J, Nielsen NV, and Kjaergaard JJ: Hemoglobin A_{Ic} and red cell oxygen release capacity in relation to early retinal changes in newly discovered overt and chemical diabetics. Metabolism 28 Suppl 1:440–447, 1979

30

Diabetic Retinopathy

Paul Henkind, M.D., Ph.D.
Joseph B. Walsh, M.D.

INTRODUCTION

Retinopathy remains one of the major clinical problems of the diabetic patient. The ophthalmoscopically visible features such as microaneurysms, deep retinal hemorrhages, exudates, and new vessel formation are well known to clinicians. While not specific to diabetes, such lesions can be intimately associated with the disorder when they occur bilaterally, symmetrically, and show progression with time. While retinopathy may be the first clinical sign of diabetes, more frequently it is seen several years after onset of other symptoms, and only rarely is it totally absent in a diabetic of long standing.

LOSS OF VISION

Visual loss in diabetes mellitus most frequently develops as a result of intraretinal hemorrhage and exudation in the macular region. Profound visual disturbance is usually secondary to bleeding from retinal or optic disc neovascularization. In the latter instance, blood enters the vitreous cavity, either behind a collapsed vitreous or it admixes with the vitreous, and is only slowly resorbed. Resorption may take many months or years and recurrent bleeding often ensues.

Macular Edema: Within the past decade, ophthalmologists have recognized that many diabetics can have substantial loss of central vision as a result of macular edema. In such instances, it is postulated that there is a breakdown of the blood-retinal barrier with resultant accumulation of intraretinal fluid. The normal architecture of the retina is distorted and neuronal elements may be damaged. Initially the damage is reversible; later it may become permanent. This process occurs slowly, often without ophthalmoscopically visible hemorrhages and exudates. The first symptom noted by the patient is metamorphopsia—or visual distortion. Careful ophthalmoscopy may reveal macular edema evidenced as a "wetness" of the posterior pole with blunting of normal markings, including loss of the foveal reflex. Untreated, this condition often leads to progressive visual impairment. In a study of 247 untreated eyes with macular edema followed a mean of two years, 4.5 percent had improved vision, 57 percent were unchanged, and 38.5 percent had poorer vision.[1] Laser photocoagulation of the leaking sites demonstrated by fluorescein angiography may be beneficial. Among 265 treated eyes, 25 percent showed improved vision, 65 percent remained stable, and only 10 percent had diminished acuity.[1] A randomized double-blind controlled study of diabetic maculopathy is presently being conducted by the National Eye Institute.

BLOOD/RETINAL BARRIER

In 1975, Cunha-Vaz and colleagues[2] demonstrated, by vitreous fluorophotometry in humans, that there can be a significant disturbance in the blood-retinal barrier of diabetics prior to any clinically visible fundus lesions. More recently this same group[3] reported a series of 25 diabetic patients with "normal" fundi by ophthalmoscopy and fluorescein angiography who were studied over a period of 39 months. The results showed that breakdown of the blood-retinal barrier increased with the duration of the diabetic disease and was most marked in patients with poor metabolic control. This is one of the first scientific demonstrations of the value of diabetic control in stabilizing the blood-retinal barrier.

PROLIFERATIVE RETINOPATHY

It is postulated that proliferative retinopathy develops as a result of the liberation of a biochemical factor from hypoxic retina. The diabetic fundus prone to develop this complication shows, by fluorescein angiography, large areas of poor or absent retinal capillary perfusion. It has also been recently suggested that, in addition to a biochemical factor, the retinal vessels themselves must be diseased before they will start to proliferate.[4] The new vessels that grow out of the retinal or optic nerve vascular network possess thin walls which do not have a normal blood-retinal barrier. Thus, they are "leaky" to fluorescein, and presumably leak many molecules usually restricted from leaving normal retinal vessels. Such new vessels are prone to bleed, resulting in vitreous hemorrhage.

Current management of diabetics mandates careful observation of the fundus at periodic intervals. If new vessels are detected or suspected, then fluorescein angiography is indicated. The presence of such vessels requires immediate attention and treatment. Management is by panretinal photocoagulation, using either the xenon (white light) coagulator or argon laser. With this treatment modality, several thousand retinal burns are created during several treatment sessions. The theory is that such therapy converts hypoxic or metabolically deranged retina into totally anoxic retina incapable of liberating a vasculogenic factor. Initially, the neovascular tufts themselves are not directly coagulated; they often regress with adequate treatment. Remaining tufts may be directly obliterated by photocoagulation. The efficacy of such treatment has been documented by the Diabetic Collaborative Study of the National Eye Institute. According to the results of the Collaborative Study,[5] more than a quarter of affected untreated eyes lost vision compared to approximately 10 percent of treated eyes. Panretinal photocoagulation has also been found to be efficacious in the treatment of iris neovascularization, a dread complication which can cause intractable hemorrhagic glaucoma in the diabetic.

VITRECTOMY

Once vitreous hemorrhage occurs, it is no longer possible to perform photocoagulation of the retina. Also, if there is significant intravitreal fibrosis with traction on the retina, photocoagulation may be associated with an increase in the fibrosis and traction on the retina, leading to its detachment. Vitrectomy— entering the vitreous cavity with cutting instruments—can clear the vitreous hemorrhage and also cut traction bands that cause traction detachment of the retina. In one study of diabetic vitreous hemorrhage treated by vitrectomy, 66 percent of the cases showed some improvement in visual acuity.[6] In 7 percent of the cases, visual acuity declined. Some of the causes of decreased visual acuity were rubeosis iridis (iris neovascularization) leading to secondary glaucoma, traction detachment of the retina, or even endophthalmitis. In those cases with diabetic vitreous hemorrhage and detachment of the retina treated with vitrectomy, 50 percent of the patients showed some improvement of vision, and 14 percent of these cases had diminished visual acuity. In cases of vitreous hemorrhage, lack of visualization of the retina can often be overcome by the use of ultrasonography, and retinal function can be measured by electroretinography and the visual evoked response. Vitrectomy is beneficial in selected cases; the complications in diabetes remain high, and clarification of proper indications must await a double-blind study currently being performed by the National Institutes of Health.

PITUITARY ABLATION

There is a small group of juvenile diabetics who have what has been referred to as a malignant or accelerated phase of proliferative retinopathy. In these cases, there is a marked increase of neovascularization of the retina with a rapid downhill course that, in many cases, is not responsive to photocoagulation. In these cases, pituitary ablation may be an effective method of maintaining visual acuity.[7]

CONCLUSION

In patients with diabetic retinopathy, the major reason for diminished visual acuity is a slow process related to accumulation of edema and edema residues at the posterior pole of the eye. Photocoagulation may reduce the edema. With diabetic retinitis proliferans, panretinal photocoagulation may be beneficial. Once vitreous hemorrhage and/or traction on the retina has occurred, vitrectomy offers some benefit in improving or stabilizing the visual acuity, but the complications of this technique, particularly in diabetics, remains high. In the small group of juvenile diabetic patients with a florid onset of diabetic proliferative retinopathy, pituitary ablation may offer significant maintenance of visual acuity. Good control of the diabetic state seems essential to reduce the time of onset and severity of the retinopathy.

References

1. Patz A, Schatz H, Berkow JW, et al: Macular edema—An overlooked complication of diabetic retinopathy. Trans Amer Academ of Ophthal 77:34, 1973
2. Cunha-Vaz J, Abreu JR, Campos AJ, et al: Early breakdown of the blood-retinal barrier in diabetes. Br J Ophthal 59:649, 1975
3. Cunha-Vaz J, Fonseca JR, Abreu JF et al: A follow-up study by vitreous fluorophotometry of early retinal involvement in diabetes. Amer J Ophthal 86:467, 1978
4. Henkind P: Ocular neovascularization. Amer J Ophthal 85:287, 1978
5. Diabetic Retinopathy Study Research Group. Photocoagulation treatment of proliferative diabetic retinopathy: the second report of the Diabetic Retinopathy Study findings. Ophthal 85:82, 1978
6. Peyman GA, Huamonte FU, Goldberg MF, et al: Four hundred consecutive pars plana vitrectomies with the vitrophage. Arch Ophthal 96:45, 1978
7. Valone JA and McMeel JW: Severe adolescent onset proliferative diabetic retinopathy, the effect of pituitary ablation. Arch Ophthal 96:1349, 1978

31

Diabetic Neuropathy

Max Ellenberg, M.D.

The importance of diabetic neuropathy derives from its remarkable frequency and its clinical impact. The scope of involvement is widespread, with virtually every system at risk. Although peripheral neuropathy is by far the most common expression, visceral neuropathy is highly significant. Neuropathy in diabetes offers a specific and important diagnostic challenge to the clinician and plays a definitive role in differential diagnosis. The problem is heightened by the fact that any and all of the diabetic neuropathic syndromes may be the initial clinical manifestation of diabetes in the absence of covert manifestations of carbohydrate metabolic disorders.

There has been considerable controversy over the basic aspects of this complication, including pathology, pathogenesis, etiology, metabolic and electrophysiological implications, and the clinical course.

Pathology: The vasa vasorum have been shown to be involved in some cases. Another established pathological finding is ischemic infarction. The motor endplate may be altered in diabetic neuropathy in the early stages of juvenile diabetes. The most common finding is segmental demyelination of peripheral nerve fibers. Since the myelin sheath is formed by spiral folding of the Schwann cell surface membrane, the implication is that diabetic neuropathy may result from an interference with the metabolic activity of the Schwann cell. The location of the pathology varies markedly and may be in the spinal cord, posterior root ganglion, or the peripheral nerves. All these changes have been described as occurring independently and in combination. An intriguing and as yet unexplained observation is the marked discrepancy between the severity of the pathologic findings and the relative paucity of the clinical findings in many instances.[1]

Metabolism: There are definite metabolic aberrations underlying nerve affection in diabetes. Involvement of the sorbitol pathway in the intermediate metabolism of diabetic neural tissue has been demonstrated. In the animal treated with alloxan, the isolated nerve response to a significant elevation in the blood sugar is increased formation of sorbitol and its retention within the nerve fibers. Most exciting, this impairment is reversible in the experimental animal with lowering of the blood sugar to normal levels;[2] however, this observation has yet to be demonstrated in man.

Depletion of myoinositol has been suggested as an underlying cause of diabetic neuropathy. It may well prove to be a reflection of the deterioration that ensues.

Electrophysiology: In addition to the established abnormalities seen in clinical neuropathy, measurements of motor nerve conduction velocity, as well as electromyography and sensory perception in man, have shown abnormalities present at the early onset of diabetes, including juvenile diabetes. Sensory nerve conduction may be impaired at the onset of diabetes and may be the most sensitive index of peripheral neuropathy. Although these measurements suggest early involvement of the nervous system in diabetes, one must note that these abnormalities are not accompanied by clinical symptoms, that the relationship to the eventual development of the clinical syndrome of diabetic neuropathy has not been established, and that, actually, most juvenile diabetics do not develop diabetic neuropathy until many years later. Furthermore, the improvement reported in motor nerve conduction velocity following the institution of good control more likely reflects the associated alteration of hydration and electrolyte concentrations in the perineural milieu than any change in nerve pathology, the latter probably not being present at this stage.

Clinical: The diversity of observation is even more in evidence in the clinical aspects of diabetic neuropathy encompassing a polymorphous group of syndromes, which range from an acute onset with a short duration and reversibility to an insidious onset that is inexorably progressive and entirely irreversible. The symptoms also exhibit the widest range of manifestations.

The diverse findings, as outlined above, instead of being contradictory, indicate that there are different kinds of neuropathies in diabetes. Thus, there is no such entity as diabetic neuropathy; rather, there are *diabetic neuropathies.* This is an important concept that explains so many of the diverse hypotheses and controversial arguments in this field. Consequently, no single generalization or generalizations can explain all the manifestations of the varying diabetic neuropathies.

Clinical Manifestations: The clinical syndromes associated with diabetic neuropathy have been amply detailed and described in the literature. It is important to recognize that new entities have been recorded and that many advances have been made in reevaluating known entities so that better clinical appraisal, treatment, and prognosis can be achieved. Among these are the asymmetric neuropathies, including the truncal mononeuropathies and diabetic amyotrophy. A newly described syndrome is diabetic neuropathic cachexia. Diabetic gastropathy, esophageal neuropathy, and, more recently, autonomic nerve involvement of the cardiovascular neurogenic reflexes have been documented. The neuropathic pathogenesis accounting for the increased frequency of impotence in the diabetic male and retrograde ejaculation has been established. A more fundamental understanding and therapy for some of the older known neuropathic syndromes in diabetes have been achieved. For example: pathogenesis of the neuropathic ulcer has been elucidated, leading to improved treatment; neuropathy of the upper extremity has been more clearly defined; the significance of absent deep reflexes, as well as bilateral interosseous atrophy of the hand as a clue to the existence of unrecognized diabetes, has been appreciated; the improved therapy of neuropathic arthropathy; a realization of the spontaneous self-limited clearing of the mononeuropathies, especially external oculomotor paralysis; the improved therapy resulting from the elucidation of the basic pathophysiology of the neurogenic paralytic bladder, as well as recognition of the asymptomatic incipient neurogenic bladder and its implications in the increased frequency of urinary tract infection.[3,4]

The Autonomic Nervous System: Briefly summarized, the cardiovascular reflexes maintain physiological homeostasis by reflecting the constant flux on demand imposed by external environmental influences. These reflexes are mediated via the autonomic nervous system. Thus, autonomic neuropathy in diabetes may have a profound effect in impeding or even eliminating the ability to respond. The impairment of these basic reflexes involves precisely those areas where arteriosclerotic changes are most prominent in the diabetic; i.e., the brain, heart, and foot. The inability to respond, and thus maintain, homeostasis suggests the possibility that these features superimposed on the existing severe arteriosclerosis may play a role in the precipitation of, or be a contributory determinant to, the vascular events which are so common in diabetes and which are the chief cause of morbidity and mortality in this disease.[5]

Therapy: In peripheral neuropathy, phenytoin and carbamazepine have been used with a measurable degree of success, although they are clearly not panaceas. Since depression is part of the syndrome of peripheral neuropathy, the use of an antidepressant is helpful. The Charcot joint is improved considerably by the prolonged use of a walking cast. The neuropathic ulcer is treated by a number of orthopedic appliances, the best of which is probably an inner space sole which alleviates the pressure on the ulcer site. It is important to reemphasize that the mononeuropathies are self-limiting and spontaneously reversible in most instances and may recover in approximately three months. Diabetic gastropathy frequently responds to the use of metoclopramide. At least half the cases of diabetic diarrhea are helped by the use of a broad spectrum antibiotic. The neurogenic paralytic bladder is successfully treated by conservative medical measures in many instances and, if these fail, then a relatively simple surgical procedure consisting of destruction of the internal vesical sphincter produces a dramatic result. Retrograde ejaculation will occasionally respond to the use of antihistamines which have a sympathomimetic action. This failing, the centrifugation of a catheterized postmasturbation urine specimen and the insertion of the separated sperm into the uterine canal may result in pregnancy. Diabetic impotence can be helped by two surgical procedures, one of which is the implantation of a silicone prosthesis into the corpora cavernosa and the other is the implantation of a silicone elastic prosthesis with a fluid reservoir, all of which is controlled by a pump located in the scrotum. Orthostatic hypotension is helped by 9-alpha-fluorohydrocortisone or the use of an Air Force antigravity suit.[3]

Therefore, the diagnosis of the syndromes of diabetic neuropathy, as manifested clinically, is more than an academic exercise, since most carry, if not a cure, at least some specific therapeutic modality that can be offered to the patient.

References

1. Dolman CL: The morbid anatomy of diabetic neuropathy. Neurology 13:135, 1962
2. Gabbay KH, O'Sullivan JB: The sorbitol pathway. Diabetes 17:239, 1968
3. Ellenberg M: Diabetic autonomic neuropathy: role in vascular events. NY State J Med 78:2214, 1978
4. Rundles RW: Diabetic neuropathy. Medicine 24:111, 1945
5. Ellenberg M: Diabetic neuropathies: clinical aspects. Metabolism 25:1627, 1976

32

Renal Impairment in Diabetes Mellitus

Philip D. Lief, M.D.

While diabetes mellitus is a truly multisystem disease, the renal manifestations are particularly important for several reasons. First, nephropathy affects a sizeable proportion of patients with diabetes, especially in the younger age group. Second, diabetic nephropathy assumes great clinical significance since it is associated with substantial morbidity and mortality. Third, recent experimental and clinical evidence has suggested that proper control of carbohydrate metabolism may slow or even reverse some of the specific renal lesions in diabetes, offering hope that these complications may some day be prevented.

In this review, we shall consider some renal diseases which are either specific or nonspecific for the diabetic, focusing on clinical and differential diagnostic features and on management.

SPECIFIC DIABETIC NEPHROPATHY

Within 20 years of the onset of diabetes, clinical and pathologic evidence of renal disease may be found in nearly all patients, especially in the juvenile group.[1] The most specific pathologic entity, nodular glomerulosclerosis, was described by Kimmelsteil and Wilson in 1936.[2] This lesion, an eosinophilic nodule at the periphery of the glomerulus, has a laminated appearance on PAS staining. The nodules are of progressively increasing size, are deposited in the endothelial or intracapillary cells, and may eventually distort or obliterate the capillaries of the glomerulus. A less pathognomonic, but much more frequent, lesion is the diffuse glomerulosclerosis described by Bell.[3] In this lesion, PAS positive material is deposited diffusely in the walls of the capillaries and in the mesangium, with progressive narrowing and eventual obliteration of vessels.

Both lesions, but particularly diffuse glomerulosclerosis, are associated with a characteristic clinical syndrome.[1,4,5] Very early in the course, glomerular filtration rate may be supranormal, and urinary albumin excretion may be increased, particularly with exercise. As time passes, there is a slow but inexorable decline in GFR but with progressive increase in urinary protein excretion. While considerable variation exists among individuals, abnormal proteinuria is generally noted 15–18 years after the onset of diabetes, and renal insufficiency within 2–4 years of that. A significant number of patients develop hypertension, usually after the onset of renal insufficiency, and the full nephrotic syndrome occurs with great frequency (70–90 percent).

The diagnosis of diabetic nephropathy is usually clear, with the typical features occurring in a patient with a prior history of documented, long-standing diabetes, usually with some evidence of diabetic retinopathy. However, in some patients, the absence of retinopathy or the lack of a history of diabetes may lead to consideration of other forms of renal disease, particularly idiopathic membranous glomerulopathy. Occasionally, renal biopsy may be required to distinguish these conditions. However, in contrast to the slow rate of progression and frequent remission of nephrosis in membranous nephropathy, diabetic nephropathy progresses relentlessly, with worsening of the clinical and chemical features of the disease. End-stage uremia occurs within 2–4 years of the onset of clinical signs in nearly all patients.

Treatment of the renal manifestations of diabetes may be considered in two phases. In the early stages of the disease, salt and water restriction and an appropriate diuretic regimen may help to control the edema and congestion associated with the nephrotic syndrome. Additionally, antihypertensive therapy should be employed when indicated.

In the later stages when severe renal insufficiency ensues, appropriate dietary restrictions and, ultimately, substitution therapy with dialysis or transplantation (vide infra) may be required.

NONSPECIFIC CONDITIONS

Although they are not always specifically attributable to diabetes, there are a number of conditions which commonly affect renal function in the diabetic.[6] First, neurogenic bladder dysfunction can be demonstrated in more than 80 percent of patients with neuropathy. The condition may dispose either to acute urinary retention or to moderate, but persistent, obstructive uropathy. A proper index of suspicion and prompt correction of obstruction can prevent acceleration toward renal failure. Second, because of the multiple factors in intrinsic susceptibility to infection, glycosuria, and decreased renal medullary blood flow, urinary tract infection is quite common in diabetes. This complication can also lead to loss of kidney function and, therefore, should be diagnosed and treated appropriately. Third, when infection and obstruction occur together, renal papillary necrosis, an ischemic infarction of the renal medullae and papillae is more likely. In this syndrome, patients develop flank pain, fever, oliguria or anuria, and may suffer total loss of renal function. A fourth, and important, renal complication occurring with increased frequency in diabetic patients is acute renal failure caused by radiographic contrast media.[7] While a variety of factors, including dehydration, uricosuria, albuminuria, Tamm Horsfall proteinuria, nephrotoxicity of contrast media, and allergy have been suggested as potential causes, the precise etiology of this complication is unknown. Management is similar to that of any form of acute renal failure. The prognosis for recovery is good in patients who have good baseline renal function; however, significant long-term impairment of function occurs in some patients, particularly those with already advanced nephropathy.

SUBSTITUTION THERAPY

Both dialysis and transplantation have been employed in the care of diabetic patients with end-stage renal failure.[8,9] Analysis of these treatments will be discussed in Chapter 33. Results with hemodialysis or peritoneal dialysis have been fair, with mortality greater than 30 percent per year and substantial morbidity from progression of vascular and retinal disease. Renal transplantation, though much less widely employed, appears to offer a somewhat better prognosis, though complications in this group are related to surgery, vascular disease, immunosuppression, and infections. Since neither form of substitution therapy is ideal, improvement in the fate of patients with diabetic renal disease appears to rest with developments in blood glucose control or in areas as yet unexplained.

References

1. Goldstein DA and Massry SG: Diabetic nephropathy. Nephron 20:286, 1978
2. Kimmelstiel P and Wilson C: Intercapillary lesions in the glomeruli of the kidney. Am J Path 12:83, 1936
3. Bell ET: A postmortem study of vascular disease in diabetics. Arch Pathol 53:444, 1952
4. Kussman MJ, Goldstein H, and Gleason RE: The clinical course of diabetic nephropathy. JAMA 236:1861, 1976
5. Mogensen CE: Renal function changes in diabetes. Diabetes 25, Suppl 2:872, 1976
6. Arieff AI: Kidney, water and electrolyte metabolism in diabetes mellitus. *In* The Kidney, WB Saunders Co, Philadelphia 1976
7. Diaz-Buxo JA, Wagoner RD, Hattery RR, et al: Acute renal failure after excretory urography in diabetic patients. Ann Int Med 83:155, 1975
8. Johnson WJ: End-stage renal disease in the diabetic. Mayo Clinic Proc 52:335, 1977
9. Zancke H, Woods JE, Sterioff S, et al: Renal transplantation in patients with diabetes mellitus—revisited. Transplantation Proc 11:55, 1979

33

Kidney Transplantation As Treatment For the Renal Complications of Diabetes

Frederick C. Goetz, M.D.

My purpose is to describe a new phase in the life of the diabetic patient—what it is like to survive end-stage diabetic glomerulosclerosis by means of a kidney transplant.

The report will be based largely on the series with which I am most familiar, that under the care of the surgical and medical services of the University of Minnesota Hospitals in Minneapolis. I will add comparisons with other large series in the United States and Scandinavia, as well as a summary of world experience in transplantation and dialysis for kidney patients.

RELUCTANCE TO TRANSPLANT THE DIABETIC PATIENT

Although 2,500 or more new cases of end-stage diabetic glomerulosclerosis probably occur each year in the United States alone, transplantation units have been slow to respond to this enormous need. Our own series began formally in 1969, but by 1972 only 19 cases had been recognized by the world-wide transplantation registry, providing a trivial 0.3 percent of the cumulative experience of more than 5,000 transplants reported in that year, the ninth year of the registry.

Why has there been such reluctance to meet what appears to be a pressing need? Three arguments, all reasonable, have usually been raised against the proposal to transplant a kidney into a diabetic patient:

1. Diabetic patients with renal failure are poor surgical risks; they will have a small chance of surviving the process of transplantation itself.

2. Even if they survive the procedure, they will be seriously handicapped by other major problems, especially blindness.

3. There is also a possibility that the diabetic lesion may recur rapidly and destroy the transplanted kidney.

The conclusion was drawn by many groups that transplanting the diabetic patient would thus be a futile exercise and a waste of a kidney.

On consideration, we rejected these arguments as unproven hypotheses and planned a trial of transplantation in advanced diabetic patients.

GENERAL DESCRIPTION OF THE TRIAL

Beginning in mid-1969, patients with advanced kidney failure presumed due to diabetic kidney disease were offered kidney transplantation. In the first six months, five patients were given new kidneys. The number has increased year by year; it is now up to about 70 per year, with a cumulative total over ten years of 300 patients actually transplanted one or more times.

Almost all of the subjects are, by conventional clinical evidence, youth-onset, insulin-dependent diabetic subjects. The mean age at transplantation is 31 (range 18–64); duration of diabetes is usually 15–20 years. At first, transplantation was offered when the serum creatinine concentration had reached 10 mg/dl or more; the creatinine clearance was at 10 percent of normal or less. In the last five years, the criteria have been modified so that patients are now transplanted more commonly when the serum creatinine is only at about 6 mg/dl or creatinine clearance below 20 percent of normal.

SURVIVAL

The series is now large enough so that cumulative survival figures for at least the first four years have a very small standard error; this allows some useful comparisons with the experience with nondiabetic recipients to be made.

Table 33-1 shows that somewhat more than 60 percent of all diabetic subjects in this series survived for at least four years. This figure by itself is encouraging, although it is clearly not as great as survival of nondiabetic cases.

Table 33-1. Cumulative Survival of Adult Diabetic and Nondiabetic Patients After Kidney Transplant.
(University of Minnesota, 1969-1979.)

Donors	Diabetic Patients			Nondiabetic Patients		
	No. of patients at zero time	Percent surviving		No. of patients at zero time	Percent surviving	
		At 1 yr.	At 4 yrs.		At 1 yr.	At 4 yrs.
HLA-identical siblings	55	95	85	73	98	98
Living non-HLA identical	141	80	60	173	90	85
Cadaver	109	75	60	216	80	70
All cases	305	80	65	462	90	80

Some interesting points of difference appear when the diabetic cases are considered according to the source of the donated kidney. When the source is a living sibling with perfect matching by tissue typing (HLA identical), which is true in about 1/6 of our diabetic cases, the survival is extremely good and is only slightly below that of nondiabetic cases. When the source is a living relative who is not closely matched (HLA non-identical), as in 1/2 of our cases, the survival is considerably less good—and not clearly better than the remaining 1/3 of cases who received their kidneys from an unrelated cadaver donor.

It appears that, for the diabetic as for the nondiabetic uremic patient, availability of a donor who is not only living but is HLA-identical (inevitably a sibling) gives the best chance for prolonged survival.

Survival beyond four years is less clearly documented because the number of patients is fairly small; however, two of the original group of five patients have survived for ten years and continue to do well. There does not appear to be any great change in mortality after 4–5 years. The greatest risk of death is in the first year or 18 months.

CAUSES OF DEATH

Causes of death in the Minnesota series are indicated in Table 33-2. The two major problems are, clearly, cardiovascular disease and infection. Cardiovascular causes include, especially, documented myocardial infarction and unexplained sudden death, with evidence of advanced coronary disease at postmortem. Infections are of all kinds: bacterial, yeast, fungi, and virus. In recent years, viral infection—especially cytomegalovirus (CMV)—is a major threat to life. Most commonly, signs of infection appear 2–12 months after transplantation and, fortunately, often are relatively mild. However, fatal cases have been observed as long as five years after transplantation. Other causes include dialysis-related deaths in patients who have received a cadaver kidney, with temporary renal shutdown after transplantation.

Table 33-2. Causes of Death in Kidney Transplant Recipients.

	Minneapolis— 418 Nondiabetic Cases*	Minneapolis— 132 Diabetic Cases*	Scandinavia— 146 Diabetic Cases**
Cardiovascular	10 deaths	12 deaths	35 deaths
Sepsis	59 deaths	21 deaths	23 deaths
Dialysis and other	21 deaths	11 deaths	21 deaths
All cases	90 deaths	44 deaths	79 deaths

*Data adapted from Sutherland, et al (7).
**Data adapted from Joint Scandinavian Report (3).

For comparison, causes of death are also shown as taken from a recent large series compiled in Scandinavia.[3] The highest mortality in this Scandinavian diabetic series is attributable to more cardiovascular- and dialysis-related deaths; these, in turn, may be related to the preponderance of cadaver-donor kidneys reported from Scandinavia. Use of living related donors has been relatively rare in Europe up to the present. For the approximately 1/5 of the Scandinavian cases who received a kidney from a living donor, the survival appears to be just as good as that in the Minnesota series.

When diabetic and nondiabetic survival is compared within the Minnesota experience, the cardiovascular deaths—not infection—appear to account for most of the increased mortality for the diabetics.

THE KIDNEY AFTER TRANSPLANTATION INTO THE DIABETIC PATIENT

The most important statement that can be made is that the *function* of the transplanted kidney shows no signs of a progressive decline—for as long as ten years after transplantation. Two of our 1969 patients have now reached the ten-year mark. One of them maintains a normal serum creatinine at 1.3 mg/dl and a creatinine clearance of about 75 ml per minute, an excellent value for a single kidney. The other showed a moderate decline in kidney function within one year after transplantation, with evidence of fairly marked rejection on biopsy. Her serum creatinine level, however, has remained stable at 2.0 to 2.5 mg/dl for the subsequent nine years. The course of these two patients is representative of the whole group, aside from a small number of technical failures which have led to transplantation of a second kidney for a few.

Most of the patients have remained free of proteinuria, although at six to ten years, slight but persistent proteinuria is appearing in the urine of some. Hypertension, in general, is well-controlled after transplantation, although many patients require fairly heavy medication to accomplish this.

Only one subject has passed rapidly through what might be thought of as an accelerated course of diabetic nephropathy in less than three years after transplant, including a phase of full-blown nephrotic syndrome. He has now received a second kidney transplant and the course has not been repeated.

In contrast to the absence of changes in kidney function, definite changes in kidney morphology have been found. In biopsies taken at 2–4 years, more than 90% of biopsies in more than 20 patients show characteristic changes in the glomeruli and tubules. These include: hyalinosis of both afferent and efferent arterioles; thickening of both capillary and tubular basement membrane; and adherence of both albumin and immune globulin to glomerular and tubular basement membrane, as revealed by immunofluorescent methods. Thickening of the capillary basement membrane appears to be not specific to the diabetic transplanted kidney and is seen also in nondiabetic cases. The other changes, however, appear to be nearly specific for diabetes.[8] No classical Kimmelstiel-Wilson nodules have been recognized, however, even 8 years after transplantation (a single biopsy at this stage is available so far). Thus, it appears clear that changes consistent with diabetes develop after transplantation, but the overall course, fortunately, is a gradual one.

THE EYES

All but a very few of the patients selected for transplantation showed significant or serious retinopathy—usually the proliferative form—at the time of transplantation (Table 33-3). Careful prospective observation of ophthalmologists, especially Dr. Robert Ramsay, have confirmed the initial impression of Dr. C. M. Kjellstrand that vision stabilizes in the first six months to one year after kidney transplantation. It has not been considered ethical to withhold other treatments, especially photocoagulation, so that clear assignment of the benefit solely to improvement in kidney function cannot be made with certainty. However, a small number of eyes that have not received photocoagulation treatment have done as well as the photocoagulated eyes. Overall, as long as 10 years after transplantation, most of the patients retained useful vision in at least one eye.

Table 33-3. Vision in 134 Eyes of Diabetic Patients Before and After Kidney Transplantation.

Visual acuity (meters)	Baseline (No. of eyes)	Final* (No. of eyes)
Good (6/15 or better)	66	69
Impaired (6/21 to 6/30)	14	13
Poor (6/60 or worse)	54	52

*After 1 to 7 years; median, 3 years.
Adapted from Ramsay, et al (5).

The appearance of the retinae is a strikingly uniform progression to a quiescent, involutional stage. Massive hemorrhage becomes infrequent or absent. Function is still abnormal, however, and this can be brought out by specific testing, such as for color vision. It is possible that a very slow further attrition of vision is going on, possibly through progressive ischemia of the retina. For the present, however, most of the patients who have had some vision at the time of transplantation are able to maintain it for many years.

It should be underscored that we have not ruled out transplantation, even in the presence of complete blindness, so that some patients labor under this handicap from the time of transplantation.

NEUROLOGICAL CHANGES

The explanation for the severe muscle weakness often developing late in the course of diabetic kidney disease must certainly be complex, although it tends to be discussed under the heading of "peripheral neuropathy." Almost certainly it has both diabetic and uremic components. In any case, the return of excellent or even normal function in the first six months to one year after kidney transplantation is one of the most gratifying aspects of the clinical course. It is *not* accompanied by parallel improvement in objective measurements such as motor or sensory nerve conduction velocity.

Symptoms due to autonomic neuropathy may also improve. Especially striking is the disappearance of diarrhea and incontinence of stool, even when it had an apparently typical "diabetic" pattern, with the worst symptoms at night. Occasional observations of upper gut motility by barium study still show a delay in emptying. At the same time, symptoms of poor gastric emptying have usually disappeared. Again, it appears that there is a uremic, as well as a diabetic, component in these symptoms, but the precise details of the disturbance and its relief remain to be worked out.

Bladder emptying may improve to some extent, but this is variable. Surprisingly, an occasional patient has managed to do well for as long as 2–3 years, with occasional self-catheterization as the price of continued bladder atony.

Postural blood pressure drops are often much worse immediately after transplantation, especially if there has been a preceding nephrectomy because of especially severe hypertension. Fortunately, severe symptoms of postural blood pressure drop can usually be relieved by cutting back on drugs, increasing salt intake, and so on.

OTHER VASCULAR DISEASE

Nonfatal strokes, progressive congestive heart failure, and nonfatal myocardial infarction certainly occur, but less commonly than one might have expected. More obvious disability is due to vascular disease of the limbs. Not surprising is the frequency of loss of one leg or (fortunately, rarely) both. More surprising has been the development of lesions in the *upper* extremity. More than 20 fingers and two hands have been amputated because of progressive painful ulceration. The explanation for this problem, which is certainly extremely unusual in the spontaneous course of diabetes, is not yet clear.

WHAT KIND OF LIFE?

The patient and families of prospective diabetic transplant recipients naturally want to know the overall picture of life which may lie ahead of them.

It should be pointed out to them that perhaps as many as 1/3 of the patients surviving transplantation have some degree of handicap, either from blindness or loss of a limb. But the remaining 70 percent are doing reasonably well (see Table 33-4).

Table 33-4, based on an assessment by Lois Recker, R.N., and Marvin Haymond, Social Service, shows that a majority of diabetic patients can return to an active life, although activity does not necessarily include earning money.

Overall, about 70 percent of our patients have a chance of surviving for at least five years, and 70 percent of those are doing "well." We wish the results were even better than this, but they are better than we expected at the beginning.

Table 33-4. Vocational Status of 82 Survivors Out of 125 Diabetic Kidney Transplant Patients.

Status 6 months after transplantation	No. of patients	Percentage of total
Active		
Work full-time	25	
Work part-time	4	
Active at home or in avocation	27	
Student	5	
Subtotal	61	74
Inactive		
Disabled (blindness, amputation)	16	
Poor motivation, unemployed	4	
Subtotal	21	26
TOTAL	82	100

Adapted from Haymond, et al. (6).

WORLD EXPERIENCE —DIALYSIS VS. TRANSPLANTATION FOR DIABETIC PATIENTS

The experiences of the Mayo Clinic and Joslin Clinic with kidney transplantation are quite compatible with ours. Although world experience is still small in proportion to the magnitude of the problem, it is uniform in showing the relatively good outlook for the diabetic patient who has survived the "first tumultuous year"[9] after transplantation. This is especially true if the donor is a closely-related and well-matched relative. In fact, Kjellstrand has estimated that current figures suggest that those surviving after one year share a prospect of 50 percent survival time ($t_{1/2}$) of as long as 12 years! In contrast, chronic hemodialysis, although current techniques have much improved the outlook for survival, still does not appear to offer better than an approximately 50 percent survival chance at 3 years. There is a suggestion from cumulative data that the percentage of diabetic patients dying on dialysis remains the same year after year.

FINAL COMMENTS

Both hemodialysis and transplantation are costly methods of saving lives, but it seems inescapable that the diabetic patient has as much right to these as anyone else with chronic renal failure. In fact, our commitment to the youth-onset diabetic patient clearly began with the introduction of insulin treatment more than 50 years ago. What is clearly needed is a commitment also to the continued search for better understanding of the causes of diabetic renal disease and, ultimately, for simpler and cheaper treatments.

ACKNOWLEDGMENTS

The clinical data summarized here are based on the study of patients on the medical and surgical services of the University of Minnesota Hospitals. Dr. John Najarian, Dr. Carl Kjellstrand, Dr. Jose Barbosa, and Lois Recker, R.N. have been especially close collaborators throughout; Justine Willmert, R.N. and Lois Bartell, R.N., Transplant Nurse Coordinators, have organized the overall care of the patients with a high standard of quality. Many other colleagues have also contributed to their care.

References

1. Najarian J, Sutherland D, Simmons R, et al: Kidney transplantation for the uremic diabetic patient. Surg Gynecol Obstet 144: 682–690, 1977
2. Najarian J, Sutherland D, Simmons R, et al: Ten year experience with renal transplantation in juvenile onset diabetics. Annals Surg (In Press)
3. Joint Scandinavian Report: Renal transplantation in insulin-dependent diabetics. Lancet 2: 915–917, 1978
4. Zincke H, Woods J, Sterioff S, et al: Renal transplantation in patients with diabetes mellitus—revisited. Transplant Proc 11: 55–59, 1979
5. Ramsay R, Knobloch W, Barbosa J, et al: The visual status of diabetic patients after renal transplantation. Am J Ophthalmol 87: 305–310, 1979
6. Haymond M, Recker L, Willmert J: Vocational rehabilitation status of 125 diabetic transplant recipients. Dial & Transplant 8: 52–56, 1977
7. Sutherland D, Kjellstrand C, Simmons R, et al: Renal transplantation in the diabetic. Minnesota Medicine 59: 766–771, 1976
8. (a) Mauer S, Barbosa J, Vernier R, et al: Development of diabetic vascular lesions in normal kidneys transplanted into patients with diabetes mellitus. N Engl J of Med 295: 916–920, 1976
   (b) Mauer S, Miller K, Goetz F, et al: Immunopathology of renal extracellular membranes in kidneys transplanted into patients with diabetes mellitus. Diabetes 25: 709–712, 1976
9. Kjellstrand C, Goetz F, Najarian J: Transplantation and dialysis in diabetic patients. (In Preparation, 1979)

34

Diabetic Peripheral Vascular Disease

Marvin E. Levin, M.D.

Peripheral vascular (P-V) disease in the diabetic is common and expensive. Approximately 30 percent of all diabetics eventually develop P-V disease, and 20 percent of all diabetics admitted to the hospital are for foot problems resulting from P-V disease and/or diabetic neuropathy. Fifty to 70 percent of all nontraumatic amputations in the United States occur in diabetics, although only 3 percent of the diabetic population are amputees at any one time.[1] This is due to the early death of these patients from heart attack and stroke. The monetary cost of a period of hospitalization ultimately resulting in amputation can run from five to seven thousand dollars, and the annual cost for diabetic-related P-V disease in this country easily exceeds one hundred million dollars per year.[1] Add to this the cost of time lost from work, probable loss of job, disability pay, and loss of gross national product, and it is evident that the financial aspects of diabetic foot lesions can be astronomical.

RISK FACTORS

Risk factors in P-V disease vary from series to series. In the Framingham Study, the strongest risk factor for intermittent claudication was smoking. This was followed by hyperglycemia, hypercholesterolemia, and hypertension.[2] Others have found that hypertension had only a minimal effect on P-V disease. The frequency of hyperlipoproteinemia has been high in most clinical studies of diabetic P-V disease.[3] Whether hypercholesterolemia or hypertriglyceridemia or both represent the greatest risk has not been totally resolved.

Age is an extremely important factor in diabetic P-V disease. It is rare to see significant clinical P-V disease prior to age fifty. Duration of diabetes also appears to be a significant factor. Nilsson found severe calcifications to be present in 4.8 percent of nondiabetic controls, in 8.7 percent of short duration diabetics and 17.9 percent in long duration diabetics.[4]

Hyperglycemia as a major risk factor still remains a matter of some controversy. A number of animal and human studies have suggested a direct relationship between the presence of hyperglycemia and diabetic complications. However, the effects of blood sugar and its association with P-V disease must be interpreted not only with the degree of hyperglycemia and its duration but with the presence or absence of lipid abnormalities, age, sex, and, to a degree, genetic and racial factors. It should also be noted that, while there is apparently a close association between hyperglycemia, retinopathy, and nephropathy, there is poor correlation between these diabetic complications and P-V disease, indicating that factors other than hyperglycemia per se are operative in the development of diabetic P-V disease.

PATHOPHYSIOLOGY

Macroangiopathy: Macroangiopathy includes not only the large blood vessels such as the femoral, popliteal, dorsalis pedis, and posterior tibials, but the small arterioles as well. Although the exact pathophysiology in the development of macroangiopathy is unknown, the following steps now seem to be an accepted series of events.[5]

The first step in the development of macroangiopathy consists of endothelial damage from lipid and/or blood pressure effects. This is followed by platelet adherence and aggregation, which seems to be accelerated in the diabetic. Platelets have a stimulatory effect on smooth muscle proliferation. These muscle cells from the media then proliferate into the intima and lumen of the vessel. Clot or plaque formation then consists of deposits of lipid, platelets, muscle cells, and debris.

A number of studies have shown that prostaglandins may play an important role in ischemia and thrombus formation as well as in the inhibition of these events. Prostaglandin G_2 is formed from arachidonic acid and is converted to thromboxane A_2 and to prostacyclin. Thromboxane A_2 is formed in platelets and results in increased platelet aggregation and vasoconstriction, while prostacyclin decreases platelet aggregation and causes vasodilatation. Prostacyclin is formed in the endothelial lining of the vessels. Damage to the endothelium conceivably interferes with local prostacyclin synthesis; furthermore, the injury could lead to the exposure of collagen to platelets. These events would produce increased platelet deposition accompanied by unopposed thromboxane A_2 synthesis, which would further enhance platelet aggregation, local vasoconstriction, and contribute to ischemia.[6]

The pathophysiology of plaque and thrombus formation differs slightly, if at all, in the diabetic as compared with the nondiabetic. The changes in the vessel media and intima are qualitatively the same in both groups, although quantitatively greater in the diabetic. However, P-V disease in the diabetic differs from in the nondiabetic in a variety of other ways. In the diabetic, the process is more common than in the nondiabetic. It appears at a younger age and advances more rapidly. In the nondiabetic, the ratio of P-V disease in male to female is 30:1, while in the diabetic it is reduced to 2:1. In the diabetic, there are multisegmental occlusions in the vessels with diffuse mural changes proximally and distally, whereas in the nondiabetic the occlusions most often involve a single segment with a relatively normal adjacent arterial tree. In the diabetic, there is involvement of the collaterals and of the small blood vessels. This extensive involvement makes vascular surgery significantly more difficult in these patients than in the nondiabetic. Once the process begins in the diabetic, both lower extremities are usually involved; in the nondiabetic, the lesions are more likely to be unilateral. Other differences also exist between the two groups with regard to the vessels involved. The vessels most frequently involved in the diabetic are the tibials, peroneals, and small distal vessels, whereas the femoral and iliac vessels tend to be more involved in the nondiabetic. Large and small vessel disease does not necessarily progress at the same rate. It is not uncommon for small vessel disease to be far advanced compared with disease in the larger vessels. This explains the finding of palpable dorsalis pedis and posterior tibial pulses in one-third of the patients with gangrene of the toes or patchy areas of gangrene of the foot.

One other important difference between the diabetic and the nondiabetic is the effect of infection on microthrombi formation. In the nondiabetic, infection leads to an increase in vessel dilation, heat, and redness. However, in the diabetic, infection frequently results in microthrombi formation adding to the ischemic process. For example, infection in the web of the toes can be accompanied by microthrombi in the vessels supplying blood to the toes, leading to gangrene of the toes.

Microangiopathy: The major angiopathic lesion and the hallmark of diabetic vascular disease is the thickened capillary basement membrane (BM). This thickening increases with the duration of diabetes and may be related to the degree of blood sugar control, although this has not been substantiated. In addition, the greatest degree of BM thickening is found in the most dependent parts of the body. Thus, the capillaries of the foot and leg have the thickest BM. The exact pathologic significance of this thickened BM is unknown. However, it has been demonstrated that this thickened membrane has an increased permeability to fluid and protein. There is also some evidence that it might inhibit the egress of the leukocyte into the interstitial fluid, thus decreasing the defense against bacterial infection.

CLOTTING FACTORS

A variety of clotting abnormalities have been implicated in diabetic P-V disease. These include increased fibrinogen level, decreased fibrinolytic activity, increase in Von Willebrand factor, and a tendency for an increased platelet adhesiveness and aggregation. Currently, platelets occupy center stage in the pathogenesis of both large and small blood vessel disease.

Platelets: Recent information now suggests that abnormal platelet adhesiveness and aggregation may be critical factors in the genesis of vascular lesions.[7] Platelet adhesiveness refers to the ability of platelets to adhere to foreign surfaces such as glass or fiberglass. Platelet aggregation refers to the ability to adhere to each other to form "white thrombi." Increased platelet adhesiveness and aggregation have been demonstrated in diabetics.[7] From a therapeutic point of view, it has been shown that the platelet aggregations seen in diabetics are reversible with the use of acetylsalicylic acid. The mechanism by which aspirin may accomplish this is unknown, but recent evidence suggests that aspirin may act by inhibiting the synthesis of prostaglandin G_2, thus decreasing thromboxane A_2. The addition of dipyridamole (Persantine) therapy may be more effective than aspirin alone in preventing platelet aggregation. However, more research is necessary to establish that aspirin and dipyridamole are beneficial and that they should be used in diabetics with P-V disease.

SIGNS AND SYMPTOMS OF VASCULAR INSUFFICIENCY

Listed in Table 34-1 are the signs and symptoms associated with ischemia of the lower extremity. Although intermittent claudication classically begins with pain in the calf, it may be manifested by pain in the foot when the vascular occlusion is low, or it may appear in areas as high as the thigh, hip, or buttocks when the vascular occlusion is in the iliac vessels. Pain compatible with intermittent claudication must always be differentiated from similar pain caused by motion. Such pain may be due to arthritis, or may be muscular or radicular in origin. Rest pain is an ominous sign of severe vascular insufficiency and is an indication for angiography and possible vascular surgery. Rest pain or nocturnal pain of vascular insufficiency can be clinically differentiated from nocturnal pain of diabetic neuropathy; neuropathic pain is frequently relieved by walking, whereas that of vascular insufficiency is aggravated by walking.

Diabetic P-V disease is frequently associated with diabetic peripheral neuropathy, although one or the other may be the predominant clinical feature. The persistence of the neuropathic

Table 34-1. Signs and Symptoms of Vascular Disease in the Diabetic Foot and Leg.

Intermittent claudication
Cold feet
Rest pain
Absent pulses
Blanching on elevation
Delayed capillary filling
Persistent or dependent rubor
Atrophic skin changes
Atrophy of subcutaneous tissue
Ulceration
Infection
Gangrene

ulcer is due primarily to recurrent physical stress to the ulcer site, but a poor vascular supply is also a major factor in delayed healing and infection. Furthermore, poor response to antibiotics is frequently the result of poor delivery of the antibiotic to the infected site because of vascular insufficiency.

An excellent clinical evaluation of the competency of the circulation can be made by physical examination, noting the strength of the pulses, the coldness of the skin, atrophy of the subcutaneous tissues, the presence or absence of hair on the foot, the degree of blanching on elevation of the extremity, and delay or persistence of dependent rubor. It must be kept in mind that patients with varicose veins may have abnormal signs of rubor on the basis of the venous insufficiency.

LABORATORY DIAGNOSIS IN PERIPHERAL VASCULAR DISEASE

Doppler: The best device for the noninvasive evaluation of the competency of the peripheral vascular tree is the use of the ultrasonic flow meter based on the Doppler effect. The Doppler is used either to measure blood flow velocity or for the measurement of blood pressure in the lower extremity. The Doppler probe may be used as a sensitive electronic stethoscope to assess the systolic pressure at any point in the limb. This permits simple quantitation of the presence of arterial occlusive disease. In the presence of peripheral occlusive disease, the systolic pressure at the ankle will be below that of the arm. When the ankle pressure is 50 percent below that of the arm, it is an indication for angiography. The Doppler can also be used to measure blood flow velocity. The normal arterial velocity signal is multiphasic, with a prominent systolic component and one or more diastolic sounds. Distal to an arterial obstruction, the arterial velocity signal is attenuated with a less prominant systolic sound and absence of discrete diastolic sounds. The Doppler probe can thus be used to assess arterial blood flow velocity along the course of the artery. The area of stenosis or occlusions can thus be readily determined from the audio signal alone.

Angiography: Despite the fact that P-V disease in the diabetic primarily involves the small vessels, there is always the possibility that a proximal stenotic lesion is superimposed on distal diabetic vascular disease. Therefore, one cannot always assume that P-V disease in the diabetic is all at the small-vessel level. Thus, small-blood vessel disease may be aggravated by segmental occlusion of major vessels between the aorta and popliteal artery bifurcation. Grafting bypass procedures or endarterectomy from the common femoral to the popliteal artery may provide sufficient blood supply to prevent extension of gangrenous changes as well as aid in the healing of persistent diabetic ulcers and/or infection.

To evaluate the vascular tree for the possibility of doing bypass surgery or endarterectomy requires angiography. It must be emphasized that angiography should not be used as a test or procedure simply to evaluate the arterial tree. Rather, it should only be used as a preoperative procedure, and a vascular surgeon should be consulted before ordering the procedure.

Indications for angiography are: (1) rest pain: rest pain is indicative of severe arterial insufficiency and is an ominous sign suggestive of the early development of gangrene; (2) abnormal Doppler pressures: a blood pressure at the ankle which is 50 percent of that in the arm is an indication of severe vascular insufficiency; (3) ulcerations and/or infections which are not responding to bed rest or vigorous antibiotic therapy; and (4) gangrene of the distal portion of the foot.

Complications of Angiography: Angiography is not a totally benign procedure. Thrombus formation can occur following injection of the dye, with resulting gangrene of the leg and amputation. Hematoma and severe bleeding can also occur at the injection site. For this reason, clotting studies should be done prior to the procedure to rule out the possibility of a bleeding tendency. Patients should not be on anticoagulation therapy. Fortunately, these complications are relatively uncommon with today's techniques.

One recently observed complication of angiography is renal shutdown. This is most likely to occur in the older patient and in the patient with preexisting renal disease, the latter being a rather common occurrence in the diabetic. The exact mechanisms resulting in renal shutdown are unknown. However, because concentrations of the dye in the kidney may be a factor, it is important that these patients be well hydrated for the procedure. Despite hydration, renal shutdown can still occur. Caution should, therefore, be exercised in the use of contrast material in patients with pre-existing renal disease and with elevated blood urea nitrogen (BUN) and creatinine values. The patients receiving angiography should be followed closely after the procedure with serial creatinine and BUN determinations. Should shutdown occur, care must be exercised in limiting fluid intake so as to avoid fluid overload. Fortunately, most cases of renal shutdown secondary to contrast material will resolve within a few days to a week. Only rarely has shutdown been permanent.

AMPUTATION IN THE DIABETIC

Mortality: The outlook for the diabetic undergoing amputation has always been poor. In the pre-antibiotic era, the principal cause of in-hospital mortality in patients with gangrene was toxemia and infection with a mortality rate of close to 50 percent. Despite the medical improvements of recent years, the in-hospital mortality for the diabetic undergoing major amputation is still close to 20 percent, with mortality due mostly to postoperative cardiovascular events. The long-term outlook for the diabetic amputee is also poor. There is a mean survival rate of 65 percent at three years, but only a 40 percent survival rate at the end of five years. Because of the high mortality in this group of diabetics, many do not live long enough to undergo an amputation of the remaining leg. For those who do, the outlook is very poor. On the average, 40 percent will have an amputation of the remaining leg in one to three years and 56 percent in three to five years.

Treatment: Although a variety of medical treatments have been proposed, none has proved to be of any significant or consistent value. Among these has been the use of a wide variety of peripheral vasodilators. Since the major vascular lesion is not a vasospastic one, but rather an anatomical narrowing of the vessels, oral peripheral vasodilators are of little or no value. Sympathectomy is rarely of benefit. The involvement of the autonomic nervous system has, in effect, resulted in an autosympathectomy in many of these patients. The use of antiplatelet drugs such as dipyridamole and/or aspirin may prove to be helpful, but at this time is still experimental. Cigarette smoking must be avoided. Finally, control of blood sugar, blood pressure, and the correction of hyperlipemia and/or hypercholesterolemia are therapeutic measures which can be taken and which should be vigorously pursued until more specific forms of therapy become available.

References

1. West KM: Specific morbid effects (Complications). *In* Epidemiology of Diabetics and its Vascular Lesions. New York, Elsevier, 1978, pp. 351–441
2. Gordon T, Kannel WB: The Framingham Study: Predisposition to atherosclerosis in the head, heart and legs. JAMA: 661–666, 1972
3. Newell RG, Bliss BP: Lipoproteins and the relative importance of plasma cholesterol and triglycerides in peripheral arteriole disease. Angiology 24:297–302, 1973
4. Nilsson SE, Nilsson JE, Frostberg E, et al: Kristianstad Survey II: Studies in a representative adult diabetic population with special reference to comparison with an adequate control group. Acta Med Scand 496 (Suppl):1–42, 1967
5. Ross R and Glomset JA: The pathogenesis of atherosclerosis. N Engl J Med 295:402–425, 1975
6. Needleman P, Kaley G: Cardiac and coronary prostaglandin synthesis and function. N Engl J Med 298:1122–1128, 1978
7. Sagel J, Colwell JA, Crook L, et al: Increased platelet aggregation in early diabetes mellitus. Ann Intern Med 82:733–738, 1975

35

The Foot in Diabetes Mellitus

Paul W. Brand, F.R.C.S.

Diabetes is today the commonest cause of amputation of the foot in civilian life. Experience at a large urban diabetic clinic has shown that the amputation rate can be reduced by 50 percent if the physicians and clinic staff undertake regular foot inspections of all diabetics and advise about management before the foot gets into serious trouble. As a background to such a foot management program, the physician needs to understand the pathology and sequence of events that commonly lead to amputation. There are five factors in such a sequence: vascular, neuropathic, mechanical, infective, and metabolic.

The common sequence of events is:

1. The diabetic may have a reduced peripheral circulation, adequate for regular use but inadequate for the extra blood supply needed to combat gross infection.
2. The patient has diminished sensation—not total anesthesia, but a changed threshold of perception of pain and pressure.
3. He or she then suffers a break in the skin from external mechanical force, often associated with improper footwear.
4. In the absence of pain, the patient continues to walk on this open wound, pressing on the infected tissues and

spreading the infection until it becomes a gross cellulitis and osteomyelitis.

5. Now feeling ill, and with pus in his shoe, the patient goes to a surgeon or to an emergency room. The surgeon finds that he is a diabetic, checks his glucose level, and finds him out of control (perhaps due to the infection). He assumes that such a foot is a danger to the limb or even to the life of the patient, and amputates below or above the knee.

It is at stages 3 and 4 that early intervention can often prevent the need for amputation and restore the patient to a normal life. We will now consider each of the five factors in turn, looking at these from the point of view of management.

VASCULAR FACTOR

The pathology of the small vessels is well known, and the changes in basement membrane are significant. However, there is not much we can do about them except to keep the disease under good control. The large vessel changes are sometimes localized enough to be amenable to vascular surgery. It should be the responsibility of the clinic team to keep a record of the major pulses around the foot. A Doppler machine is a good way to quantify the status of the major vessels. Whereas, for questions of vascular surgery, very precise information is needed, for the basic management of foot problems, it is simpler and more useful to rely on the temperature reactions of the peripheral tissues to give evidence of the adequacy of their circulation. In a cool room, if a foot is warm, it has an adequate blood supply. Routine foot examinations should be done by a nurse, therapist, or technician who will stay with the job and become experienced at it and who will have a skin thermometer or radiometer to use for temperature measurement.

At first examination and at subsequent routine checkups, the patients should sit for a few minutes with shoes and socks removed, and then the therapist should pass his own hands over all surfaces of both feet and take and record the temperature of the coolest and the warmest parts. If the distal foot seems unusually cool, the patient may put on slippers and walk for a few minutes and then be retested. Another way to challenge the circulation is to put a tourniquet above the knee and keep it on for five minutes and take the distal temperature after release. One benefit of taking this routine baseline temperature is that it enhances the value of subsequent checkups that may reveal a "hot spot" associated with mechanical damage (see "Mechanical Factor").

NEUROPATHIC FACTORS

Every diabetic of long standing has some sensory neuropathy and it is most commonly in the feet. Whereas the detailed evaluation of sensation is useful and interesting, it is not strictly necessary as a routine for foot care. It is probably enough to ask the blindfolded patient to distinguish the blunt, from the sharp, end of a pin. I have found a simple assessment of sweating to be an excellent way to identify feet which are at risk. Feet that can sweat rarely suffer trophic problems.

MECHANICAL FACTOR

All diabetics should be advised about footwear; even those with sensitive feet may become insensitive at a later stage, without being aware of the change. Moreover, I see no reason why even healthy people should abuse and distort their feet at the call of fashion or vanity. If five million diabetics start rejecting harmful shoes, perhaps the industry will get a message that will help us all.

Shoes should fit well around the heel and be roomy at the toes. Leather shoes with low or moderate heels, sandals, or clogs are all acceptable. No new shoe should be worn more than two or three hours at a time for the first few days, and I advise all diabetics to change their shoes mid-day and when they get home in the evening.

If feet are insensitive, and especially if they have a previous history of injury or ulceration, we advise using an extra-depth shoe (Treadeasy by P.W. Minor or Mason Shoes, Alden, or Scholl). The in-sole that comes with the extra-depth shoe may be removed and replaced with a custom molded in-sole of Plastazote, Pelite, AliMed, or with a simple soft Spenco in-sole (double thickness). In case of deformed feet or after recurrent ulceration, it may be necessary to use special modifications, such as a rigid sole with a rocker.

Patients who have diminished sensation should be taught to inspect their feet daily when they go to bed, looking for blisters, patches of redness, or calluses that may need to be rubbed down (after soaking) with pumice stone. The patient may also learn to feel for hot spots which will indicate areas of excessive stress that need to be attended to either by walking less or by shoe modifications to relieve pressure and friction.

INFECTIVE FACTOR

The single most critical part of foot care in diabetes is to convince the patient and the staff that even the smallest wound or ulcer is an emergency. In the absence of pain, diabetics will usually continue walking on their ulcerated feet, hoping they will heal. Even doctors do not take seriously a problem that the patient does not complain about. At the early stage, these little wounds will heal easily IF THE FEET ARE RESTED. It is not the lack of vascular supply, in most of the cases, that prevents healing and allows spreading infection. It is walking on an open wound, permitted by lack of pain. Patients must be taught and trained and urged to report the most trivial and insignificant wound, or else to go to bed at home and use crutches until it heals. We usually use bed rest and antibiotics if the wound looks acute and has much swelling and discharge or if there is fever. As soon as the acute stage has passed and swelling has diminished, we like to get the patient up and walking a little, but without subjecting the wounded part to weight bearing—even for a single step. In the absence of pain, it is rare for a patient to be able to remember to keep his foot up, even if he or she uses crutches. We get much better success by using a total contact plaster cast with a "heel" or rocker under the center of the foot. A therapist or technician should be trained to apply these casts, with padding only around the ankle and a strip of felt down the front to facilitate cast removal. The cast must be changed as soon as it becomes even a little loose (as swelling diminishes). For patients who cannot have a cast, we sometimes provide a half sandal strapped to the foot. It is made of Plastazote and molded to fit the back half of the foot and keep the injured part two inches off the floor. This allows the patient to hobble around the house while the ulcer is healing.

THERAPEUTIC FACTOR

If, in spite of all precautions, a wounded foot shows signs of spreading infection and gangrene, or if the foot remains cool or cold in the wounded area, this suggests that the blood supply is inadequate and surgical intervention may be necessary, perhaps amputation. The physicians at the diabetic clinic should develop a good relationship with an orthopedic surgeon and a vascular surgeon to whom problem cases are referred. There should be full understanding and agreement about the collaborative management of the diabetic foot, so that patients are not exposed to contradictory advice. Patients need to understand that their foot problems are part of their disease, and that they should take the advice of their diabetic clinic doctors when they need a surgeon and when buying their shoes.

Any sizeable diabetic clinic should consider the establishment of a foot care unit with permanent staff and with established links to a podiatrist, a good orthotic shoemaker, a vascular surgeon, and an orthopedic surgeon.

36

The Heart in Diabetes

Harvey C. Knowles, Jr., M.D.

INTRODUCTION

Disease of the heart is the most common form of overt vascular disease and cause of mortality in the middle-aged, stable-type diabetic. Inasmuch as this patient outnumbers by six to one or more the younger insulin-dependent diabetic who particularly is at risk for small vessel diseases of the eyes and kidneys, disease of the heart becomes the most common complication of the total diabetic population.[1] Recent reviews on the heart in diabetes have been those monographs on diabetes and the heart edited by Scott and Zoneraich.[2,3]

For purposes of discussion, three types of cardiac disorders will be presented. One of these, atherosclerosis of the coronary arteries, or coronary heart disease (CHD), has been recognized as a problem in diabetes for half a century. The other two types have attracted attention only in recent years, however. These include the concept of a myocardiopathy of uncertain cause and disturbances related to autonomic neuropathy.

CORONARY HEART DISEASE

Epidemiology

In older studies, at autopsy, CHD was found, on the average, two and one-half times more commonly in the diabetics than in control groups without known diabetes. In living diabetics, prevalences have been reported of 26 to 42 percent in groups of all ages and of 10 to 20 percent in noninsulin-dependent type diabetics at the time of diagnosis of diabetes.

Pathology

There have been numerous studies of the gross and light microscopical changes of the larger arteries and myocardium in diabetic patients coming to autopsy. In earlier investigations, no differences were noted in the gross pathology of CHD between diabetics and controls. Furthermore, there were no differences in the location and size of the infarcts, thromboembolism, mural thrombi, or rupture. Goldenberg, et al.[3] described the sequelae of CHD seen in diabetics coming to autopsy. Hypertension appeared to increase the risks of CHD, embolization, and transmural rupture compared to controls. Additionally, infarcts in diabetics were less well healed, which led the authors to suggest that small artery disease might be present also in the diabetic heart.

Extensive studies of the extra- and intramural portions of the right coronary, right descending anterior, and right circumflex arteries in older diabetics and controls have recently been performed, including observations on structure, calcium, fat, collagen deposits, and polysaccharide staining.[4,5] In the diabetics, the distal parts of the extramural coronary arteries contained excess hyaline, PAS positive material, and fat in the intima, and more calcium was noted in both the proximal and distal portions of the arteries.

Pathogenesis

The development of CHD in diabetics is poorly understood. The risk factors for atherosclerosis—namely, smoking, hypertension, and hyperlipidemia—appear to be the same for the diabetic as for the nondiabetic. The cumulative risk of CHD increases with duration of diabetes, but other factors may play a role since CHD occurs beyond that expected from risk factors alone. In population surveys, the prevalence of CHD has been found to increase as levels of blood sugar rise following glucose challenge. Recently, a new area of circulating lipid physiology has attracted attention.[6] It is possible that decreased levels of high-density lipoprotein cholesterol may be a better predictor of atherosclerosis than levels of triglycerides or cholesterol. This apolipoprotein has been reported to be decreased in the noninsulin-dependent diabetic when control is unsatisfactory. Its relation to control in the insulin-dependent juvenile diabetic, however, has been uncertain. Finally, the rapid progression of CHD in renal failure is particularly apparent in the diabetic treated for end-stage kidney disease.

Course

Certain aspects of myocardial infarction in the diabetic differ from those in the nondiabetic. Signs and symptoms are listed in Table 36-1. Of note is the absence of chest pain in a quarter to a third of patients, which may be related to autonomic sensory neuropathy. Obesity, hypertension, and the development of congestive heart failure with the attack are commonly noted. Risk factors for immediate mortality have been analyzed and, with the exception of uncontrolled diabetes and duration of diabetes, no conclusion could be drawn for the relative influence of factors such as shock and congestive heart failure. Survival rates in diabetics, both immediate and 5 years after an episode of acute myocardial infarction, are approximately one half that found in nondiabetics.

Treatment

In general, the treatment of CHD in the diabetic differs little from that in the nondiabetic. Although it would seem wise to avoid hypoglycemia and its catecholamine response in the insulin-treated patient, there is no certain evidence that hypoglycemia has an unfavorable effect in CHD, either in the course of the disorder or during acute infarction.

The role of coronary bypass in the treatment of intractable angina is uncertain, though reports on small numbers of cases indicate it may be of benefit.

Table 36-1. Diabetic Myocardial Infarction
*(Percentage of signs and symptoms)**

	Soler '75 (N=285)	Tansey '77 (N=89)	Partamian '65 (N=258)
Chest pain	67		76
Hypertension		43	55
Obesity		56	42
Angina		31	39
Failure (old)	13		25
Failure (new)		45	67
Shock	3		26

*Frequency in 793 nondiabetics with myocardial infarction.

CARDIOMYOPATHY

Several studies in recent years have led to the concept that a cardiomyopathy of uncertain cause may exist in diabetes.[7] Congestive failure not explainable by CHD or other causes led investigators to suggest that some form of cardiomyopathy existed in diabetes which could be due to small vessel disease or a metabolic process. More invasive techniques, including the measurement of left ventricular function by systolic time intervals, as well as echocardiograms, gives credence to the concept of a cardiomyopathy probably related to small blood vessel disease. Histological studies, however, have provided conflicting data for the existence of small vessel disease.

Regan, et al.[8] conducted extensive studies in diabetic patients without significant occlusive coronary artery disease lesions by angiography and without heart failure. They found an elevation of left ventricular and diastolic pressures and reduction of stroke volume consistent with cardiomyopathy. They observed no luminal narrowing of the intramural vessels but did note, however, interstitial PAS positive material and collagen accumulation. These findings, plus a lack of change in lactate on atrial pacing and accumulation of myocardial triglycerides and cholesterol, led these investigators to suggest a diffuse, extravascular abnormality rather than an obstructive lesion as the cause of the myopathy.

CARDIAC NEUROPATHY

For some time, two events have been noted—namely, the occurrence of elevated pulse rates, which may be quite fixed, and the absence of sinus arrhythmia on respiration. Beat-to-beat variation has been found to be diminished in diabetics after deep breaths, which suggested that vagal denervation existed. In addition, decreased reflex bradycardia after the Valsalva maneuver, a poor response to carotid pressure, and a decreased sympathetic response to tilting have also been observed. Furthermore, the pulse response to orthostatic hypotension has been investigated, the results of which suggest that a rapid pulse could be caused by vagal weakness and uninhibited sympathetic activity, and a no pulse response by a decline in sympathetic activity. Bennet, et al.[9] also studied several means to best demonstrate the occurrence of autonomic control of the heart and concluded that a single deep breath was the best challenge. All these observations indicate that the heart may function as if there were partial or even complete denervation, and parasympathetic activity can be lost to a greater extent than sympathetic activity.

The clinical effects of autonomic neuropathy on cardiac disease may explain the occurrence of painless myocardial infarction in the diabetic. Faerman, et al.[10] examined the myocardial autonomic nerves in diabetic patients with silent myocardial infarcts and found lesions similar to those observed in diabetic autonomic neuropathy in other areas. Other clinical effects of cardiac autonomic neuropathy in the diabetic include unexplained cardiorespiratory arrests and orthostatic hypotension.

In summary, the heart in diabetes is at high risk for atherosclerosis, may be afflicted with a cardiomyopathy of uncertain cause, and may be affected by autonomic neuropathy. Coronary heart disease is the most frequent serious complication suffered by the diabetic. It occurs about twice as often as in the nondiabetic. The gross pathology of large vessels differs little from that of CHD in nondiabetics. CHD in the diabetic may develop in relation to factors other than the known risk factors for CHD. Also, the course of CHD in the diabetic may differ in that there may be no pain with acute infarction, and the five year survival is decreased. There may be a diabetic cardiomyopathy as evidenced by congestive failure of unknown cause, functional studies, and possible abnormality of small vessels. Neuropathy results in decreased autonomic activity, particularly of parasympathetic—and to some extent—sympathetic innervation, and has been reported even to lead to cardiac arrest.

References

1. Bennett PH, Entmacher PS, Habicht JP, et al: Diabetes Data, DHEW Publication No (NIH) 78-1468, 1977
2. Scott R: Clinical Cardiology and Diabetes. Futura Publishing Co, Inc, Mt. Kisco, New York, In Press
3. Zoneraich S: Diabetes and the Heart. Charles C Thomas, Pub, Springfield, Illinois, 1978
4. Ledet T: Histological and histochemical changes in the coronary arteries of old diabetic patients. Diabetologia 4:268–272, 1968
5. Crall FV, Roberts WC: The extramural and intramural coronary arteries in juvenile diabetes mellitus. Analysis of nine necropsy patients ages 19 to 38 years with onset of diabetes before age 15 years. Am J Med 64:221–230, 1978
6. Miller GJ and Miller NE: Plasma-high-density lipoprotein concentration and development of ischemic heart disease. Lancet 1:16–20, 1975
7. Kannel WB and McGee DL: Diabetes and cardiovascular disease. The Framingham study. JAMA 241:2035–2038, 1979
8. Regan TJ, Lyons MM, Ahmed SS, et al: Evidence for cardiomyopathy in familial diabetes mellitus. J Clin Invest 60:885–899, 1977
9. Bennett T, Farquhar IK, Hosking DJ, et al: Assessment of methods for estimating autonomic nervous control of the heart in patients with diabetes mellitus. Diabetes 27:1167–1174, 1978
10. Faerman I, Faccio E, Milei J, et al: Autonomic neuropathy and painless myocardial infarction in diabetic patients. Diabetes 26:1147–1158, 1977

37

Gastrointestinal Manifestations of Diabetes Mellitus

William McBride, M.D., F.R.C.P. (C)
Howard M. Spiro, M.D.

To a large extent, gastrointestinal abnormalities of diabetes are the result of structural, hormonal, and neural disorders which interact in complex ways, particularly in patients with long-standing diabetes. The physiological interdependence of the pancreas and the gut in normal digestive processes is underlined by the manifestations of diabetes in all parts of the gut.

ACUTE GASTROINTESTINAL SYMPTOMS IN DIABETIC KETOACIDOSIS

The nausea, vomiting, and anorexia of diabetic ketoacidosis probably result from gastric atony and stasis. Reduced gastric motility leading to distention is the result of multiple factors: (1) reversible autonomic dysfunction has been demonstrated in patients with diabetic acidosis and acute gastric stasis, but needs further documentation;[1] (2) hyperglycemia per se may be important, as gastric emptying of protein and fat are also delayed in normal subjects with induced hyperglycemia; (3) many gastrointestinal peptide hormones, such as glucagon, relax the stomach and delay emptying, but their role, if any, in the genesis of acute gastric atony of diabetic ketoacidosis is not known.

Table 37-1. Gastrointestinal Manifestations of Diabetes Mellitus

---

Acute symptoms of diabetic ketoacidosis (DKA)
    Gastric atony with distention
    Acute abdominal pain
    UGI bleeding
General symptoms
    Chronic or episodic abdominal pain
    Thoracic radiculopathy
Esophagus
    Abnormal peristalsis—asymptomatic
Stomach
    Atrophic gastritis
    Pernicious anemia
    Impaired gastric secretion
    Gastroparesis diabeticorum
Intestines
    Diabetic diarrhea
    Constipation
Pancreas and gallbladder
    Pancreatic insufficiency
    Pancreatic autoimmunity
    Pancreatic carcinoma
    Cholecystitis with cholelithiasis
    Emphysematous cholecystitis

Gastric atony and distention may contribute to the abdominal pain common in patients with diabetic ketoacidosis. Abdominal pain usually subsides when metabolic events return to normal. When abdominal pain persists, the physician should search for an acute abdominal disorder. Hyperamylasemia suggests pancreatitis. Unfortunately, pancreatitis is not easy to prove in such patients with diabetic ketoacidosis because more than half of such patients may show amylase elevations, usually in the range of 200–800 Somogyi units, even without conclusive evidence of pancreatitis. Such a rise in amylase has been associated with a rapid rise of blood sugar to over 500 mg% and is probably of nonpancreatic origin, since elevations in diabetic patients with ketoacidosis have represented primarily an increase of salivary-type amylase, while pancreatic amylase remains within normal limits.[2]

Hematemesis is another common gastrointestinal event in diabetic ketoacidosis. One-third of 30 autopsied subjects with diabetic coma had had clinical evidence of upper gastrointestinal bleeding, but only in about 1/3 were lesions found at autopsy and consisted mainly of erosions or capillary hemorrhage. Gastritis is presumably the cause of such upper gastrointestinal bleeding in most patients. Bleeding from peptic ulcer and varices or Mallory-Weiss tears is relatively rare. The role of back diffusion of hydrogen ion in the gastritis of diabetics has not been investigated, but the low acid output of many diabetics suggests that other mechanisms may be responsible.

GENERAL SYMPTOMS

Diabetics may complain of chronic or episodic abdominal pain, usually of "neuropathic" origin. The abdominal pain has a girdle distribution, is often associated with nausea and vomiting, and may last hours or days. An important contribution to the understanding of such abdominal pain has been made in diabetics in whom electromyographic studies have demonstrated thoracic radiculopathy.[3] The pain in these patients was upper abdominal, sometimes with paresthesias, and was associated with nausea and significant weight loss to suggest a malignant process. The pain subsided in all patients over a span of 6–20 months as they gradually regained weight. The exact importance of this mechanism should become clear as more clinicians attempt to document it in their diabetic patients who have perplexing abdominal pain.

ESOPHAGUS

Despite the many radiological and manometrical esophageal abnormalities in diabetics, the esophagus usually functions well enough to make esophageal complaints rare. About 80 percent of patients with peripheral neuropathy show abnormal esophageal motility, most commonly decreased primary peristalsis and increased frequency of tertiary contractions. Abnormal esophageal motility may also be found in as many as 20 percent of diabetics without peripheral neuropathy.[4]

THE STOMACH

Gastric atrophy, often with parietal cell antibodies, is common in diabetics. The frequency of pernicious anemia, with its expected intrinsic factor antibodies, is also increased. These abnormalities are most common in insulin-dependent diabetics.[9]

Gastric analysis in diabetic patients has given conflicting results, but generally suggests that long-standing diabetics have lower acid levels than normal, possibly secondary to vagal neuropathy.[6] Fluctuating metabolic events, such as hyperglycemia and hyperglucagonemia, both of which inhibit gastric acid, might account for the inconsistent results, but it seems likely that the contribution of other peptide hormones may be equally important. For example, gastric inhibitory peptide, an enteric hormone that inhibits gastric acid secretion and stimulates insulin in response to glucose, is released in diabetic patients given oral glucose and may contribute to the low acid levels in some diabetics.[5]

Chronic gastric atony in some patients with longstanding diabetes has been associated with upper abdominal discomfort, vomiting, and a clinical picture of gastric outlet obstruction; it may also be found in many asymptomatic patients. Indeed, unrecognized delayed gastric emptying may contribute to the poor control of blood sugar level in some diabetics. Studies using radioactive labeled physiological meals have demonstrated abnormalities in the gastric emptying of liquids and solids in three of twelve diabetics; the three patients with delayed emptying had peripheral neuropathy, but three others who also had peripheral neuropathy showed normal gastric evacuation.[7] The role of metoclopramide, a dopamine depleter which stimulates esophageal and gastric emptying, has shown great promise in alleviating gastric emptying problems in such patients, but it has not yet been released by the FDA for general use.

THE SMALL INTESTINE

Most gastrointestinal complaints of diabetics arise from disordered small intestinal function. Diabetic diarrhea characteristically occurs in young, brittle diabetics with severe peripheral neuropathy, nephropathy, and retinopathy. The diarrhea is

chronic, often postprandial, nonbloody, liquid, and it characteristically occurs at night. Fecal incontinence, particularly during
sleep, is not uncommon. Spontaneous remissions and relapses
occur, often regardless of therapy.[8] Steatorrhea, with loss of
10–40 percent of ingested fat, is sometimes present; hydroxyla-
tion of fatty acids by colonic bacteria may be an important contribution to the diarrhea, as hydroxy fatty acids interfere with
colonic absorption of water and electrolytes. Bacterial overgrowth in the small intestine itself as a result of sluggish small
bowel motility may also be responsible for diarrhea in some
diabetic patients. Both forms of diarrhea and steatorrhea may
respond to temporary administration of antibiotics such as tetracycline.

Radiological studies in such patients show barium retained
in the stomach, dilated loops of small bowel, and a slow transit
through the small intestine. Biopsy of the small intestine in patients with diabetic diarrhea generally shows a normal mucosa,
but, rarely, flat villi unresponsive to a gluten-free diet have been
seen. An interesting association of diabetes with celiac disease
has been highlighted in the observation that diabetes is more
frequent than expected in children with celiac disease, occurring
in 4–6 percent of one series.[9] On the other hand, studies of large
numbers of adults with celiac disease have not confirmed an
increased incidence of diabetes, possibly as a result of the different genesis of diabetes in the young and in the middle-aged.

Therapy of diabetic diarrhea, beyond the attempt to treat
bacterial overgrowth with antibiotics and the exclusion of celiac
sprue by trying a gluten-free diet, has not advanced beyond the
symptomatic measures used for so long. Whether metoclopramide will prove of value in speeding up small intestinal motility
remains to be seen.

THE COLON

Constipation is the most common colonic complaint of diabetics
and is severe in about 20 percent. Colonic neuropathy has not
yet been identified by colonic motility studies, although massive
colonic dilatation has been seen in such diabetics.[8] Treatment
for constipation in diabetics does not differ from that in non-

diabetics, but, as in any circumstance, the wary clinician will always consider another cause.

THE PANCREAS

It has become increasingly clear over the past decade that diminished exocrine pancreatic function is characteristic of insulin-dependent diabetic patients. In 80 percent of 20 juvenile-onset diabetics, the output of bicarbonate, trypsin, and amylase in response to intravenous secretion and CCK-PZ, (cholecystokinin-pancreozymin) was reduced, in direct relation to the duration of the diabetes.[10] Similar decreases in trypsin output in insulin-dependent diabetics were correlated with the degree of beta cell dysfunction. Evidence of severe pancreatic insufficiency has been identified in 23 percent of 107 consecutive adult African diabetics; steatorrhea was present in 23, and 14 of 16 subjects who underwent CCK-PZ stimulation of the pancreas showed abnormal exocrine secretion. The cause for such exocrine pancreatic insufficiency in diabetics is not known. Repeated infarcts and subsequent fibrosis have been postulated. Recent evidence has suggested that diabetes in juveniles can be viral-induced. Viral injury to the islets of Langerhans in such patients might extend to the exocrine portion of the pancreas as well, perhaps causing the pancreatic insufficiency often seen in insulin-dependent diabetics. In such insulin-dependent diabetics, the pancreas is a source of antigen which may be associated with the development of diabetes. The presence of islet cell antibodies (ICA) in insulin-dependent diabetics in three large series of 1848 patients was 29 percent; in contrast, in 54 noninsulin-dependent diabetics, their prevalence was only 6.3 percent.[11] The titers gradually decreased with time; the specific role of circulating ICA in diabetics has yet to be defined, but the impression exists that antipancreatic autoantibodies correlate with the progression of islet cell dysfunction and may provide the link between the viral infection and the subsequent diabetes and even chronic pancreatitis.

Patients who develop diabetes as a complication of chronic pancreatitis obviously have exocrine pancreatic insufficiency, but their diabetes also differs from the idiopathic variety in the lesser amounts of insulin required, a lesser tendency to develop ketoacidosis, and a relative rarity of cardiovascular and neuropathic complications. In patients with chronic pancreatitis, glucagon secretion is impaired in response to aminogenic stimulation, in contrast to the hyperglucagonemia of adult-onset diabetics; such lowered glucagon levels may account for the differing clinical manifestations of diabetes in the patient with chronic pancreatitis.

Acute pancreatitis is associated with glucose intolerance in about 1/3 of patients and disappears when the attack subsides, although glucose intolerance may persist in an occasional patient. The levels of glucagon are much greater in such patients than in normal persons and are probably responsible for the hyperglycemia of acute pancreatitis.

Alpha cell pancreatic tumors that secrete large amounts of glucagon, the so-called "glucagonoma," have been increasingly reported. Such patients have diabetes, diarrhea, and necrotizing skin lesions, the dermatitis being a clue to the diagnosis. In 47 reported cases, the tumors were sufficiently localized to be resected in 15, sometimes with cure.[12] Clearly, in the diabetic with a perplexing skin rash, the clinician will do well to exclude the possibility of such a tumor.

The association between glucose intolerance and pancreatic carcinoma is well known. Carcinoma of the pancreas accounts for at least 12 percent of all carcinomas in diabetic patients. With the increasing incidence of pancreatic carcinoma in recent decades, the incidence of this tumor has increased to 10 percent of all carcinomas. In a recent study of 100 patients, 59 percent of the patients had fasting hyperglycemia, although the number of patients with established diabetes before the carcinoma developed is not known.[13] It is likely that the incidence of pancreatic carcinoma complicating diabetes mellitus is underestimated, since, in any group of patients with pancreatic carcinoma and glucose intolerance, it is difficult to prove that the hyperglycemia is not a consequence of the tumor itself. In any event, the physician should be concerned about the possibility of pancreatic carcinoma in any diabetic patient with weight loss, abdominal pain, and change in insulin requirement.

THE GALLBLADDER

Gallstones are more common in diabetics than in normals; at autopsy the incidence of gallstones is approximately 30 percent in diabetics as compared to 20 percent in nondiabetic patients. Recently it has been suggested that gallstones may be a clue to an underlying somatostatinoma. Because of the high operative mortality of 20 percent in diabetics with acute cholecystitis and an impressive 50 percent incidence of postoperative complications, we recommend that elective cholecystectomy be performed in any diabetic with asymptomatic gallstones.

Twenty percent of cases of emphysematous cholecystitis—an infection of the gallbladder wall with gas-producing organisms, usually without cholelithiasis—occurs in diabetics, particularly men. Obstruction of the cystic artery with secondary infection has been implicated as a cause of this unusual form of cholecystitis. Antibiotics and cholecystectomy are the recommended treatment.

CONCLUSIONS

The diabetic patient suffers from functional abnormalities of the gastrointestinal tract which often cause great concern. Esophageal motility is commonly abnormal in patients with peripheral neuropathy, but usually causes no symptoms. Gastric dilation with stasis can occur in diabetic ketoacidosis but can be present chronically. Gastric atrophy and pernicious anemia occur frequently in diabetics.

Intestinal complications of diabetes include diabetic diarrhea and constipation. Pancreatic insufficiency is common in insulin-dependent diabetics, as is evidence of pancreatic autoimmunity. Carcinoma of the pancreas is associated with glucose intolerance and should be suspect in any diabetic with unexplained abdominal pain. Surgical cure of diabetes is possible if glucagonoma is the underlying cause.

Finally, cholelithiasis is more frequent in diabetics, and cholecystitis is associated with a great morbidity and mortality in the diabetic. Elective cholecystectomy is indicated in any diabetic with gallstones.

References

1. Scarpello JHB and Sladen GE: Progress report: Diabetes and the gut. Gut 19:1153–1162, 1978
2. Warshaw AL and Feller ER: On the cause of raised serum amylase in diabetic ketoacidosis. Lancet 1:929–931, 1977
3. Longstreth GF and Newcomer AD: Abdominal pain caused by diabetic radiculopathy. Ann Int Med 86:166–168, 1977
4. Hollis JB, Castell DO and Braddom RL: Esophageal function in diabetes mellitus and its relation to peripheral neuropathy. Gastroenterology 73:1098–1102, 1977
5. Ross SA, Brown JC and Dupre J: Hypersecretion of gastric inhibitory polypeptide following oral glucose in diabetes mellitus. Diabetes 26:525–529, 1977
6. Feldman M, Corbett DB, Ramsey EJ, et al: Abnormal gastric function in longstanding insulin dependent diabetic patients. Gastroenterology 77:1247, 1979
7. Campbell IW, Heading RC, Tuthill P, et al: Gastric emptying in diabetic autonomic neuropathy. Gut 18:462–467, 1977
8. Katz LA and Spiro HM: Gastrointestinal manifestations of diabetes. N Engl J Med 275:1350–1361, 1966
9. Walsh CH, Cooper BT, Wright AD, et al: Diabetes mellitus and coeliac disease: A clinical study. QJ Med 47:89–100, 1978
10. Frier BM, Saunders JHB, Wormsley KG et al: Exocrine pancreatic function in juvenile onset diabetes mellitus. Gut 97:685–691, 1976
11. Kaldany A: Autoantibodies to islet cells in diabetes mellitus. Diabetes 28:102–105, 1979
12. Higgins GA, Recont L, and Fischman BA: The glucagonoma syndrome: surgically curable diabetes. AJ Surgery 137:142–148, 1979
13. May RE and Strong R: Acute emphysematous cholecystitis. BJ Surg 58:453–460, 1971

38

Skin Manifestations of Diabetes Mellitus

Robert S. Gilgor, M.D.
Gerald S. Lazarus, M.D., F.A.C.P.

Thirty percent of patients with diabetes mellitus (DM) develop a skin disorder which may act as an indicator for the development of DM or which may complicate the course of the diabetes. Furthermore, certain skin problems are far more threatening to the diabetic than nondiabetic patient, and these problems require prompt, aggressive management to prevent serious complications.

CUTANEOUS INDICATORS OF DIABETES

Microangiopathic Skin Disorders

The characteristic microangiopathy of diabetes is associated with the development of diabetic dermopathy, necrobiosis lipoidica diabeticorum (NLD), diabetic bullae, and granuloma annulare. The microangiopathy is characterized histologically by deposition of PAS positive glycoprotein in the thickened basement membrane of capillaries, arterioles, and venules and by abnormal configuration of capillary loops. The vessels may proliferate in the upper dermis and demonstrate enlarged endothelial cells or an increased number of endothelial cells.[1,2]

DIABETIC DERMOPATHY

Diabetic dermopathy is one of the most common clinical findings in diabetes. Dermopathy is observed in over sixty percent of male diabetics and approximately thirty percent of female diabetics. Most patients are over the age of thirty years, and over fifty percent will have associated retinopathy, nephropathy, or neuropathy. Similar lesions may be seen in patients without diabetes, probably secondary to trauma. The histopathology shows microangiopathy in the capillaries and arteriolar walls of the superficial and deep dermis.

The lesions are multiple, discrete, 5–12 mm, flat-topped, dull, red papules that may have a central dell. They are especially prominent on the extensor aspects of the legs, but they are also observed on the forearms, thighs, and over the lateral malleolus of the foot. Usually 4–5 lesions appear symmetrically and simultaneously. Lesions are usually asymptomatic. Over a period of several years, they heal completely or they may leave a thin hyperpigmented, atrophic, sometimes slightly depressed area. These lesions cannot be induced by trauma. There is no treatment described for this problem.[3]

DIABETIC BULLAE

Diabetic bullae (Bullosis diabeticorum) was described first as phlyctenar lesions of the feet in diabetics because these blisters clinically resemble burns. Blisters often occur in patients with long-standing diabetes who have neuropathy. They are characterized by the rapid onset of unilateral or bilateral tense, serous-filled, 0.5–3 cm blisters, usually on the plantar surface of the toes, soles, or margins of the feet. They have also been noted on the dorsum of the toes, as well as on the legs and upper extremities. The blister base is not inflamed and there is no pain associated with the blister. Patients at bed rest have been noted to develop these lesions, so they are not necessarily caused by trauma. Arterial pulses are usually normal. The lesions usually heal in two to six weeks without scarring, although scarring may occur on occasion.[4]

NECROBIOSIS LIPOIDICA DIABETICORUM (NLD)

NLD is an uncommon finding in diabetic patients, occurring in 0.1 to 0.3 percent of diabetics. However, necrobiosis is very strongly associated with diabetes; sixty-five percent of persons with NLD have overt diabetes mellitus and another twenty-five percent have either an abnormal GTT or a very strong family history of diabetes mellitus. NLD is seen three times more commonly in women than in men and is observed on the legs in about eighty-five percent of patients. Fifteen percent of patients with NLD develop lesions on their upper extremities (hands, fingers, forearms), abdomen, or head. Seventy-five percent of patients with NLD are less than forty years of age. Diabetes is usually present for over a year before NLD appears (62 percent). Concomitant onset of NLD and diabetes (within one year) occurs in twenty-four percent of NLD patients. Approximately sixteen percent of patients with NLD have spontaneous clearing, with an average time of resolution of twelve years.

The lesions of NLD are round or oval, sharply defined, firm plaques with a glazed porcelain-like sheen. Larger plaques may be more irregularly shaped and oblong. Borders are frequently elevated and the center may be depressed. Lesions of recent onset are red to brown in color, but they soon develop a yellowish hue. Over a third of necrobiotic lesions will ulcerate, especially after trauma; ulcers are painful and slow to heal. Consequently, lesions of NLD should be protected from trauma. The appearance and the course of necrobiosis is similar in nondiabetics, well-controlled diabetics, or poorly controlled diabetics.

The histopathology shows a peculiar change in the collagen called necrobiosis. The collagen bundles throughout the dermis, but especially in the lower dermis, show amorphous degeneration with disorganization. A palisading granuloma is usually noted in necrobiosis associated with diabetes, whereas a histiocytic epithelioid cell response is more often seen in patients without diabetes.

A promising new treatment for necrobiosis is the long-term use of low-dose salicylates (600 mg morning and evening) in combination with dipyridamole (50 mg QID). Patients have responded to this combination with healing of ulcerations within three weeks. Topical steroids under occlusion and intralesional ster●ds have also been reported to be beneficial. We have used a regimen of salicylates and dipyridamole in combination with topical fluorinated steroids (Valisone cream 0.1%) under occlusion twelve hours per day for a period of one month with good success. After one month, we switch to 1% hydrocortisone cream topically and continue the systemic therapy. Fluorinated steroids should not be used in ulcerated areas since vasoconstriction may be so intense that the base of the ulcer sloughs.[5]

GRANULOMA ANNULARE (GA)

Diffuse granuloma annulare is a rare disease characterized by flesh-colored to red, ring-shaped papules over the trunk and proximal extremities. Histologically, there is necrobiosis similar to that seen in NLD, but it is usually located higher in the dermis. This uncommon generalized variant in older patients with GA may be associated with DM.[6]

Vascular Insufficiency and Gangrene in Diabetes

Atherosclerosis occurs approximately ten years earlier in diabetics than in the general population. Atherosclerosis is manifested in the lower extremities by intermittent claudication, coolness of the feet, paresthesias, numbness, pain, sensory loss, and loss of peripheral pulses. The neurological findings may be related to vascular occlusion of the nerves with neuropathy. The skin of the legs and feet becomes anhidrotic or hypohidrotic secondary to atrophy of the sweat glands. This is occasionally associated with hyperhidrosis of the head, face, neck, axillae, upper back, and trunk. The skin of the legs and feet becomes thin, cool, smooth, hairless, and shiny. Nails are thick, lusterless, and discolored. A waxy pallor is noted on elevating the feet and a bluish mottling is noted on dependency. Capillary filling is delayed. Vascular insufficiency, infection, and neuropathy are the three major factors underlying the development of gangrene. Gangrene is probably fifty times more prevalent in diabetics over the age of forty-five years than in nondiabetics of the same age. In the diabetic foot, gangrene may develop under a corn, callus, or ingrown nail or from bacterial invasion of tinea pedis or areas of trauma. Ulcerations of the foot in diabetics are frequently infected with aerobic and anaerobic bacteria and five to six species of bacteria may be found. The cardinal sign of danger to the diabetic is erythema in a patient with diabetic peripheral vascular disease and neuropathy.

The management of diabetic gangrene is influenced by the temperature of the affected foot. Gangrene in the cold foot almost always results in a major amputation. Gangrene in a hot foot should be managed conservatively with removal of the obvious necrotic tissue, topical and systemic antibiotics, room temperature compresses with or without whirlpool or jet lavage.

Prophylaxis is the key to management of diabetic patients with atherosclerosis. Patients who have corns and calluses should be seen regularly to have lesions pared down. After surgical manipulation, affected areas should be treated with polysporin ointment to decrease friction and control the number of bacteria. Various orthopedic devices (adhesive foam rubber, metatarsal pads) should be prescribed to decrease excessive pressure on specific areas of the foot. Sometimes surgical procedures to remove bunions or other orthopedic deformities are indicated. Certainly all diabetics should be given written instructions in caring for their feet and told not to go barefoot, not to expose their feet to heat or cold, and not to smoke. They should powder their feet daily and should examine their feet morning and evening. New shoes should be soft and carefully fitted. Any minor disturbance of the foot should be reported to the physician. The nails should be trimmed straight across. Tinea pedis and tinea unguium in a diabetic should be treated with systemic griseofulvin until the fungal infection is clear. Griseofulvin micro fine at a dose of one gram per day (500 mg with meals twice daily) for up to one and one-half years may be necessary to clear tinea infections of the nail. Patients should be instructed that any problem with the foot is potentially serious and could lead to bacterial infection and gangrene.[7,8]

Cutaneous Infections in Diabetics

There is controversy as to whether diabetics have an increased incidence of bacterial infections on their skin. Certainly there is no question that diabetics who do get skin infections have more trouble controlling the infection, more difficulty with their diabetes during the infection, and more problems with recurrence of bacterial infections. Dermatophyte infections of the skin are probably not increased in incidence in diabetics. Diabetics in good control do not carry an increased number of pathogens in their skin or in their nasal flora. By contrast, monilial paronychia and monilial vulvovaginitis have an increased frequency in diabetics. Patients with severe, extensive erythrasma also have an increased incidence of diabetes. Resistant venereal warts may also be more common in diabetic females. Mucormycosis, protothecosis, melioidosis, and perianal gangrene secondary to amebic dysentery, are some unusual infections which seem to occur more frequently in diabetics. Severely ill diabetics may also carry gram-negative organisms on their skin more frequently than does a healthy control population.

Diabetics frequently are obese and prone to develop intertrigo and moniliasis in areas of skin apposition. Monilial infections are characterized by flat, beefy red central areas with overhanging white edges and satellite pustules or papules. Most monilial infections will respond to topical treatment with nystatin cream, miconazole, or clotrimazole lotion. Sometimes one-half strength clear Castellani's paint can be used as a drying and peeling agent to prevent recurrences, or simple powdering of the area to keep it dry may be helpful. The severity of candidal infections seems to correlate with the control of the diabetes.[9]

Pruritus

Pruritus in the anogenital area associated with candidal infections is probably increased in diabetics. In addition, pruritus may be present on the lower extremities secondary to the dryness. Generalized pruritus is poorly documented in its association with diabetes.

Carotenemia

Carotenemia is yellow discoloration of the skin due to accumulation of carotene in the stratum corneum. Ten percent of diabetics have yellowing of the skin; this is most often seen on the palms, soles, over bony prominences, in the nasolabial fold, on the rims of the nostrils, the rims of the ears, and the forehead. Carotene is not deposited in the sclera; hence the conjunctivae are clear. Blood levels of carotene must exceed 0.2 to 0.7 mg/ml for carotenoderma to become evident. Carotene is excreted, in part, by the sebaceous glands and reabsorbed by the stratum corneum, hence the tendency for location on the rims of the nostrils and nasolabial folds. The thickness of the stratum corneum on the palms and soles is the reason for the accentuation of the color in these areas. The carotenemia may be due in part to increased intake of leafy and yellow vegetables (fruits and tomatoes), but it is also related to impaired conversion of carotene to Vitamin A in the diabetic liver.

Xanthomas

Eruptive xanthomas are noted in 0.1 percent of diabetics. They are usually associated with either the onset of diabetes or poor control of the diabetes. Xanthomas are more common in men. Pruritus or tenderness may be associated with the development of sudden crops of multiple, yellowish, 2–5-mm papules with surrounding pink halos on the extensor aspects of the extremities, buttocks, dorsum of the hands, and dorsum of the feet. Multiple eruptive xanthomas may coalesce, forming tuberous xanthomas. Lipemia retinalis and hepatosplenomegaly are frequently associated. Lesions usually clear completely as the diabetes improves, although, rarely, xanthomas may heal with atrophy and pigmentation.

Lipodystrophy

Lipodystrophy (atrophy of fat), appearing as coin-sized or palm-sized depressions in normal skin, has been noted in as many as twenty-five percent of diabetics using insulin. The lesions are especially common on the arms and thighs of children and women. Lesions usually occur six months to two years after insulin has been injected repeatedly at the same site. Rarely, atrophy has been reported in distant sites. Lipohypertrophy may similarly occur. Clinically and histologically, this overgrowth of fat simulates a lipoma. Both of these conditions clear spontaneously over years simply by rotating sites of insulin administration.

Acanthosis Nigricans (AN)

AN is associated with several different unique syndromes seen in diabetes. One syndrome occurs in younger females with signs of virilization, accelerated growth rate, hirsutism, multiple skin tags, polycystic ovaries, clitoral enlargement, and coarse features. Most patients are black. There is a marked decrease in insulin binding on monocyte membrane receptors without an elevation of anti-insulin antibodies. Clearly related to this is the syndrome of Lawrence-Seip or total lipoatrophy. Patients with this autosomal recessive disorder manifest complete loss of fat, usually noted at birth, and later develop hepatomegaly, hyperglycemia, insulin resistance, hyperlipidemia, hypertriglyceridemia with xanthomas, hypermetabolism, hyperpigmentation, clitoral or penile enlargement, hirsutism, absence of ketosis, acanthosis nigricans, and cardiomegaly. Younger subjects may have increased height, advanced bone maturation, prominence of muscles, and abdominal protruberance. Neuropathy, retinopathy, nephropathy, and susceptibility to infections are rare. This syndrome is considered to be a diencephalic syndrome with disturbance of hypothalamic transmitters. Recently, fenfluramine has been reported to give dramatic improvement in this syndrome.

Another syndrome seen in diabetes with acanthosis nigricans is noted in older females with circulating antibodies to the insulin receptors. There is an associated alopecia, arthralgia, increased salivary gland size, elevation of gammaglobulin, proteinuria, leukopenia, positive antinuclear antibody, and elevated antiDNA antibodies, and, sometimes, hypocomplementemia and glomerulonephritis.[10]

There are also a number of diseases or clinical findings which have been associated with diabetes. These are listed below for completeness.

Achard-Thiers syndrome
Cushing's syndrome
Dupuytren's contractures
Hemochromatosis
Kaposi's sarcoma
Kyrle's disease
Lipoid proteinosis
Multiple skin tags
Porphyria cutanea tarda
Purpura and pigment—lower extremities
Rubeosis
Scleroderma adultorum
Stomatitis
Vitiligo
Werner's syndrome

References

1. Goebell F, et al: Muscle capillary basement membrane thickness in lipotrophic diabetes. Resp Exp Med 171:271–6, 1977
2. Pardo V, et al: Electron microscopic study of dermal capillaries in diabetes mellitus. Lab Invest 15:1994–2005, 1966
3. Binkley G, et al: Diabetic dermopathy—A clinical study. Cutis 3:955–958, 1967
4. Bernstein J, et al: Bullous eruption of diabetes mellitus. Arch Derm 115:324–325, 1979
5. Muller S, et al: Necrobiosis lipoidica diabeticorum. Arch Derm 93:272–281, 1966
6. Rhodes E et al: Granuloma annulare. Brit J of Derm 78:532, 1966
7. Williams H, et al: Gangrene of the feet in diabetes. Arch Surg 108:609, 1974
8. Lithner F, et al: Skeletal lesions of the feet in diabetics and their relationship to cutaneous erythema with or without necrosis of the feet. Acta Med Scand 200:155–161, 1976
9. Savin J: Bacterial infections in diabetes mellitus. Brit J of Derm 91:481, 1974
10. Kahn C, et al: The syndromes in insulin resistance and acanthosis nigricans. New Eng J Med 294:739, 1976

39

Dental Aspects of Diabetes Mellitus

Robert Gottsegen, D.D.S.

Diabetes mellitus has been implicated in a variety of pathological conditions of the oral cavity and dental structures, ranging from dry mouth and increased incidence of moniliasis to loss of all the teeth because of aggressive periodontitis. Symptoms related to the oral and dental structures frequently furnish valuable clues to the possible presence of diabetes. Of special clinical interest, however, are the different ways in which the two major dental diseases, caries and periodontal disease, are influenced by diabetes mellitus and, in turn, influence it. The most obvious example, perhaps, is the interaction between acute dental infection and uncontrolled diabetes, wherein each condition intensifies and worsens the other.

CARIES

Of the two major dental diseases, dental caries has not been found to be any more prevalent nor more severe in either children or adults who have diabetes when compared with their nondiabetic counterparts.[1] Microbial plaque and sugar in the diet are the two etiological agents of dental caries and, when these factors are controlled in the diabetic child, the caries reduction is the same as in the nondiabetic. Furthermore, the protective effect of fluoride is the same for both groups.

PERIODONTAL DISEASE

With regard to periodontal disease, however, the relationship to diabetes is complex, not well understood and still in considerable dispute. The prevailing view is that diabetes can somehow alter the periodontal tissue* response to local noxious agents towards more severe disease.[2]

It has been conclusively demonstrated that gingivitis and periodontitis, which are the most common periodontal diseases and which are so ubiquitous that they affect virtually all population groups and all socioeconomic classes, are caused by bacteria. Microorganisms in the oral cavity selectively localize to specific sites on teeth where they settle, adhere, and colonize as microbial plaque, both supra or subgingivally. Inflammation of the gingivae and subsequent destruction of the connective tissue of the periodontal tissues including bone resorption are caused either directly by bacterial products or are mediated by destructive elements in the immunological response.[5] It is generally agreed that diabetes does not initiate gingivitis and periodontitis, but most studies seem to indicate that it can adversely modify their course.

Since gingivitis and periodontitis are bacterial infections,[5] they must be regarded with the same concern and awareness of interactions as other infections in the diabetic patient, such as those of the skin, lungs, or urinary tract. Acute dental infection may increase the insulin requirement and may precipitate frank ketoacidosis. The converse relationship also holds—that ketoacidosis predisposes to infection and elevated blood glucose may favor it. A reasonable hypothesis to explain the progressive periodontal breakdown in some diabetics is that, in the presence of poor diabetic control, periodontal infection may become more active and aggressive episodically, corresponding to swings in the blood chemistry, thus resulting in incremental but cumulative irreversible breakdown of the periodontal tissues.

Chronic gingivitis-periodontitis is age related, becoming progressively more prevalent and more advanced with increasing age, thus resembling the frequency distribution of

---

*The periodontal tissues are the supporting and surrounding tissues of the teeth, the gingiva, periodontal ligament, and alveolar bone.

noninsulin-dependent diabetes and adding to the difficulty of establishing correlations.

In general, epidemiological studies corrected for variables such as age and oral hygiene tend to show that neither the amount of plaque nor gingivitis is related to diabetes. However, with increasing age, the periodontal destruction, i.e., the amount of bone resorption around the teeth and the loss of periodontal attachment, is slightly greater in diabetics than in controls presumed to be nondiabetic on the basis of normal two-hour postprandial blood glucose.

There is evidence in some reports which seems to show that periodontal disease is correlated with duration and complications of diabetes, particularly microvascular complications,[2,4] but other clinical studies do not confirm this. Similarly, there is conflicting evidence concerning the presence of microangiopathy in the gingivae of diabetics.[6,7]

CLINICAL CONCERNS

The same constraints and precautions which apply to other surgery in the diabetic patient also apply to dental surgical procedures. Extractions, other oral surgery, or periodontal manipulation should not be performed until the diabetes (glycemia?) has been brought under control. Acute abscesses, however, require immediate drainage. Complete regulation of the diabetes may not be possible while dental infection is still present, but the glycemia can be reduced. Dental treatment may then be instituted under medical monitoring. With removal of hopeless teeth and elimination of dental and periodontal infection, the insulin requirement may be lowered and fluctuating uncontrollable sugar levels may be brought to a more manageable state. In this way, the treatment of periodontal disease may facilitate the practical regulation of diabetic patients.

Since dental disease may make mastication painful or difficult, the patient may then select foods which are easier for him to handle but which may be dietetically improper, thus thwarting efforts at good systemic management. Hasty extraction of the teeth as a simple solution to the dental problems in diabetic patients is not desirable, since dentures may not be well tolerated in this group and may further complicate the nutritional difficulties. It is wiser not to hasten the consummation of the edentulous state in the diabetic patient but rather to make every effort to preserve a healthy, functioning natural dentition so that proper foods may be chewed efficiently and comfortably.

References

1. Cohen MM: Clinical studies of dental caries susceptibility in young diabetics. J Am Dent A 34:239, 1947
2. Gottsegen R: Dental and Oral Aspects of Diabetes Mellitus, Chapter 36 *In* Diabetes Mellitus: Theory and Practice, Ellenberg M and Rifkin H (eds), McGraw-Hill, New York, 1970
3. Glavind L, Lund B, and Loe H: The relationship between periodontal state and diabetes duration insulin dosage and retinal changes. J Periodont 39:341–347, 1968
4. Firestone AJ and Boorujy SR: Diabetes Mellitus and periodontal disease. Diabetes 16:336–340, 1967
5. Tanzer JM: "Microbiology of Periodontal Disease," Section 3 *In* International Conference on Research in the Biology of Periodontal Disease, June 1977, American Academy of Periodontology, Chicago, Ill
6. McMullen JA, Legg M, Gottsegen R, et al: Microangiopathy within the gingival tissues of diabetic subjects with special reference to the prediabetic state. Periodontics 5:61–69, 1967
7. Listgarten MA, Ricker FH, Jr, Laster L, et al: Vascular basement lamina thickness in the normal and inflamed gingiva of diabetics and non-diabetics. J Periodont 45:676–684, 1974

SPECIAL PROBLEMS AND RELATED
CLINICAL ISSUES

40

Adverse Drug Interactions of Clinical Importance to Diabetics

Holbrooke S. Seltzer, M.D.

With the ever increasing number of new drugs being developed and released for clinical use, it is not surprising that a parallel increase of adverse drug interactions between two or more concurrently administered agents is being reported. In 1977 the Medical Letter listed 168 drug combinations that yielded adverse effects,[1] and by 1979 the list had grown to 198 drug combinations.[2]

The purpose of the present review is to consider the mechanisms whereby drugs interact to yield undesired effects; the factors that predispose to drug interactions; and the principal drug interactions that either make diabetes worse or cause dangerous hypoglycemia. It should be pointed out that many potentially adverse drug interactions, based on animal studies, have not occurred in clinical practice.[3,4]

MECHANISMS OF DRUG INTERACTIONS

Two or more drugs given concurrently or within a short time period can either potentiate or antagonize the therapeutic effect of the primary drug, or they may produce a totally different effect than that of either agent alone. They may do this by altering the absorption, distribution, metabolism (biotransformation), or excretion of the primary agent.[5]

Changes in Absorption. Since most drugs are given by mouth, drug interactions affecting absorption usually occur within the gastrointestinal tract, with one drug altering the absorption of another by changing the amount available for absorption. For example, antacids containing calcium or magnesium form insoluble complexes with tetracycline, which decreases the amount of the antibiotic absorbed. Also, drugs that decrease gastric emptying rate, such as codeine or atropine, depress the rate of absorption of simultaneously administered drugs and ingested food.

Changes in Distribution. Following absorption, many drugs are bound to plasma proteins for transport to their sites of action. Such a protein-bound drug is metabolically inactive, but serves as a drug reservoir which becomes pharmacologically active when dissociated from the binding protein to replace the fraction of unbound circulating drug that is metabolized. Moreover, certain drugs bind more strongly to the same plasma proteins than do other drugs, thus displacing the latter into the circulation in the free form and increasing their metabolic activity. A prime example of such a strongly bound agent is phenylbutazone, which can displace salicylates, sulfonamides, sulfonylureas, and the oral coumarin anticoagulants (bishydroxycoumarin and warfarin) from plasma proteins. The addition of phenylbutazone to the therapy of a patient on maintenance dosage of sulfonylurea or an oral anticoagulant, for example, might result in excessive hypoglycemia or bleeding, respectively.

Changes in Metabolism (Biotransformation). The pharmacologic activity of one agent may be markedly increased or decreased in the presence of, or by the addition of, another drug. The most alarming example of this interaction is the hypertensive crisis set off in patients taking monoamine oxidase inhibitors (MAOI)* who inadvertently ingest tyramine-containing foods like matured cheese (e.g., cheddar) or certain wines, or

---

*Monoamine oxidase inhibitors (MAOI): tranylcypromine, isocarboxazid, pargyline, phenelzine, others.

who take across-the-counter "cold medicines" containing sympathomimetic amines like phenylephrine or phenylpropanolamine. Another important mechanism by which one drug markedly alters the metabolic activity of another is by induction, i.e., stimulation, of drug-metabolizing enzymes. The marked induction of hepatic microsomal enzymes by barbiturates must particularly be kept in mind, since by increasing the degradation of such agents as oral anticoagulants, corticosteroids, digitoxin and phenothiazines** by the liver, they decrease the pharmacologic effects of maintenance dosages of these agents and require increased amounts for the same therapeutic effect.

Changes in Renal Excretion. Almost all the factors that modify urinary excretion of drugs produce a decrease in rate which, in turn, leads to increased duration of drug action. These alterations in excretory rate may result from changes in the rate of glomerular filtration, tubular reabsorption or tubular secretion. For example chlorpropamide and digoxin, which are excreted unchanged into the urine, will exert greater hypoglycemic and digitalis effects, respectively, if excessive treatment with thiazide or loop diuretics causes decreased glomerular filtration rate.

FACTORS PREDISPOSING TO DRUG INTERACTIONS

Clinically significant drug interactions are potentially more likely to occur if two or more are taken simultaneously or close together, if taken for several days or longer, or if given to patients with underlying hepatic or renal disease. Undefined genetic differences, which cannot be identified in advance, may also affect drug metabolism and interactions.[6]

Drug interaction can occur when an agent is added to or deleted from a previously effective therapeutic program. For this reason, when an interaction is known to affect dosage requirements and one of the drugs is stopped, a modified dose of the

---

**Phenothiazines:* chlorpromazine, promazine, prochlorperazine, thioridazine, fluphenazine, others.

second drug may be required. For example, the dosage of bishydroxycoumarin or warfarin may need reduction when a barbiturate or equally potent hepatic microsomal enzyme-inducer is stopped or decreased. In addition, patients on monoamine oxidase inhibitors should not only beware of foods containing tyramine (certain cheeses, Chianti wine, beer), but should also avoid across-the-counter diet control pills or nasal decongestants that contain sympathomimetic amines.

PRINCIPAL DRUG INTERACTIONS AFFECTING CARBOHYDRATE TOLERANCE

The following sections describe the most common drug interactions that might unbalance a stable blood sugar maintenance program in diabetics by causing hyperglycemia or hypoglycemia, respectively. In addition, there are many other adverse drug interactions of clinical importance to diabetic patients; for a complete list of the latter, the reader is referred to the especially pertinent review by Avery.[3]

Drug Interactions That Make Diabetes Worse:

Glucocorticosteroids: Glucocorticoids like hydrocortisone and its derivatives, especially when given chronically in large doses, aggravate both subclinical and overt diabetes by increasing hepatic glucose output via gluconeogenesis. Diabetic patients requiring prolonged high doses of corticosteroids usually require insulin therapy, since both diet alone and diet plus sulfonylurea are ineffective.

Oral contraceptives: Long term use of oral contraceptives ("birth control pills") mildly impairs glucose tolerance in non-diabetics, and may bring subclinical diabetes above the clinical horizon. Since most overt diabetics in the child-bearing age are insulin-dependent women, insulin requirements may increase but the diabetes itself will not be harder to control. The diabetogenic mechanism is presumably increased peripheral insulin resistance.

Oral diuretics: Oral diuretic agents, especially the salt-losing thiazides (chlorothiazide, hydrochlorothiazide, trichlormethiazide, others) sometimes aggravate diabetes by causing both extracellular and intracellular potassium depletion. Of these diuretics, chlorthalidone, which is a slightly modified thiazide molecule, is the most potent potassium-wasting agent. Maturity-onset diabetics who are well controlled on diet and a sulfonylurea agent, may develop severe hyperglycemia on chronic thiazide therapy; when this happens, serum potassium levels are usually low, but they may be normal. Treatment consists of correction of potassium deficits by giving oral potassium supplements,[7] and/or by switching to furosemide, a "loop diuretic" which usually does not cause significant potassium loss. Finally, the combined use in an adult-onset diabetic of chlorpropamide as the oral hypoglycemic agent and a thiazide diuretic for treatment of hypertension has caused symptomatic hyponatremia in several patients.[8]

Diazoxide: Diazoxide is also a thiazide, but is a salt-retaining agent instead of a salt-losing one. As such, it does not cause potassium depletion. However, it is a powerful blocker of insulin secretion,[9] and chronic oral dosage is used to treat inoperable insulin-secreting tumors. Clinically, however, it is mainly given as one or more acute intravenous boluses to control dangerous hypertension. Because of this therapeutic limitation, it is not a clinically important diabetogenic agent.

Sympathomimetic agents: Besides the prototype drugs epinephrine and norepinephrine, other clinically important sympathomimetic agents are amphetamines, ephedrine, phenylephrine and phenylpropanolamine. The latter three agents are found in many common, across-the-counter remedies for colds, cough and "sinus trouble." These epinephrine-like agents cause hyperglycemia by stimulating glycogenolysis, and also by blocking insulin secretion. To prevent worsening of diabetes, medicines containing these agents should be avoided.

Nicotinic acid: Large amounts of nicotinic acid, which are usually given chronically to treat hypercholesterolemia, occasionally aggravate glucose intolerance or existing diabetes by causing hepatocellular dysfunction. A typical dosage causing such abnormal liver function tests is Nicalex®, 2–3 gm daily. Under such circumstances, nicotinic acid should be stopped and cholestyramine or colestid used instead.

Drug Interactions Causing Severe Hypoglycemia in Diabetic Patients:

Alcohol: The worst clinical combination predisposing to irreversible hypoglycemic coma is insulin-plus-alcohol; this is typified by an insulin-dependent diabetic who is also a chronic alcoholic.[10] Chronic alcohol intake blocks hepatic glucose output, which normally protects against both fasting and postprandial hypoglycemia. Against this background, insulin-induced hypoglycemia is made irreversibly worse by failure of the alcoholic liver to release hepatic glucose via glycogenolysis. Actually, in all insulin-dependent diabetics, even moderate alcoholic intake must be accompanied by adequate carbohydrate intake to prevent alcohol-induced hypoglycemia.

Bishydroxycoumarin: The anticoagulant bishydroxycoumarin prolongs the metabolic activity of tolbutamide and has caused severe hypoglycemic coma in at least six patients.[10, 11] This possibility can be avoided by using warfarin instead of bishydroxycoumarin when anticoagulation is needed in patients on any of the sulfonylureas,* especially tolbutamide.

Phenylbutazone: This anti-inflammatory agent displaces sulfonylureas from protein binding sites, and thereby prolongs their hypoglycemic activity. At least 14 cases of severe drug-induced hypoglycemia have been reported by the co-administration of a sulfonylurea and phenylbutazone in maturity-onset diabetics.[10,11] In maturity-onset diabetics on sulfonylurea therapy, indomethacin should be used instead of phenylbutazone as an anti-inflammatory agent. Since oxyphenbutazone-plus-sulfonylurea can likewise cause hypoglycemia, it should also be avoided in sulfonylurea-treated patients.

Sulfonylureas: tolbutamide, chlorpropamide, acetohexamide, tolazamide.

Salicylates: Large doses of salicylates (e.g., 4 grams or more daily given to patients with rheumatoid arthritis) have a primary hypoglycemic effect themselves, and they also displace sulfonylureas from protein binding sites. At least five cases of severe hypoglycemia have been reported in patients receiving both a sulfonylurea and large doses of salicylate or acetaminophen.[10, 11] On the other hand, ordinary sporadic amounts of salicylate, as for a headache, pose no such danger.

Sulfonamides: The combination of a sulfonylurea (tolbutamide or chlorpropamide) and one of three sulfonamides has caused seven cases of drug-induced hypoglycemia.[10] Four incidents were caused by the co-administration of either sulfonylurea and sulfisoxazole for urinary tract infections; two cases by co-administration with sulfaphenazole; and one case by co-administration with sulfadimidine (only the first of these three sulfonamides is used in the United States). The sulfonamides prolong metabolic activity of sulfonylureas by displacing them from protein-binding sites. A different antibacterial agent should obviously be used in diabetic patients on sulfonylureas.

Propranolol: This beta-adrenergic blocking agent prevents the rapid hepatic glycogenolytic response that normally corrects insulin-induced or spontaneous hypoglycemia. Severe hypoglycemia has therefore occurred in at least four insulin-dependent diabetics who also received from 40 to 200 mg of propranolol daily.[10, 11] Prevention includes periodic blood sugar monitoring and, when propranolol is needed in insulin-requiring diabetics, use of the lowest effective dosage.

GENERIC AND TRADE NAMES OF DRUGS

1. Acetaminophen—Tempra, Tylenol.
2. Acetohexamide—Dymelor.
3. Amphetamines—Benzedrine, Desoxyn, Dexamyl, Dexedrine.
4. Bishydroxycoumarin—Dicoumarol.
5. Chlorothiazide—Diuril.
6. Chlorpromazine—Thorazine.
7. Chlorpropamide—Diabinese.
8. Chlorthalidone—Hygroton.
9. Cholestyramine—Questran.
10. Colestid—Colestipol.
11. Diazepam—Valium.
12. Diazoxide—Proglycem, Hyperstat (IV only).
13. Digoxin—Lanoxin.
14. Epinephrine—Adrenalin.
15. Fluphenazine—Prolixin, Permitil.

16. Furosemide—Lasix.
17. Hydrochlorothiazide—Hydrodiuril.
18. Indomethacin—Indocin.
19. Isocarboxazid—Marplan.
20. Nicotinic acid—Nicalex, Nicobid, Nicolar, others.
21. Norepinephrine—Levophed.
22. Oral contraceptives—Enovid, Ovulen, Norinyl, others.
23. Pargyline—Eutonyl.
24. Phenelzine—Nardil.
25. Phenylbutazone—Butazolidin.
26. Phenylephrine—Component of Duo-Medihaler, others.
27. Phenylpropanolamine—Component of Allerest, Dimetapp, Ornade, Robitussin, others.
28. Phenytoin—Dilantin.
29. Prochlorperazine—Compazine.
30. Promazine—Sparine.
31. Propranolol—Inderal.
32. Salicylate—Aspirin.
33. Sulfisoxazole—Gantrisin.
34. Sulfadimidine—Diazil, Sulmet (not used in U.S.A.)
35. Sulfaphenazole—Orisulf (not used in U.S.A.)
36. Thioridazine—Mellaril.
37. Tolazamide—Tolinase.
38. Tolbutamide—Orinase.
39. Tranylcypromine—Parnate.
40. Trichlormethiazide—Naqua, Metahydrin, others.
41. Warfarin—Coumadin.

References

1. Adverse interactions of drugs. Medical Letter 19:5–12, 1977.
2. Adverse interactions of drugs. Medical Letter 21:5–12, 1979.
3. Avery, GS: Drug interactions that really matter: a guide to major importance drug interactions. Drug 14:132–146, 1977.
4. Antidiabetic drug interactions. *In* Drug Interactions, Third Edition, Chap. 13, Hasten, P.D., ed. Philadelphia, Lea and Febiger, 1975, pp. 56–69.
5. Drug Interactions. *In* Pharmacology. Drug Actions and Reactions, Levine R.R., ed. Boston, Little, Brown and Company, 1973, pp. 278–291.
6. Scott, J, and Poffenbarger, PL: Pharmacogenetics of tolbutamide metabolism in humans. Diabetes 28:41–51, 1979.
7. Rapoport, MI, and Hurd, HF: Thiazide-induced glucose intolerance treated with potassium. Arch. Internal Med. 113:405–408, 1964.
8. Fichman, MP, Vorherr, H, Kleeman, CR, and Telfer, N.: Diuretic-induced hyponatremia. Ann. Int. Med. 75:853–863, 1971.
9. Seltzer, HS, and Allen, EW: Hyperglycemia and inhibition of insulin secretion during administration of diazoxide and trichlormethiazide in man. Diabetes 18:19–28, 1969.
10. Seltzer, HS: Drug-induced hypoglycemia. A review based on 473 cases. Diabetes 21:955–966, 1972.
11. Seltzer, HS: Severe drug-induced hypoglycemia: a review. Comprehensive Therapy 5:21–29, 1979.

41

Employability of the Diabetic

Gerald J. Friedman, M.D., F.A.C.P.

THE PROBLEM

The need for enlightened employment attitudes towards diabetics is underlined by the increasingly large number of diabetics in the United States. There are six million *known* diabetics and an additional four million undiagnosed at this time. With six hundred thousand *new* cases being diagnosed annually and the disease increasing six percent per year, opportunities must be available for diabetics to be gainfully employed and to receive fair and equal treatment in their jobs.

Well-controlled, properly supervised, cooperative diabetics without serious complications are "good-risk" employees capable of safe and efficient service in appropriate jobs for which they are vocationally qualified and have the physical, mental, and educational capabilities.

Guidelines have been published for job placement and employability of diabetics.[1-3] Recent publications have stressed employment opportunities and protection for diabetics,[4] as well as career choices.[5-7]

CAREER CHOICES FOR DIABETICS

The choice of a career depends upon many factors (i.e., educational requirements, need for new workers in the chosen field, working conditions, etc.). Aside from those jobs where there is an element of danger for the diabetic, his co-workers, or the public, there are few jobs in any field that cannot be filled successfully by the diabetic. For diabetic patients seeking employment, education and training are of great importance. Diabetics with unique capabilities essential for industry or government face little difficulty in obtaining employment.

The Department of Vocational Rehabilitation in each state can help diabetics seeking careers by assigning trained counselors to obtain medical, psychological, social, educational, and job training services—if funds are available. Several affiliates of the American Diabetes Association have their own Vocational and Counseling Services to aid diabetics in career planning.

Noninsulin-dependent diabetics rarely have any employment restrictions.

Insulin-dependent diabetics face some restrictions in employment, based mainly on the fear that some jobs may be dangerous because of potential hypoglycemic reactions. The Federal Government does not allow insulin-dependent diabetics to enter the military service or become licensed pilots; nor does it permit them to drive commercial vehicles in interstate or foreign commerce.

Jobs as police or fire officers or as airplane stewards or stewardesses are unwise choices for insulin-dependent diabetics because of the long and erratic working hours and the emergencies which can develop.

DISCRIMINATION AGAINST DIABETICS

Discrimination against diabetics still exists, but is far less common today that it was just a few years ago. Federal regulations, as well as many state and local laws, have made it illegal for most employers (or schools) to reject a diabetic on the basis of his disease alone. As long as diabetics are capable of performing the jobs sought and present no hazard to themselves or others, they cannot be denied employment.

Title V of the Rehabilitation Act passed in 1973 entitles all qualified "handicapped" to equal job opportunities and treatment. Whether the patient or the physician considers the diabetic "handicapped" does not matter since the regulations go beyond customary medical usage and consider diabetes a "handicap." Thus, diabetics are entitled to share the benefits of the Affirmative Action programs demanded by law.

The law requires employers to hire *qualified* diabetics and promote them on the same basis as nondiabetics. Discrimination on the basis of the diabetes is prohibited. The applicant's qualifications (by experience or training) to do a particular job must be the sole consideration in hiring, training, and promoting.

Rights of Diabetics under the Federal Rehabilitation Act of 1973

1. *Section 101:* (Vocational Rehabilitation *State* Plan). Covers State Rehabilitation Agencies. Each agency must try to hire qualified handicapped people (which includes diabetics) and promote those who are qualified. (Enforced by the Rehabilitation Service Administration)

2. *Section 501:* (Employment of the Handicapped Individuals). Covers departments and agencies in the *executive* branch of the Federal Government. All of these agencies must try to hire and promote qualified handicapped people. Each agency's plan must be approved each year. (Enforced by the United States Civil Service Commission)

3. *Section 503:* (Employment under Federal Contracts). Covers those with Federal Contracts for more than twenty-five hundred dollars per year. This includes about one-half of the businesses and nearly all of the major industries throughout the country. (Enforced by Office of Federal Contracts Compliance Program: Department of Labor.)

4. *Section 504:* (Nondiscrimination under Federal Grants). Covers all programs and activities receiving Federal money. This covers most schools, colleges, hospitals, health and social agencies. (Enforced by the Department of Health, Education and Welfare, Office of Civil Rights)

Many states and local governments have laws similar to the Federal Rehabilitation Act—except that they apply to all businesses.

Protocol in Cases of Discrimination

When a physician believes that a diabetic has been discriminated against because of the diabetes, the following protocol may be instituted:

1. Call the employer and discuss the situation in an effort to resolve the problem.

2. If unsuccessful, try the company's complaint process and involve the union where feasible.

3. Following this, write to the Handicapped Workers Task Force, Department of Labor, 200 Constitution Avenue, N.W., Washington, D.C. 20210.

4. If the Department of Labor does not agree with the complaint, request a review of the case.

5. If the Department of Labor does agree, they will request that corrective action be taken by the employer.

A formal complaint is the last step and should be filed with the Federal Agency involved in paying the employer, (i.e., Departments of Health, Education and Welfare, Labor, Transportation, Housing, etc.).

Discrimination Based on Possible Future Problems

An employer may not use the specter of the future to deny a qualified handicapped worker a job today. Thus, a diabetic cannot be rejected on the basis that diabetes may be a *potential future* liability.

SECOND INJURY LAWS

Many states have laws which provide industry with protection in future compensation claims when they hire applicants with "disabilities" or retain them in their employ after the development of such conditions.

Second Injury Laws encourage the employment of those with diabetes mellitus or other chronic disease.

WORK ATTENDANCE

The high incidence of cardiovascular and other complications suggests an absence risk for *all* diabetics, whether insulin-dependent or not. The severity and duration of the disease, as well as the state of control, influence this risk. However, several studies have shown that the risk of poor work attendance is no greater for the majority of diabetics than it is for nondiabetics—especially when compared with age-matched controls.[13]

Development of maximal educational capabilities, proper job selection, medical supervision, maintenance of good health, and "control" of diabetes through improved professional, public, and patient education; cooperation among labor, management, and professional staff (occupational, private and/or clinic physicians, nurses, nutritionists, etc.) should benefit the employee with diabetes as well as the employer.

SUMMARY

1. Well-controlled, well-supervised, cooperative diabetics make excellent employees. They are self-disciplined, show excellent motivation in their jobs, and often become outstanding workers in whatever position they occupy. Depending on their physical, mental, and vocational qualifications, they are entitled to the same (equal) opportunities for employment as the nondiabetic.

2. Federal, State, and local laws outlaw discrimination based solely on the diabetes.

3. If complications arise, appropriate job assignment can keep the diabetic productive. It is the physician's responsibility to inform the employer what the diabetic can do rather than what his limitations are.

4. Physicians must join efforts by the company and union to get disabled diabetic workers back to work as quickly as is consistent with good medical practice.

5. Physicians must join education efforts to change attitudes and/or behavior that block the hiring of diabetics.

6. Occupational physicians should keep supervisors and employees informed about the latest developments in medicine which affect diabetes. They should make certain that first aid and safety personnel are qualified in aiding diabetics in an emergency.

7. Adequate, *confidential* records should be maintained so that improved facts may be obtained concerning the relationship of diabetes mellitus to job capabilities and work attendance.

References

1. Friedman GJ: Employability of diabetic persons. New York State Journal of Medicine 66:1662, June 1966
2. Report of the Committee on Employment and Insurance of the New York Diabetes Association. Recommendations for determining the employability of the job applicants with diabetes mellitus. Journal of Occupational Medicine 7:20, January 1965
3. Alexander R, Tetrick L, and Friedman GJ: Physicians guidelines for the diabetic in industry. Journal of Occupational Medicine 15:802, December 1974
4. Employment Opportunities and Protections for the Diabetic. American Diabetes Association Pamphlet—1978
5. Career Choices for Diabetics. American Diabetes Association Pamphlet—1978
6. Diabetics are Desirable Workers. American Diabetes Association Pamphlet—1978
7. A Choice of Careers for the Student with Insulin-dependent Diabetes. American Diabetes Association: Southern California Affiliate, Pamphlet, 1976
8. Newsletter for Industry. Affirmative Action for Handicapped People. 4:1, June 1979
9. Goodkin G: Mortality factors in diabetes. Journal of Occupational Medicine 17:716, November 1975
10. Cohen EB and Mastbaum I: Employment of Patients with Diabetes. 57:24, March 1974
11. Tetrick L and Colwell JA: Employment of the diabetic subject. Journal of Occupational Medicine 13:380, August 1971
12. Pell S, D'Alonzo CA: Sickness Absenteeism in employed diabetics. American Journal of Public Health, 57:253, 1967
13. Moore RH and Buschbom RL: Work absenteeism in diabetics. Diabetes 23:957–961, 1974

42

Insurability and Life Expectancy of Diabetics

Paul S. Entmacher, M.D.
Gurunanjappa S. Bale, Ph.D.

INSURABILITY

The demonstrated improvement in life expectancy, as well as the better understanding of different types of diabetes, has led to a more rational and, in many instances, a more liberal approach to the underwriting of persons with diabetes who apply for life insurance. Today most insurance companies will issue insurance with no increase in premiums to diabetics who are not dependent on insulin for the control of their disease, if there are no significant complications. The findings of an extensive twenty-year follow-up of insured diabetics by Dr. George Goodkin of the Equitable Life Assurance Society[1] are still considered to be valid, however, and form the general parameters within which individual companies tend to establish their underwriting criteria. The principal findings of the Equitable study were as follows:

1. The mortality declines progressively with increasing age at the time of application.

2. The mortality increases with increasing duration of the disease until the fifteenth year, when it flattens out.

3. The mortality ratios are markedly higher for the same durations of the disease in the juvenile growth-onset diabetic than in the adult maturity-onset diabetic.

4. The age of onset of diabetes is the most significant factor in mortality and shows the highest mortality ratios at ages 14 and under.

5. Poor control shows about two and a half times the mortality of the well-controlled group.

6. Diabetics on diet alone or diet and oral medication show lower mortality ratios than do the insulin-dependent diabetics.

7. The underweight diabetic shows a higher mortality than does the standard or overweight diabetic.

8. The presence of albuminuria on examination is an extremely unfavorable prognostic sign.

Insulin-dependent diabetics are generally classified as substandard risks and charged an extra premium. Some may be declined for insurance if they have developed complications. Since mortality ratios tend to decrease with advancing age, the youngest diabetics are rated in the highest classification. Also, the ratings tend to increase with long duration of disease.

Associated impairments, such as hypertension and obesity, are considered as additive risks. All insurance company studies have shown, however, that the presence of proteinuria, presumably indicative of nephropathy, is an indication that there will be an extremely unfavorable mortality experience, and such applicants are either issued high substandard insurance or rejected. The presence of significant retinopathy is also considered to be an unfavorable prognostic indicator, but this is not true of neuropathy.

More attention is currently being given to control of the disease since there is some indication that good control may delay or prevent some complications and since measurement of glycosylated hemoglobin gives a more accurate picture of the degree of control. The Equitable study demonstrated a more favorable mortality experience among diabetics who were thought to be well controlled. Some companies are using glycosylated hemoglobin as a screening test for diabetes, but most companies continue to use glucose tolerance tests with different standards depending on age.

LIFE EXPECTANCY

Life expectancy among diabetics increased during the past several decades according to follow-up studies of diabetic patients of the Joslin Clinic (1947–51) and studies of mortality data in the states of Pennsylvania (1968–69) and Iowa (1972–73). Bale and Entmacher[2] estimated that diabetics had an expectation of life at birth of 63.4 years in Pennsylvania and 65.7 years in Iowa; at age 10, the average life expectancy was 57.0 years in Iowa and 54.9 years in Pennsylvania. Marks and Krall[3] estimated an average life expectancy of 44.3 years at age 10 among diabetic patients who attended the Joslin Clinic in 1947–51.

Table 42.1. Life Expectancy of Diabetics by Sex.
(Pennsylvania 1968–69, Iowa 1972–73, and United States 1976 and 2050)

Age (in years)	Average Years of Life Remaining							
	Pennsylvania 1968–69		Iowa 1972–73		United States			
					1976		2050	
	Male	Female	Male	Female	Male	Female	Male	Female
0	59.1	66.3	59.7	69.8	66.6	73.7	68.2	75.5
10	51.4	57.2	52.7	59.8	58.4	65.2	59.8	67.0
20	41.6	47.5	44.6	52.5	48.9	55.8	50.3	57.5
30	33.3	37.8	35.7	43.1	40.1	46.5	41.4	48.1
40	26.6	29.4	29.0	34.8	32.0	37.8	33.2	39.1
50	19.5	21.5	22.3	26.4	24.2	29.2	25.3	30.3
60	13.0	14.7	15.0	18.9	16.9	21.6	17.8	22.6
70	9.0	10.6	10.0	13.3	10.9	15.4	11.5	16.1

Note: Mortality data for the year 1976 were adjusted using ratios derived from the results of Pennsylvania, 1968–69; Iowa, 1972–73; and United States, 1955, studies involving all conditions listed on death certificates. Mortality among diabetics for the year 2050 was computed from postulated death rates in the OASDHI study. Mortality figures were not adjusted for underreporting of diabetes.
Source of basic data: Bale GS and Entmacher PS: Diabetes 26:437, 1977, for 1968–69 and 1972–73 data. United States figures for 1976 and 2050 computed in the Statistical Bureau of Metropolitan Life Insurance Company.

To further assess the longevity of diabetics, life expectancy figures have been computed for the diabetic population of the United States in 1976 and 2050. The 1976 estimates are based on mortality data obtained from the National Center for Health Statistics, while a detailed population projection[4] prepared for long-range cost estimates for the Old Age, Survivors, Disability and Hospital Insurance (OASDHI) system provided the basic data for 2050. These estimates of life expectancy among diabetics and the earlier calculations based on Pennsylvania and Iowa data are shown in the table. The life expectancy of diabetics in the United States population in 1976 was markedly higher than that in Pennsylvania and Iowa, especially at the earlier ages. For example, the expectation of life among diabetics in 1976 was higher by 6 to 8 years at age 10 and by 3 to 8 years at age 40. The expectation of life at birth in the year 2050 is estimated at 68.2 years for diabetic males and 75.5 years for diabetic females; at age 10, the corresponding figures are 59.8 for males and 67.0 for females. Compared with the expectation of life among diabetics in 1976, the figures for 2050 are slightly higher at every age and

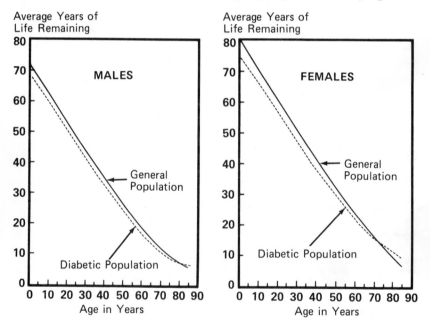

Figure 42-1. Projection of life expectancy of diabetics versus the general population. (See text for details.)

for both sexes, reflecting the lower diabetic mortality projection in the OASDHI study.

When compared with the average life expectancy for the general population of the United States in the year 2050, the expectation of life for the diabetic population is lower at every age except 80 or over for males and 75 or over for females (see Figure 42-1). The largest difference in average life expectancy occurs at birth—4.9 years for females and 3.5 years for males.

The improvement that has occurred in life expectancy is undoubtedly due to better management of the disease. The projections indicate, however, that no dramatic increase in life expectancy among diabetics can be anticipated in the foreseeable future.

References

1. Goodkin G, Wolloch L, Gottcent RA, et al: Diabetes—A twenty year mortality study. Transactions of the Association of Life Insurance Medical Directors of America 58:217–269, 1974
2. Bale GS and Entmacher PS: Estimated life expectancy of diabetics. Diabetes 26:434–438, 1977
3. Marks HH and Krall LP: Onset, course, prognosis and mortality in diabetes mellitus. *In:* Joslin's Diabetes Mellitus, Philadelphia, Lea and Febiger, 1971, pp. 209–254
4. United States Population Projections for OASDHI Cost Estimates, U.S. Department of Health, Education, and Welfare, Social Security Administration, Office of the Actuary, Actuarial Study No 77, June 1978, HEW Publication No (SSA) 78-11523

43

Hyperlipidemias

Sheldon J. Bleicher, M.D.

INTRODUCTION

Clinical interest in hyperlipidemia derives from the observation that it is associated with an increased risk of vascular pathology.[1] The Framingham study clearly documented the fact that hypercholesterolemia, independent of other factors such as hypertension, cigarette smoking, obesity, and diabetes, augmented substantially the risk of coronary artery disease in the male study population. Somewhat less apparent, and substantially more controversial, has been the delineation of risk to be attributed to elevated levels of plasma triglycerides. In this review, we will attempt a clinical overview of hyperlipidemia, its origin, recognition, and practical diagnosis and management.

LIPID PARTICLES

A.

The primary function of lipid particles in the bloodstream is that of fat transport, whether postfeeding (when lipid must be transported from intestines to liver and adipose storage areas) or during fasting (lipid must be recalled from adipose depots and made available to peripheral tissues, for ongoing energy requirements).[2] Dietary triglyceride (structured of three long-chain fatty acids esterified to glycerol, the structural backbone of the triglyceride molecule) is hydrolyzed in the intestinal lumen by the action of pancreatic lipase. Long-chain fatty acids and glycerol, thus released, cross the mucosal surface of the intestinal cell and are re-esterified into triglyceride within the mucosal cell. Fatty acids shorter than 10 carbons in length are *not* re-esterified—rather, they pass directly into the portal vein from the mucosal cell and are used directly by the liver for synthetic or metabolic purposes. Advantage is taken of this differentiation by the intestine, in regard to the fate of fatty acids dependent on chain length, to meet energy requirements in patients with reduced absorptive intestinal surface area, by feeding medium-chain triglyceride as dietary fat, thereby bypassing the "packaging" steps which are about to be described. Fatty acids, 12 carbons or longer, are resynthesized into triglyceride, "wrapped" in a rather bulky package along with a small quantity of structural cholesterol, phospholipid, and protein, and "exported" into the lymphatic system, thence passing up through the thoracic duct and into the circulation. Large enough to be seen under the light microscope, these *chylomicrons* are normally present for several hours after eating a meal containing fat and are composed of at least 85 percent to 90 percent triglyceride (dietary in origin). Chylomicron particles are removed from the circulation by the reticuloendothelial system (liver and spleen) or may be degraded in the circulation by lipoprotein lipase, found on endothelial cell surfaces. Lipoprotein lipase activity is dischargable from the endothelial surface into the circulation by such highly polyionic compounds as heparin, an effect recognized many decades ago by characterizing the effect of heparin on postprandial turbidity of plasma as a "clearing factor." Long-chain fatty acids, released by hydrolysis of chylomicrons, are transferred into adipose cells for storage purposes or are taken up in the liver and used for energy needs or are resynthesized into a new triglyceride-transporting particle, the *very low density lipoprotein* (VLDL) particle (also known as the pre-beta lipoprotein particle). Patients lacking the capacity to metabolize chylomicrons will be found to have enlarged livers and spleens and persistent turbidity of the plasma (on lipoprotein electrophoresis, seen to be chylomicrons (see below)). Infants with a deficiency of lipoprotein lipase will manifest rapid abdominal distention, hepato- and spleno-megaly, and abdominal pain on being fed a diet containing triglyceride. This rare disorder may lead to unnecessary surgery if the nature of the abdominal discomfort is not recognized.

B.

The second lipid-bearing particle, the VLDL particle, begins its life in the liver. The ratio of triglyceride to other constituents is much lower in this particle than in the chylomicron, but still constitutes about 50 percent of the total particle weight. Both the VLDL particle and the chylomicron are large enough to diffract light; hence, lipemia due to either of these particles is associated with opalescence or turbidity of plasma in the *fasting* state. While turbidity normally is present for several hours postprandially, it never should be seen after an overnight fast (12 or more hours), and, when present, is an immediate clue to the presence of hyperlipidemia. The VLDL particle also is attacked and digested by lipoprotein lipase, its fatty acids going to meet energy needs of virtually all tissues (probably excluding the central nervous system and the red cells). As the VLDL particle is "consumed" by hydrolysis of its triglycerides, the particle itself decreases in physical size and undergoes a change in the ratios of its constituents, experiencing a steady *relative* increase in protein, phospholipid, and cholesterol. *Intermediate density lipoprotein* particles (IDL), those sized between VLDL and LDL particles (see below), continue to be hydrolyzed and normally do not accumulate in significant quantities. Under certain circumstances, however, these IDL particles may accumulate, producing, by one or another separatory technique, a relatively heterogeneous population of particles smaller than VLDL particles but larger than the final particle of the life cycle of the VLDL, the *low density lipoprotein* (LDL) particle or betalipoprotein particle. Since many IDL particles themselves are large enough to diffract light, hyperlipidemic states associated with substantial numbers of IDL particles may be associated with opalescence or turbidity of plasma. While accumulation of

IDL particles is relatively uncommon, it may be encountered in women using estrogen-containing oral contraceptives or in patients who have blood dyscrasias, particularly those associated with the presence of abnormal circulating proteins.

C.

The LDL particle is the last step in the "life cycle" of the VLDL particle, representing the "metabolic garbage" of VLDL metabolism; it is relatively poor in triglyceride and substantially richer in protein, phospholipid, and, particularly, cholesterol and cholesterol esters (up to 40 or more percent of the total particle weight). A further consequence of extraction of triglyceride from the VLDL particle, steady shrinkage in physical size, leads to the fact that plasma heavily laden with LDL particles may be completely translucent, lacking even that hint of turbidity which suggests hyperlipidemia. A useful clinical "rule of thumb" is that opalescence in a plasma or serum specimen obtained after overnight fast suggests the presence of triglyceride content exceeding 350 milligram per deciliter, and that the presence of a clear or transparent specimen *does not* exclude the presence of either high levels of cholesterol or elevation of triglyceride levels above the upper normal value of about 170 milligrams per deciliter but below the level of 350 milligrams per deciliter.

D.

An important step in understanding the regulatory role of lipid-transporting particles has been identification of receptors for the LDL particle on cell membrane surfaces. These particles, triglyceride depleted, merge with the cell membrane at the LDL receptor and enter the intracellular space, where they are attacked and degraded. A "feedback" relationship exists between cholesterol entering the cell via this means and cholesterol produced within the cell by the nearly ubiquitous cholesterol-synthesizing system. Intracellular production of cholesterol, a critically important structural and membrane lipid, is governed or "down regulated" by the arrival of substantial amounts of cholesterol born by the LDL particle. When cholesterol biosynthesis has lost this regulation, it proceeds at a rate independent of levels of circulating LDL particles, with apparent accumulation of large concentrations of cholesterol within the tissues. The presence of LDL receptor sites on cell membranes is genetically determined, and homozygous and heterozygous deficiency states have been identified. Homozygous deficiency is recognized as "essential hypercholesterolemia," known for many years to be associated with a rapid and malignant course with regard to cardiovascular disease and characteristically associated with death before the mid-20s due to myocardial infarction or stroke. Relatively little can be done to retard or arrest the unfortunate course of illness with homozygous receptor defect, although some of the therapeutic maneuvers available are discussed below.

E.

Excess cellular cholesterol must be disposed of, and a transport system recently has been recognized which transfers cholesterol from cells to the liver, the major site of exit for cholesterol from the body. The *high density lipoprotein*[3] (HDL), or alpha-lipoprotein particle, has as its major function removal of cholesterol from various tissue sites. Rather tubular in shape and smaller than the VLDL particle, it is composed of at least 50 percent protein and substantial quantities of phospholipid, cholesterol, and cholesterol esters. As a result of its high protein content, it is the most highly charged electrically of the lipid particles and migrates most rapidly on serum lipoprotein electrophoresis. Debate continues as to how cholesterol is removed from tissues and transferred to HDL, but at least two mechanisms are defined. In one, as HDL particles travel adjacent to cell membrane surfaces, cholesterol is leached physically from the cell membrane lipid surface into the lipid-rich surface layer of HDL. A second mechanism, involving the plasma enzyme lecithin cholesterol acyltransferase (LCAT), transfers an acyl group from lecithin and esterifies the hydroxyl group of cholesterol. Cholesterol, so esterified, is markedly hydrophobic, moves towards the core of the HDL particle, and is removed from proximity to the aqueous phase of plasma. This process, repeated many times over, leads to a particle laden with a core of cholesterol-rich material; the particle itself swells and becomes more spherical, ultimately arrives at, and is removed by, the liver, and cholesterol is excreted into the biliary tract. HDL may also lower cellular cholesterol content by blocking the cellular uptake of LDL particles through the obscuring or obstructing of LDL receptor sites on cell membranes. Both of these mechanisms would lower tissue levels of cholesterol and exert a beneficial effect in regard to vascular pathology. It has been shown by several investigators that HDL concentrations are lower in patients with myocardial infarction than in age-matched controls, and the delineation of a risk-factor relationship has been observed: the risk of coronary artery disease increases substantially inversely to the concentration of HDL or, more particularly, to the ratio between LDL and HDL cholesterol fractions.[4, 5] As a result, considerable interest exists in both the determination of HDL concentrations and the means to either raise HDL or favorably affect the ratio of HDL to LDL. A caveat: at this point in time, little documentation exists to support the notion that raising HDL concentrations will favorably affect the course of vascular disease. To further confuse this area of research: the source of HDL particles remains uncertain (some evidence suggests HDL particles may derive from VLDL and chylomicron particles), and it is apparent that several subspecies of HDL particles exist, with differing apoprotein structure. Which of these several HDL types is the most relevant to reduced coronary artery disease risk, and, therefore, which is important to measure, remains unresolved. A preliminary observation of interest: at least one of these types of HDL particles is associated with a reduction of coronary artery disease risk, and the concentration of this HDL is increased by vigorous regular exercise, particularly running.

DIAGNOSIS OF LIPID ABNORMALITIES

Useful information may be obtained by drawing a blood specimen (heparinized) and allowing the plasma to sit in the refrigerator (*not* freezer) overnight. Turbidity in the plasma/serum specimen indicates the presence (see above) of over 350 milligrams per deciliter triglyceride. If the surface layer (or miniscus) of the specimen becomes creamy on standing, the presence of chylomicrons is indicated: these should never be present after an overnight fast and should suggest that the patient be questioned closely about the time of the last meal before proceeding with further analysis of that plasma or serum specimen. Turbidity uniformly distributed throughout the specimen indicates either VLDL or IDL, or both, and would tend to categorize that patient as having a defect in the production rate (excessive) or removal rate (reduced) of these two classes of particles. The presence of clear plasma does *not* exclude the presence of hypercholesterolemia (see above). The presence of both a collar of creamy material and turbidity distributed throughout the specimen suggests a combined defect leading to the accumulation of both chylomicrons and VLDL particles. By use of paper electrophoresis, Levy, Lees, and Frederickson have been able to segregate lipid disorders into several different types. The presence of chylomicronemia has been designated as Type I defect (rare); the presence of VLDL or pre-beta hyperlipidemia has been designated as Type IV defect (very common); and the combination of the two has been designated as Type V defect (common). Thus, Type V defect may be diagnosed by the presence of a creamy collar floating on turbid plasma.[6] IDL particles are associated with a rather heterogeneous band on the paper electrophoretogram, extending from the pre-beta to beta bands; hence, the designation of this abnormality (Type III) as "broad-beta disease." The beta band, in contrast to the other bands just noted, normally is present on the paper electrophoretogram, but may be markedly increased in individuals whose content of LDL particles is above normal. Of considerable importance is the recent recognition that increased beta or LDL particles may be associated with increased pre-beta or VLDL particles, this disorder now being designated as combined or mixed hyperlipidemia. This has led to the subcategorization of two types of Type II (beta or LDL particle) abnormality, namely, Type IIA, in which only beta lipoprotein is increased, and Type IIB, in which both beta lipoprotein and pre-beta lipoprotein (or LDL and VLDL particles) are increased. Both Type IIA and Type IIB appear to be associated with increased risk of coronary artery disease, this risk apparently ascribable to the increased cholesterol content of the blood. While lipoprotein electrophoretic typing may be useful to categorize individuals, it is not necessary for the practical clinical management of hyperlipidemic conditions.

MANAGEMENT OF LIPID DISORDERS

A careful history is critically important in the assessment of patients with elevated triglyceride levels: a carbohydrate-rich or ethanol-rich diet characteristically is associated with increased levels of plasma triglyceride, and reduction of either or both dietary constituents is often gratifyingly and promptly rewarded by a substantial reduction of plasma triglycerides. The endocrine status of the patient, particularly with regard to the presence of hypothyroidism (primary or secondary) or diabetes mellitus (poorly controlled), must be evaluated in diagnosing and managing hyperlipidemias. Drug therapy for hypercholesterolemia or hypertriglyceridemia should not be undertaken until the physician is convinced that the patient is neither hypothyroid nor has diabetes with poor control. Obesity contributes substantially to elevated cholesterol levels, and, by increasing insulin resistance, also to elevated triglycerides. Accordingly, weight reduction constitutes an important therapeutic modality for reduction of plasma lipids. While insurance company ideal body weight tables may guide weight reduction programs, I have found extremely helpful the "rule of thumb" of Dr. John Davidson: For five feet of height, men should weigh 106 pounds and women 100 pounds; for each additional inch of height, for men add 6 pounds and for women 5 pounds. A recommended daily calorie intake, based on ten times ideal body weight as total calories, is instituted with dietary carbohydrate reduced below 150 grams to accomplish both weight and triglyceride reduction. Strenuous efforts to reduce plasma cholesterol concentrations, even by *stringent* low-cholesterol diets, prove unsuccessful in accomplishing sustained substantial effect. Accordingly, hypercholesterolemia is better managed by other approaches, after dietary cholesterol has been reduced to prudent levels by the avoidance of large quantities of dairy and egg yolk-containing products. Both blood pressure and plasma lipid levels will respond favorably to significant weight reduction, although normalization may not be accomplished by means of weight reduction alone. A polyunsaturated-rich source of dietary fat offers potential for augmenting the dietary impact on plasma cholesterol levels, but there appears to be little added benefit when polyunsaturated to saturated fat ratios greater than 3 to 1 are attempted.

Exercise similarly may contribute to lowering plasma cholesterol concentrations. Beyond this, a regular program of exercise may increase HDL concentrations and favorably change the ratio of HDL to LDL. Caution here is advised, since many individuals with hyperlipidemia have, or are at risk of, coronary artery disease. Careful evaluation of these individuals by appropriate means is urged prior to the initiation of a graded, regular, conservative exercise program.

Intestinal bypass surgery has attracted interest as a means of managing morbid obesity, with the additional observation that plasma cholesterol concentrations were reduced. Accordingly, intestinal bypass surgery has been proposed as a means of reducing markedly elevated plasma cholesterol levels in patients with this lipid abnormality. Unfortunately, recent observations do not support the value of this procedure for patients with homozygous Type IIA (essential hypercholesterolemia, pure LDL-receptor deficiency) and, in view of the numerous undesirable side effects inherent in this procedure, it is doubtful that the technique has any place in the management of most patients with elevated cholesterol levels. When diabetes is documented, before any antilipemic drug therapy is undertaken, diabetes should be brought under control, and probably use should be made of the determination of hemoglobin A_{1C} (glycosylated hemoglobin, fast hemoglobin, hemoglobin A_1) as a means of assessing the effectiveness of a diabetes management program.

Several lipid-lowering drugs[7,8] are available to the physician, and these agents may be separated into "major" and "minor" agents. Major drugs would include bile-acid binding resins, D-thyroxine and clofibrate; minor drugs would include nicotinic acid and Sitosterol. *Nicotinic acid,* in a dose range of 1 to eventually 5 grams per day, may contribute to the reduction of cholesterol concentrations, but many patients find the side effects (bloating, belching, flush) experienced at the full therapeutic dose level to be unacceptable. Abnormal liver chemistries and deterioration of carbohydrate metabolism have been reported during the use of this agent; nevertheless, with appropriate warning and observation, the agent may prove useful as an adjunct. *Sitosterol,* available as a suspension, has far fewer side effects, generates little in the way of patient resistance, and may be a useful adjunct in the management of hypercholesterolemia. The mechanism of action of nicotinic acid is unknown, while that of Sitosterol may be to block the reabsorption of bile-acids (enterohepatic cycle), and thereby accelerate the rate of removal of cholesterol from various tissues via the HDL-liver excretory pathway. A similar mechanism, involving irreversible binding of bile-acids and their removal from the enterohepatic cycle with accelerated transfer of cholesterol to the liver by way of HDL, has been proposed as a major therapeutic mechanism of *bile-acid binding resins.* These compounds often are rejected by the patient because of gritty taste, bloating, and belching associated with their use, the fact that they must be taken before each major meal, and that they may complicate other medication schedules. (They may *not* be taken in conjunction with various ionic drug compounds, lest they bind these drugs and remove them simultaneously from the gastrointestinal tract.) For most patients, with moderate degrees of hypercholesterolemia, resins are the medical equivalent of intestinal bypass. *D-thyroxine* offers the potential for substantial reduction of plasma cholesterol concentrations by a mechanism not well understood at the present time, but which derives from the action of native thyroid hormone on cholesterol biosynthesis or removal. D-thyroxine is "sensed" by the standard radioimmunoassay for assessing blood T-4, so that patients receiving this compound may appear chemically thyrotoxic unless the physician evaluating the laboratory data is aware of the use of the medication. D-thyroxine does interract in the normal pituitary-thyroid axis and will lower TSH and 24-hour ^{131}I-neck uptake, but neither of these phenomena holds any adverse consequences for the patient. When used, the drug should be introduced at a dose level of one milligram per day and very gradually augmented to a therapeutic maximum dose of about 6 to 8 milligrams per day, given in divided fashion. The acceleration of angina should be a warning to step down the daily dose by 50 percent and hold at the reduced level for an extended period of time, unless this maneuver fails to alleviate anginal symptoms. *Clofibrate* (2 grams/day) had originally been developed as a cholesterol-lowering agent, based on the observation that it interfered with cholesterol biosynthesis, but clinical use demonstrated at least as potent an effect in lowering plasma triglyceride levels. Accordingly, it became a drug used against both lipid constituents, but recent studies, indicating undesirable consequences of chronic clofibrate usage (such as increased gallbladder disease), make it less likely that this agent will continue to have wide applicability.[9] Further, the effect of clofibrate on liver function tests and response to oral anticoagulants warrants careful consideration. In particular, reduction of coumadin-type anticoagulant dosage is needed until a stable and not excessive prothrombin time is achieved. Recently developed cholesterol-lowering drugs have not had a sufficient period of extensive clinical use to justify comments concerning either effectiveness or safety (e.g., Probucol).

These drugs may be used in combination with each other, and, in fact, it is often necessary to combine agents to achieve the desired effect. In particular, it has been useful to combine a major and a minor drug to accomplish the desired effect. Management of hyperlipidemia necessitates a combined diet-weight control-exercise-drug program, in which art plays as much of a role as does science in accomplishing the desired ends.

References

1. Goldstein JL, Schrott HG, Hazzard WR, et al: Hyperlipidemia in coronary heart disease. J Clin Invest 52:1544–1568, 1973
2. Frederickson DJ, Levy RI, and Lees RS: Fat transport in lipoproteins—an integrated approach to mechanisms and disorders. New Engl J Med 276:34–51, 1967
3. Witzum J and Schonfeld G: High density lipoproteins. Diabetes 28:326–333, 1979
4. Miller GJ and Miller NE: Plasma high-density lipoprotein concentration and development of ischemic heart disease. Lancet 1: 16–19, 1975
5. Streja D, Steiner G, and Kwiterovich PO Jr: Plasma high-density lipoproteins and ischemic heart disease. Ann Int Med 89:871–880, 1978
6. Fisher WR and Truitt DH: The common hyperlipoproteinemias. Ann Int Med 85:407–508, 1976
7. Yeshurun D and Gotto AM: Drug treatment of hyperlipidemia. Amer J of Med 60:379–396, 1976
8. Bilheimer DW: Needed: New therapy for hypercholesterolemia. New Engl J Med 296:508–509 (Edit), 1977
9. Clofibrate: a final verdict? Lancet 2: 1131–1132 (Edit), November 25, 1978

44

Hypoglycemia: Role of Counterregulatory Hormones, Pathophysiology and Diagnosis

R.A. Rizza, M.D.
J.E. Gerich, M.D.

In man, plasma glucose is so exquisitely controlled that it is usually maintained between 50 and 150 mg/dl throughout the day. Insulin is the prime hormone responsible for preventing hyperglycemia; to prevent hypoglycemia, counterregulatory hormones (glucagon, cortisol, growth hormone, and epinephrine) oppose certain actions of insulin and, in addition, promote sufficient glucose production to meet noninsulin-mediated tissue glucose needs. The plasma glucose level itself and the autonomic nervous system may also regulate hepatic glucose production.

When exogenous nutrients are not being ingested, plasma glucose is maintained stable initially because rates of glucose production approximate rates of glucose utilization. With more prolonged deprivation of exogenous nutrients (more than 72 hours), plasma glucose may decrease to 45–50 mg/dl due to a transient excess of glucose utilization over glucose production. Ultimately, plasma glucose stabilizes at a new steady state at which a diminished rate of glucose production equals a diminished rate of glucose utilization. Although hypoglycemia may occur rarely as a primary result of substrate (glycogen storage disease) or counterregulatory hormone deficiency (Addison's disease, hypopituitarism), pathologically the most common cause of hypoglycemia is insulin excess due to an insulin-secreting islet cell tumor; in this condition, hypoglycemia develops primarily due to suppression of hepatic glucose production rather than enhanced glucose utilization. Indeed, in fasting man, the brain, red blood cells, and the renal medulla are the major glucose consumers, and these tissues are not dependent upon insulin for glucose utilization.

Counterregulatory hormones may: (1) stimulate glycogenolysis and gluconeogenesis directly (glucagon, epinephrine); (2) support these processes indirectly by providing adequate enzyme activity and precursors (cortisol, growth hormone); (3) provide alternate nonglucose sources of metabolic fuel, such as free fatty acids (epinephrine, cortisol, growth hormone); (4) diminish glucose utilization (epinephrine, cortisol, growth hormone); (5) suppress insulin secretion (catecholamines); and (6) alter insulin interaction with its receptors in target organs (cortisol, growth hormone).

Counterregulatory hormones can be subdivided into those which act as acute counterregulatory agents and those which are predominantly involved in long-term glucose counterregulation. As shown in Figure 44-1, during the development of hypoglycemia following intravenous injection of insulin, plasma glucose decreases, reaching a nadir within 30 minutes, and then gradually returns to normoglycemic values. The decrease of plasma glucose is due to both an increase in glucose utilization and a decrease in glucose production. The restoration of normoglycemia is due predominantly, if not solely, to a compensatory increase in glucose production, since glucose utilization does not decrease below baseline levels.

Glucagon and epinephrine are the only counterregulatory hormones whose peripheral circulating concentrations increase coincident with, or prior to, compensatory increases in glucose production following insulin-induced hypoglycemia. This, and the fact that epinephrine and glucagon both have virtually instantaneous actions to stimulate hepatic glucose production, suggest that these hormones are the major acute glucose counterregulatory hormones. Since adrenalectomized or hypophysectomized patients maintained on glucocorticoid replacement therapy have normal glucose counterregulation following insulin administration, it seems likely that acute changes in cortisol, growth hormone, or epinephrine secretion are not essential for appropriate

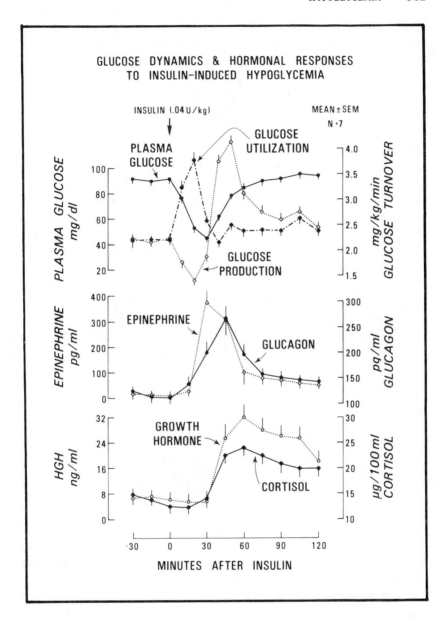

Figure 44-1. Changes in plasma glucose, rates of glucose production and utilization, and circulating levels of epinephrine, glucagon, growth hormone, and cortisol in normal man after intravenous insulin administration.

glucose counterregulation, provided there is normal pancreatic alpha cell function. Additional evidence against an acute role for growth hormone and cortisol is that increased secretion of these hormones occurs *after* compensatory increases in glucose production are already underway. Moreover, biologic effects of these hormones relevant to glucose counterregulation depend upon protein synthesis and take at least 30 to 60 minutes to occur.

Although acute changes in cortisol and growth hormone secretion are probably not important in themselves in acute glucose counterregulation, these hormones, nonetheless, play important roles in long-term glucose homeostasis by supporting adequate glycogen stores for glucagon and epinephrine to act upon, by facilitating the mobilization of alternate nonglucose substrates (glycerol, amino acids, and ketone bodies), and also by modulating insulin interaction with its receptors. This latter effect would explain why patients who chronically lack adrenal corticosteroids and growth hormone may be more sensitive to the hypoglycemic actions of insulin; deficiency of both these hormones enhances binding of insulin to its target tissues and decreases the effectiveness of glucagon and epinephrine.

A differential diagnosis of fasting hypoglycemia (plasma glucose < 45 mg/dl) in adults is given in Table 44-1. Many of these conditions can be suspected or excluded on the basis of history (known drug ingestion, pregnancy, exercise), physical examination (hepatic destruction, congestive heart failure), and routine laboratory tests (chronic renal failure, renal glycosuria, alcohol) in the context of the clinical presentation of hypoglycemia. In patients referred for diagnosis of fasting hypoglycemia, it is important to document the occurrence of hypoglycemia under conditions where appropriate hormone determinations can be obtained and where the possibility of surreptitious drug administration can be minimized.

Clinically significant fasting hypoglycemia can usually be excluded if plasma glucose levels (glucose oxidase method) exceed 45 mg/dl after a 72-hour fast during which the patient has been ambulatory. This procedure yields the fewest false positives and false negatives in the diagnoses of insulinoma, and

Table 44-1. Differential Diagnosis of Fasting Hypoglycemia In Adults.

1. Insulinoma
2. Drugs
   Insulin (therapeutic or factitious)
   Sulfonylureas (therapeutic or factitious)
   Alcohol
   Phenformin
3. Counterregulatory hormone deficiency
   Growth hormone
   Cortisol
   Glucagon
4. Extensive hepatic destruction
5. Severe congestive heart failure
6. Chronic renal failure/renal glycosuria
7. Pregnancy
8. Excessive exercise
9. Extrapancreatic tumors
10. Autoimmune (insulin antibodies)

resort to provocative tests (tolbutamide, glucagon) is generally not necessary. Oral glucose tolerance tests are useless in the diagnostic workup for fasting hypoglycemia and should be discouraged. In the extensive experience of the Mayo Clinic, 75 percent of patients with insulinoma become hypoglycemic within 24 hours of fasting, 97 percent within 48 hours of fasting, and all within 72 hours of fasting.

If symptomatic hypoglycemia develops during a fast, blood samples for insulin, proinsulin, C-peptide, insulin antibodies, cortisol, growth hormone, and a drug screen should be taken. Inappropriate plasma insulin levels and nonsuppressed C-peptide levels (> 1.5 ng/ml) in the absence of insulin antibodies in patients unlikely to be taking sulfonylureas indicate the presence of an insulin-producing tumor. Insulinomas typically release an excess of proinsulin, usually exceeding 25 percent of the fasting insulin levels. Blood may be analyzed for sulfonylurea levels to insure that these drugs have not been taken surreptitiously. The appropriateness of the plasma insulin level must be considered in the context of the prevailing plasma glucose level. To assist in this determination, use of plasma insulin/glucose ratios has been suggested; using the formula

$$\frac{\text{plasma insulin, } (\mu\text{U/ml})}{\text{plasma glucose (mg/dl)}} \quad \text{or}$$

$$\frac{\text{plasma insulin } (\mu\text{U/ml}) \times 100}{\text{plasma glucose (mg/dl)}} \quad -30,$$

respective values greater than 0.3 or 50 are considered diagnostic. An absolute plasma insulin level less than 6 μU/ml would make the diagnosis of an insulinoma extremely unlikely and warrant the search for other causes of the hypoglycemia.

Hyperinsulinemia and suppressed plasma C-peptide levels would strongly suggest surreptitious insulin administration. The presence of insulin antibodies would be confirmatory. Recently, however, an uncommon, apparently autoimmune, disorder resulting in hypoglycemia has been described; in this disorder, insulin antibodies develop without prior exposure to exogenous insulin, and hypoglycemia may occur in the presence of hyperinsulinemia and nonsuppressed plasma C-peptide levels. The latter results from interference in the C-peptide assay due to proinsulin bound to the insulin antibodies. In patients in whom this disorder is considered as an alternative to surreptitious insulin administration, it may be necessary to determine "free C-peptide levels" after extractions of plasma with polyethylene glycol to remove proinsulin bound to insulin antibodies.

Determination of plasma cortisol and growth hormone levels 30 to 60 minutes after the onset of *symptomatic* hypoglycemia can exclude the pituitary-adrenal disease as the cause for the hypoglycemia if plasma levels of these hormones exceed 20 μg/dl and 5 ng/ml, respectively. Values less than these would warrant formal evaluation of pituitary and adrenal gland function (L-dopa, ACTH, TRF tests), if the cause of hypoglycemia is otherwise not readily apparent.

After results of the above diagnostic procedures are available, the cause of fasting hypoglycemia should be evident; if not, an extrapancreatic tumor should be considered. In most instances, these tumors (fibrosarcoma, mesothelioma, adrenocortical carcinoma, hepatocellular carcinoma) are massive and usually palpable. Patients with them appear cachectic and should have appropriately suppressed plasma insulin and increased plasma growth hormone and cortisol levels during hypoglycemia. Insulinomas can often be localized by special radiological maneuvers, including celiac arteriography and computerized tomography, depending on the size of the neoplasm. Extrapancreatic tumors are frequently retroperitoneal and can be visualized by an intravenous pyelogram, ultrasonography, or computerized tomography.

Glucagon deficiency is an extremely rare cause of fasting hypoglycemia in the adult. Since suppressed plasma glucagon levels have been observed in patients with insulinoma, a decreased plasma glucagon level is, in itself, not of diagnostic significance. However, if a cause for fasting hypoglycemia still has not been identified after the above workup, infusion of arginine (20 gm over 30 minutes) can be used to assess pancreatic alpha cell function; an increase above basal levels in excess of 100 pg/ml may be considered normal.

Treatment should be directed at the underlying cause of the hypoglycemia, including surgical removal of the tumor if feasible, alcohol withdrawal in the case of alcohol-induced hypoglycemia, and replacement therapy in patients with endocrine difficulties. Administration of diazoxide or streptozotocin should be considered when an insulinoma is not surgically removable. Other chemotherapeutic agents may be indicated, particularly in patients with metastatic tumors.

References

1. Levine R and Haft D: Carbohydrate homeostasis. N Engl J Med 283:175–183; 237–246, 1970
2. Gerich J, Davis J, Lorenzi M, et al: Hormonal mechanisms of recovery from hypoglycemia in man. Am J Physiol 238:380–385, 1979
3. Rizza R, Cryer P, and Gerich J: Role of glucagon, catecholamines and growth hormone in human glucose counterregulation: Effects of somatostatin and combined α and β adrenergic blockade on plasma glucose and

glucose flux rates following insulin-induced hypoglycemia. J Clin Invest 64:62–71, 1979

4. Garber A, Cryer P, Santiago J, et al: The role of adrenergic mechanisms in the hormonal and substrate response to insulin-induced hypoglycemia in man. J Clin Invest 58:7–15, 1976
5. Landon J, Greenwood F, Stamp T, et al: The plasma sugar, free fatty acid, cortisol and growth hormone response to insulin and the comparison of this procedure with other tests of pituitary and adrenal function. J Clin Invest 45:437–449, 1966
6. Feldman J, Plonk J, and Bivens C: The role of cortisol and growth hormone in the counterregulation of insulin-induced hypoglycemia. Horm Metab Res 7:378–381, 1975
7. Merimee T and Rabin D: A survey of growth hormone secretion and action. Metabolism 22:1235–1253, 1973
8. Baxter J and Forsham P: Tissue effects of glucocorticoids, Am J Med 53:573–584, 1972
9. Kahn R, Goldfine I, Neville D, et al: Alterations in insulin binding induced by changes in vivo in the levels of glucocorticoids and growth hormone. Endocrinology 103:1054–1066, 1978
10. Soman V, Tamborlane W, DeFronzo R, et al: Insulin binding and insulin sensitivity in isolated growth hormone deficiency. N Engl J Med 299:1025–1030, 1978
11. Ginsberg D: Hypoglycemia associated with extrapancreatic tumors. Adv Int Med 12:33–65, 1964
12. Goldman J, Baldwin D, Rubenstein A, et al: Characterization of circulating insulin and proinsulin—binding antibodies in autoimmune hypoglycemia. J Clin Invest 63:1050–1059, 1979
13. Service F, Dale A, Elveback L, et al: Insulinoma—clinical and diagnostic features of 60 consecutive cases. Mayo Clinic Proceedings 51:417–429, 1976
14. Scholz D, ReMine W, and Priestley J: Hyperinsulinism: Review of 95 cases of functioning pancreatic islet cell tumors. Mayo Clinic Proceedings 35:545–550, 1960
15. Service F, Horwitz D, Rubenstein A, et al: C-peptide suppression test for insulinoma. J Lab Clin Med 90:180–186, 1977
16. Fajans S and Floyd J: Fasting hypoglycemia in adults. N Engl J Med 294:766–772, 1976

45

Transplants, Artificial Pancreas, and New Pharmacologic Advances

Philip Raskin, M.D.

INTRODUCTION

It has now been almost sixty years since the discovery of insulin by Banting and Best and their observation that this substance could reverse the severe metabolic abnormalities which occurred following pancreatectomy in the dog. However, despite almost sixty years of clinical experiences using insulin, the one crucial question which relates to the overall philosophy of the treatment of diabetes mellitus remains unanswered. That crucial question is whether or not the microvascular complications of diabetes are related, in any type of cause and effect way, to the metabolic abnormalities of the disease. In my opinion, although there is an ever increasing body of data in experimental diabetes suggesting that hyperglycemia and the microvascular disease are in some way related, there is little convincing *clinical* evidence for the view that rigid diabetic control of the metabolic abnormalities would prevent the vascular complications of the disease. However, there is also no overwhelming evidence to the contrary, i.e., that the microvascular complications of diabetes mellitus are completely independent of the hyperglycemia. My reasons for this conclusion are primarily based on the fact that, with the present modalities of treatment for diabetes mellitus, i.e., diet management, oral hypoglycemic agents, or intermittent

subcutaneous insulin therapy, it is impossible to completely restore glucose homeostasis to normal and, thus, all diabetics
rarely, if ever, have completely normal glucose levels throughout the day.

This review will be directed to those areas which offer
promise as alternatives or adjuncts to current modalities for the
treatment of the hyperglycemia of diabetes mellitus. Specific
areas to be covered include: pancreatic transplantation, islet cell
transplantation, the artificial pancreas, and, finally, a discussion
of the utility of the glucagon suppressing agent, somatostatin.

PANCREATIC TRANSPLANTATION

Except for a very rare success, clinical pancreatic transplantation has been entirely unsuccessful to date. In addition to the
multiple problems associated with immunological graft rejection
common to transplantation of any organ, transplantation of the
pancreas has presented additional special problems. These problems are related to the continuing exocrine secretory function of
the transplanted pancreas and include vascular thrombosis, pancreatitis, and digestion of host tissue by pancreatic enzymes.
Although, over the years, various surgical techniques have been
attempted, it seems clear that only those which provide for
drainage of the exocrine pancreas have a chance of success. An
important advance in pancreatic transplantation has recently
been made by Dickerman and his colleagues, who developed an
operation which allows transplantation of the body and tail of the
pancreas into a Roux-en-Y retroperitoneal limb of the recipient's
jejunum. This procedure has been utilized by Swedish workers
who treated four juvenile-onset diabetic patients without uremia.
Three of the four grafts functioned well, with resulting relatively
normoglycemia in the absence of exogenous insulin administration. The most notable success in pancreatic transplantation was
one done by Dr. Gliedman and his colleagues in New York, who
performed a pancreatic transplantation in a juvenile-onset diabetic, in which the pancreatic duct was drained into the recipient's
ureter. That patient survived for four years following the pancreatic transplantation, with persistent normoglycemia in the absence of exogenous insulin.

Despite these rare clinical successes, much more work will be required before this type of treatment will have any clinical utility.

ISLET CELL TRANSPLANTATION

Because of the many problems associated with whole or partial organ pancreatic transplantation, many workers have attempted to isolate and transplant only islet cell tissue. With present isolation techniques, it is now possible to completely separate the islet cells from the remainder of the pancreatic acinar tissue. In animals with experimental diabetes, this form of therapy has been highly successful, but in man it has been a complete failure. To date, there have been ten such attempts at islet cell transplantation in man. In all instances, hyperglycemia and glycosuria continued unabated following islet cell transplantation, although in some patients there was a temporary decrease in insulin requirements. In no patient did circulating C-peptide levels increase. The reason for this failure is straightforward enough and relates to the small amount of islet cell tissue obtained for transplantation by the isolation techniques used. In these experiments, only 0.2 to 14.5 percent of adult islet cell mass was isolated for transplantation. Until better isolation techniques are developed that will provide a larger yield of islet cell tissue, similar experiments of this nature in man appear doomed to failure.

THE ARTIFICIAL PANCREAS

In the past several years, much effort has been directed towards developing an "artificial beta cell." Such a device, if made small enough, could be totally implanted in the patient and thus function as a replacement for diseased beta cells, much in the same way that miniature pacemakers function as a replacement for diseased cardiac conduction systems. Simply put, an "artificial beta cell" is a sophisticated insulin delivery system. Development of such devices has taken two paths. The first has been the development of "closed-loop" systems, which are those in which insulin is metered out in appropriate amounts in response to a minute-by-minute measure of plasma glucose levels. Generally, if one could develop such a system and make it small enough to be totally implantable, this type could function as a replacement beta cell. Such devices have been developed and are presently available for use clinically, although they are large and must be attached to the patient via an intravenous connection. The glucose-controlled insulin infusion system (GCIIS) is one such device developed by the Life-Science Instrument Division of Miles Laboratory. The GCIIS permits computation of the proper dosage and delivery of insulin on a minute-to-minute basis based on a continuous measurement of plasma glucose concentration. Insulin delivery is calculated by means of algorithms, which relate the plasma glucose concentration and insulin dosages in a complicated mathematical way. These devices have been used in patients quite successfully for short periods of time and are capable of completely normalizing plasma glucose levels following meals, glucose ingestion, or during physical activity.

Because these "closed-loop" systems are large, complicated, and very expensive, others have been working on the development of "open-loop" systems. With these much less complicated systems, insulin delivery is preprogrammed and not dependent upon a minute-to-minute measurement of plasma glucose levels. This type of device is smaller and, although not yet small enough to be totally implanted, is sufficiently miniaturized to be portable, being carried by the patient on his/her belt or in a special harness. At present, there are several such "open-loop" insulin delivery systems under study, and most are using the subcutaneous route of insulin delivery, thus eliminating the need for an indwelling intravenous catheter. The most notable successes are those studied by Pickup and his colleagues in London and by Tamborlane, et al. at Yale. Both groups report near normalization of plasma glucose levels for up to several weeks with preprogrammed "open-loop" subcutaneous insulin delivered with a portable pump. Although not yet ready for general clinical use, the future seems bright for "open-loop" insulin delivery systems as a potential treatment for diabetics.

SOMATOSTATIN

Somatostatin is a 14 amino acid polypeptide with widespread biological activity in man, including inhibition of both insulin and glucagon secretion. The notion that somatostatin might be useful in the treatment of diabetes mellitus is based entirely upon the bihormonal theory of diabetes developed over the past several years by Unger. According to this thesis, the metabolic abnormalities of diabetes mellitus, i.e., the hyperglycemia and the hyperketonemia, are not the consequence of insulin deficiency alone but result from the combination of insulin deficiency and glucagon excess. Based on that concept, several groups have tested the utility of somatostatin on plasma glucose levels in combination with insulin therapy. Figure 45-1 shows the results of experiments carried out in four juvenile-onset diabetic patients on a diabetic diet, receiving a continuous intravenous insulin infusion. When a constant infusion of somatostatin was added to the insulin infusion, resulting in a lowering of plasma glucagon levels, plasma glucose levels fell into the nondiabetic range and postprandial hyperglycemia was eliminated. A replacement infusion of glucagon during the somatostatin and insulin infusion caused a reappearance of hyperglycemia and glycosuria.

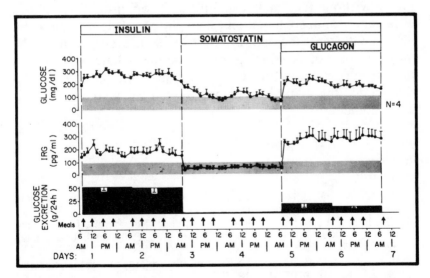

Figure 45-1. Effects of somatostatin and somatostatin plus glucagon upon the daily profiles of serum glucose and IRG levels and upon glucose excretion in 4 juvenile-type diabetic subjects receiving a continuous insulin infusion.

Although somatostatin causes abnormal platelet function when administered in very large doses to animals, there has been no indication of this occurring in man. To date, the only reported untoward effects of long-term somatostatin administration in man have been occasional nausea, vomiting, mild diarrhea, and abdominal pain.

The true efficacy of somatostatin in the treatment of diabetes remains unknown. Many experiments, like the one quoted above evaluating the use of this drug for this purpose, have yielded promising results. Whether somatostatin or one of its analogues will turn out to be the final therapeutic modality, it seems clear that attempts at pharmacological suppression of the hyperglucagonemia can be of tremendous value in the treatment of diabetes mellitus.

CONCLUSIONS

The possible future treatments of diabetes mellitus reviewed above all need considerable work before they have widespread clinical application. Of the treatments discussed, a preprogrammed subcutaneous insulin infusion, using a simple portable pump without feedback capabilities ("open-loop" system), either alone or in combination with a glucagon-suppressing agent like somatostatin (or one of its analogues), seems to have the most promise of developing into something clinically useful in the not too distant future. There is no question, however, that a "cure" for the metabolic abnormalities of diabetes mellitus is *not* imminent.

References

1. Dickerman RM, Twiest M, Crudup JW, et al: Transplantation of the pancreas into a retroperitoneal jejunal loop. Am J Surg 129:48–54, 1975
2. Gliedman ML, Tellis VA, Soberman R, et al: Long-term effects of pancreatic transplant function in patients with advanced juvenile-onset diabetes. Diabetes Care 1:1–9, 1978
3. Lillehei RC, Ruix JO, Aquino C, et al: Transplantation of the pancreas. Acta Endo Suppl 205:303–318, 1976
4. Najarian JS, Sutherland DER, Matas AJ, et al: Human islet transplantation: a preliminary report. Trans Proc 9:233–236, 1977

5. Pickup JC, Keen H, Parson JA: Continuous subcutaneous insulin infusion: an approach to achieving normoglycemia. Brit Med J 1:204–207, 1978
6. Santiago JV, Clemens AH, Clarke WL, et al: Closed-looped devices for blood glucose control in normal and diabetic subejcts. Diabetes 28:71–84, 1979
7. Tamborlane WZ, Sherwin RS, Genel M, et al: Reduction to normal of plasma glucose in juvenile diabetes by subcutaneous administration of insulin with a portable infusion pump. New Engl J Med 300:573–578, 1979
8. Raskin P: The treatment of diabetes mellitus: the future. Metabolism 28:780–796, 1979
9. Raskin P, Unger RH: Effects of hyperglucagonemia and its suppression in the metabolic control of diabetes. New Engl J Med 299:433–436, 1978
10. Unger RH: Diabetes and the alpha cell. Diabetes 25:136–151, 1976
11. Raskin P, Pietri A, Unger RH: Changes in glucagon levels and A-cell function after 4–5 weeks of glucoregulation by portable insulin infusion pumps. Diabetes 28:1033–1035, 1979

46

The Future of Diabetes

George F. Cahill, Jr., M.D.

Ten years ago any forecast made by those working in diabetes research would have included an optimistic description of pancreatic transplantation and possibly a similarly rosy prediction about the development of a mechanical device which could assume the closed-loop feedback role of the normal islets controlling glucose homeostasis. Also, the microvascular abnormalities appeared to be related to the genetic predisposition to diabetes as well as to the metabolic derangements secondary to the insulin deficiency, but the relative contributions of each were debated.

Today, pancreatic transplantation has "peaked out" due to the logistics in obtaining fresh, histocompatibility-matched glands and the need for immuno-suppression after the transplantation. The development of mechanical pancreas awaits a sensing device that is stable and accurate and compatible with living tissues. However, the recent success of open-loop delivery systems which administer insulin continuously with increased rates in association with meals has made development of the sensing system all the more a necessity.

Where next? Not forecast a decade ago were two relatively simple advances in our hypotheses of the initial pathogenic sequences in the beta cell deficiency in diabetes, as well as the microvascular and perhaps some aspects of the macrovascular and neuropathic complications. Insulin-dependent (juvenile-onset or Type I) diabetes appears to be secondary to a viral-autoimmune interaction destroying the beta cells, usually completely, after several years. Noninsulin-dependent (maturity-onset or Type II) diabetes appears to be secondary to an age-related and genetically-determined insufficiency of beta cell viability and function, with perhaps an obesity and inactivity-related peripheral unresponsiveness to what insulin is produced. In both, excess glucose is becoming more and more the culprit for the microangiopathy, possibly also for the neuropathy, and via its effects on platelets and other functions such as red cell stiffness, may be contributing to the macroangiopathy as well.

With these newer concepts of the pathogenesis and the mass of data in their support, insulin-dependent diabetes appears to be now in the research domain of the immunologist and virologist. With the concept that the environmental input or trigger is a virus, but like many other processes such as post-streptococcal glomerulonephritis or, possibly, multiple sclerosis or lupus erythematosus, with the destruction of the host's tissue being due to hereditary immune perversion, prevention appears more and more feasible. T-cell lymphocytes survey all the cells in the body and recognize self and nonself. Certain T cells help in recognizing and ejecting foreigners (helpers) and others keep this in moderation (suppressors). Still others have the nefarious role of destroying the foreigners (killers) or in helping B cell lymphocytes produce antibodies; thus, an immune interruption or even prevention can be predicted, but it is far too speculative to say when these will be practical.

Concerning the noninsulin-dependent diabetic beta cell deficiency, approaches to its prevention or reversal are more difficult. It falls into the realm of cell biology and could even be analogous to the prevention of gray hair or of menopause or baldness, these being similar genetically-programmed senescent processes. On the other side, however, if one could amplify the effect of insulin on cells, the relative deficiency of beta cell function in this type diabetic could be overcome. Weight loss, dietary restriction, and exercise can all do this; so, theoretically, could the medical researcher, if he knew the underlying mechanisms.

Rejuvenating the beta cells themselves might be a more difficult process, but, for both types of diabetes, one should not underestimate the tremendous power of molecular biology. Even five years ago the concept of transferring genetic information from one cell to another, let alone from one organism to another, was an imaginative dream. Today even undergraduate students are performing experiments involving cloning techniques. Could not the genome of one's own cells be made to direct a new group of functioning beta cells to appear, obviating the need for transplantation and immunosuppression? The genome contains all the plans for insulin production as well as its control. How are these plans called into operation? Or, to use the proper genetic terminology, how are the genomes for insulin production, storage, and release derepressed and integrated?

Concerning the microvascular complications, the data, both experimental and now clinical, implicate glucose more and more as the culprit. Yet glucose is a normal component in the nondiabetic, and the nondiabetic does not develop retinopathy and nephropathy! Like pack-years to the smoker, hyperglycemic-years roughly correlate with the complications. If glucose reacting via the hemoglobin A_{1c} type reaction with various proteins as the basis, as some are currently hypothesizing, the knowledge as to the reversibility of the process or, more accurately, of the remodeling of the same lesion which must be occurring in the nondiabetic but at a slower rate, will help to clarify the mechanisms and possibly lead to prevention or reversibility. Every clinician has seen diabetic retinopathy become spontaneously quiescent with even some degree of resolution with accompanying visual improvement. Even the nephropathy, which usually is progressive and predictable, may become stabilized, and, in both the retinopathy and nephropathy, there is no clinical reason for this change in course. Also, in about 1/5 of diabetics, retinopathy is not a major problem in spite of many hyperglycemic years. Why are these more or less protected? Again, optimistically, with the rapid increase of knowledge now occurring, physiologic or pharmacologic approaches may be feasible, as is being currently assessed with the concept that formation of one of the byproducts of hyperglycemia, the polyalcohol, sorbitol, may be inhibited by drugs, or another polyalcohol, myoinositol, which may be deficient in diabetes, may be supplemented.

In summary, prophesizing is best left to prophets, but, in looking over the past decade, the current status of diabetes and diabetes research was not predicted by even the most imaginative. With this as basis for this brief chapter, what will happen over the next decade will be surprising, and it is not beyond reason to think that insulin-dependent diabetes will be prevented or reversed early in the course of the disease, and, subsequently, that new approaches to glucose homeostasis via biological or mechanical developments will prevent the specific complications. Aging, a large proportion of the macroangiopathy, and noninsulin-dependent diabetes, all appear more difficult to approach, but we have had many surprises, and who knows?

INDEX

Sorbitol, 115
  in diabetic neuropathy, 260
Stat-Tek, 168
Steatorrhea, 307
Steroids, in necrobiosis lipoidica
  diabeticorum, 316
Stomach. *See* Gastric entries
Streptococcus pneumoniae, 216
Streptozotocin, in experimental
  diabetes, 13
Substance P, neurogastrointestinal
  activity, 59
Sulfonamide-sulfonylurea interaction,
  333
Sulfonylureas, 129–135
  and bishydroxycoumarin
    interaction, 332
  clinical studies, 134–135
  complications from use, 132
  contraindications to use, 131
  in diabetic surgical patient, 230
  indications for use, 130–131, 134,
    135
  insulin receptors and, 69–70
  pharmacology and mechanism of
    action, 129–130
  and phenylbutazone interaction,
    332
  salicylate interaction, 333
  "second generation," 133
  -sulfonamide interaction, 333
  therapy failure, 131–132
Surgery
  anesthesia, 226
  in complicated diabetes, 230
  IV insulin infusion, constant,
    229–230
  patient management on day of
    operation, 226–229
  in patient on oral hypoglycemics,
    230
  patient preparation, 225–226
Sweeteners. *See specific agent*
Sympathomimetic agents,
  hyperglycemia and, 331

T

Target cell, 63
Therapy, based on
  insulin-glucagon-somatostatin

interaction, 52
2-Thiobarbituric acid (TBA) test, 243
Thromboxane A_2, 283
Thrombus, pathophysiology, 283
Thyrotropin releasing factor (TRF),
  neurogastrointestinal activity, 60
D-Thyroxine, in hyperlipidemia, 356
Tolazamide, 129
Tolbutamide, 129
  and bishydroxycoumarin
    interaction, 332
Tolinase. *See* Tolazamide
Transplantation
  islet cell, 369
  pancreas, 368
  renal, 268
TRF. *See* Thyrotropin releasing
  factor
Triglyceride, 348, 349, 350
  in insulin deficiency, 22–23
Twins, identical. *See* Monozygotic
  twins
Type I diabetes. *See*
  Insulin-dependent diabetes mellitus
Type I hyperlipidemia, 353
Type II diabetes. *See*
  Noninsulin-dependent diabetes
  mellitus
Type IIA hyperlipidemia, 353
Type IIB hyperlipidemia, 353
Type III hyperlipidemia, 353
Type IV hyperlipidemia, 353
Type V hyperlipidemia, 353

U

UDGP. *See* University Group
  Diabetes Program
Ulcers, leg, 214
Ultralente insulin, 118
Ultrasonography
  in fetal monitoring, 171–172
  in peripheral vascular disease, 286
University Group Diabetes Program
  (UDGP), 133
Urinalysis, glycosuria, 104
Urinary tract infection, 215, 267

V

Vascular disease
  conjunctiva, 249–250